MEDICAL
INTELLIGENCE
UNIT

Immunogenetics of Autoimmune Disease

Jorge Oksenberg, Ph.D.
Department of Neurology
University of California, San Francisco
San Francisco, California, U.S.A.

David Brassat, M.D., Ph.D.
Department of Neurology
University of California, San Francisco
San Francisco, California, U.S.A.
and
INSERM U563
Toulouse-Purpan, France

LANDES BIOSCIENCE / EUREKAH.COM
GEORGETOWN, TEXAS
U.S.A.

SPRINGER SCIENCE+BUSINESS MEDIA
NEW YORK, NEW YORK
U.S.A.

Immunogenetics of Autoimmune Disease

Medical Intelligence Unit

Landes Bioscience / Eurekah.com
Springer Science+Business Media, LLC

ISBN: 0-387-36004-2 Printed on acid-free paper.

Springer Science+Business Media, LLC, 233 Spring Street, New York, New York 10013, U.S.A.
http://www.springer.com

Please address all inquiries to the Publishers:
Landes Bioscience / Eurekah.com, 810 South Church Street, Georgetown, Texas 78626, U.S.A.
Phone: 512/ 863 7762; FAX: 512/ 863 0081
http://www.eurekah.com
http://www.landesbioscience.com

Printed in the United States of America.

9 8 7 6 5 4 3 2 1

Library of Congress Cataloging-in-Publication Data

A C.I.P. Catalogue record for this book is available from the Library of Congress.

CONTENTS

EDITORS

Jorge Oksenberg
Department of Neurology
University of California, San Francisco
San Francisco, California, U.S.A.
Chapter 1

David Brassat
Department of Neurology
University of California, San Francisco
San Francisco, California, U.S.A.
and
INSERM U563
Toulouse-Purpan, France
Chapter 1

CONTRIBUTORS

Yoshiyuki Ban
Department of Medicine
Division of Endocrinology,
Diabetes and Bone Diseases
Mount Sinai Medical Center
New York, New York, U.S.A.
Chapter 4

Lisa F. Barcellos
Division of Epidemiology
School of Public Health
University of California
Berkeley, California, U.S.A.
Chapter 2

Regine Bergholdt
Steno Diabetes Center
Gentofte, Denmark
Chapter 3

Pia Bernasconi
Neurology IV Department
Immunology and Muscular
Pathology Unit
National Neurological Institute
Milan, Italy
Chapter 8

Dorothée Chabas
Faculté de Médecine Pitié Salpêtrière
Fédération de Neurologie
Hôpital Pitié-Salpêtrière
Paris, France
Chapter 5

Isabelle Cournu-Rebeix
Faculté de Médecine Pitié Salpêtrière
Fédération de Neurologie
Hôpital Pitié-Salpêtrière
Paris, France
Chapter 5

Bertrand Fontaine
Faculté de Médecine Pitié Salpêtrière
Fédération de Neurologie
Hôpital Pitié-Salpêtrière
Paris, France
Chapter 5

Mehmet L. Guler
Johns Hopkins University
School of Medicine
Baltimore, Maryland, U.S.A.
Chapter 10

Sven Hagnerud
Department of Integrative
Medical Biology
Section for Histology and Cell Biology
Umeå University
Umeå, Sweden
Chapter 9

David U.R. Hedelius
Department of Integrative
Medical Biology
Section for Histology and Cell Biology
Umeå University
Umeå, Sweden
Chapter 9

Davinna Ligons
Johns Hopkins University
School of Medicine
Baltimore, Maryland, U.S.A.
Chapter 10

Renato Mantegazza
Neurology IV Department
Immunology and Muscular
Pathology Unit
National Neurological Institute
Milan, Italy
Chapter 8

Michael F. McDermott
Clinical Science Building
St. James's University Hospital
Leeds, U.K.
Chapter 3

J. Lee Nelson
Program in Human Immunogenetics
Clinical Research Division
Fred Hutchinson Cancer
Research Center
Division of Rheumatology
University of Washington School
of Medicine
Seattle, Washington, U.S.A.
Chapter 6

Per-Arne Oldenborg
Department of Integrative
Medical Biology
Section for Histology and Cell Biology
Umeå University
Umeå, Sweden
Chapter 9

Mattias Olsson
Department of Integrative
Medical Biology
Section for Histology and Cell Biology
Umeå University
Umeå, Sweden
Chapter 9

Flemming Pociot
Steno Diabetes Center
Gentofte, Denmark
Chapter 3

Allison Porter
Program in Human Immunogenetics
Clinical Research Division
Fred Hutchinson Cancer
Research Center
Seattle, Washington, U.S.A.
Chapter 6

John D. Rioux
Inflammatory Disease Research
Broad Institute of MIT and Harvard
Cambridge, Massachusetts, U.S.A.
Chapter 7

Noel R. Rose
Johns Hopkins University
School of Medicine
Baltimore, Maryland, U.S.A.
Chapter 10

Silke Schmidt
Department of Medicine
Center for Human Genetics
Duke University Medical Center
Durham, North Carolina, U.S.A.
Chapter 2

Marcela K. Tello-Ruiz
Inflammatory Disease Research
Broad Institute of MIT and Harvard
Cambridge, Massachusetts, U.S.A.
Chapter 7

Yaron Tomer
Department of Medicine
Division of Endocrinology,
Diabetes and Bone Diseases
Mount Sinai School of Medicine
New York, New York, U.S.A.
Chapter 4

Emily C. Walsh
Inflammatory Disease Research
Broad Institute of MIT and Harvard
Cambridge, Massachusetts, U.S.A.
Chapter 7

Kai W. Wucherpfennig
Department of Cancer Immunology
and AIDS
Dana-Farber Cancer Institute
and
Department of Neurology
Harvard Medical School
Boston, Massachusetts, U.S.A.
Chapter 1

PREFACE

Autoimmunity is the downstream outcome of a rather extensive and coordinated series of events that include loss of self-tolerance, peripheral lymphocyte activation, disruption of the blood-systems barriers, cellular infiltration into the target organs and local inflammation. Cytokines, adhesion molecules, growth factors, antibodies, and other molecules induce and regulate critical cell functions that perpetuate inflammation, leading to tissue injury and clinical phenotype. The nature and intensity of this response as well as the physiological ability to restore homeostasis are to a large extent conditioned by the unique amino acid sequences that define allelic variants on each of the numerous participating molecules. Therefore, the coding genes in their germline configuration play a primary role in determining who is at risk for developing such disorders, how the disease progresses, and how someone responds to therapy.

Although genetic components in these diseases are clearly present, the lack of obvious and homogeneous modes of transmission has slowed progress by preventing the full exploitation of classical genetic epidemiologic techniques. Furthermore, autoimmune diseases are characterized by modest disease risk heritability and multifaceted interactions with environmental influences. Yet, several recent discoveries have dramatically changed our ability to examine genetic variation as it relates to human disease. In addition to the development of large-scale laboratory methods and tools to efficiently recognize and catalog DNA diversity, over the past few years there has been real progress in the application of new analytical and data-management approaches. Further, improvements in data mining are leading to the identification of co-regulated genes and to the characterization of genetic networks underlying specific cellular processes. These advances together with increasing societal costs of autoimmune diseases provide an important impetus to study the role of genomics and genetics in the pathogenic disregulation of immune homeostasis. In this book, we hope to provide a broad overview of current knowledge on how allelic diversity influences susceptibility in a wide variety of autoimmune diseases. Understanding the genetic roots of these disorders has the potential to uncover the basic mechanisms of the pathology, and this knowledge undoubtedly will lead to new and more effective ways to treat, and perhaps to prevent and cure.

There are approximately 30 recognized autoimmune diseases, affecting 10% of the population. With the aid of novel analytical algorithms, the combined study of genomic and phenotypic information in well-controlled and adequately powered datasets will refine conceptual models of pathogenesis, and a framework for understanding the mechanisms of action of existing therapies for each disorder, as well as the rationale for novel curative strategies.

Jorge Oksenberg, Ph.D.
David Brassat, M.D., Ph.D.

Chapter 1

HLA and Autoimmunity:
Structural Basis of Immune Recognition

Kai W. Wucherpfennig

Abstract

The MHC region on human chromosome 6p21 is a critical susceptibility locus for many human autoimmune diseases. Susceptibility to a number of these diseases, including rheumatoid arthritis, multiple sclerosis and type 1 diabetes, is associated with particular alleles of HLA-DR or HLA-DQ genes. Crystal structures of HLA-DR and HLA-DQ molecules with bound peptides from candidate autoantigens have demonstrated that critical polymorphic residues determine the shape and charge of key pockets of the peptide binding site and thus determine the interaction of these MHC molecules with peptides. These data provide strong support for the hypothesis that these diseases are peptide-antigen driven. In HLA-DR associated autoimmune diseases such as rheumatoid arthritis and pemphigus vulgaris, key polymorphic determinants are primarily localized to the P4 pocket of the binding site and determine whether the pocket has a positive or negative charge. Peptide binding studies have demonstrated that these changes in the P4 pocket have a significant impact on the repertoire of self-peptides that can be presented by these MHC class II molecules. In HLA-DQ associated diseases such as type 1 diabetes and celiac disease, the β57 polymorphism is critical for peptide presentation since it determines the charge of the P9 pocket of the binding site. The crystal structure of HLA-DQ8 demonstrated that the P9 pocket has a positive charge in HLA-DQ molecules associated with type 1 diabetes, due to the absence of a negative charge at β57. Striking structural similarities were identified between the human DQ8 and murine I-A^{g7} molecules that confer susceptibility to type 1 diabetes, indicating that similar antigen presentation events may be relevant in humans and the NOD mouse model. Recent studies in the NOD mouse indicated that I-A^{g7} can promote expansion in the thymus of a CD4 T cell population which recognizes a peptide ligand that stimulates a panel of islet-specific T cell clones. MHC class II molecules that confer susceptibility to an autoimmune disease may thus promote positive selection of potentially pathogenic T cell population in the thymus and later induce the differentiation of these cells into effector populations by presentation of peptides derived from the target organ.

General Structural Features of MHC Class II Molecules

The peptide binding site of MHC class II molecules is formed by the N-terminal domains of the α and β chains, with each chain contributing approximately half of the floor as well as one of the two long α helices that form the peptide binding site (Fig. 1).[1,2] The binding site is open at both ends so that peptides of different length can be bound, explaining why nested sets of peptides have been identified for a given epitope in peptide elution studies.[1,3,4] Peptides are typically bound with a high affinity and a long half-life ($t_{1/2}$ of several days or even weeks) and mass spectrometry experiments have demonstrated that at least several hundred different

Immunogenetics of Autoimmune Disease, edited by Jorge Oksenberg and David Brassat.

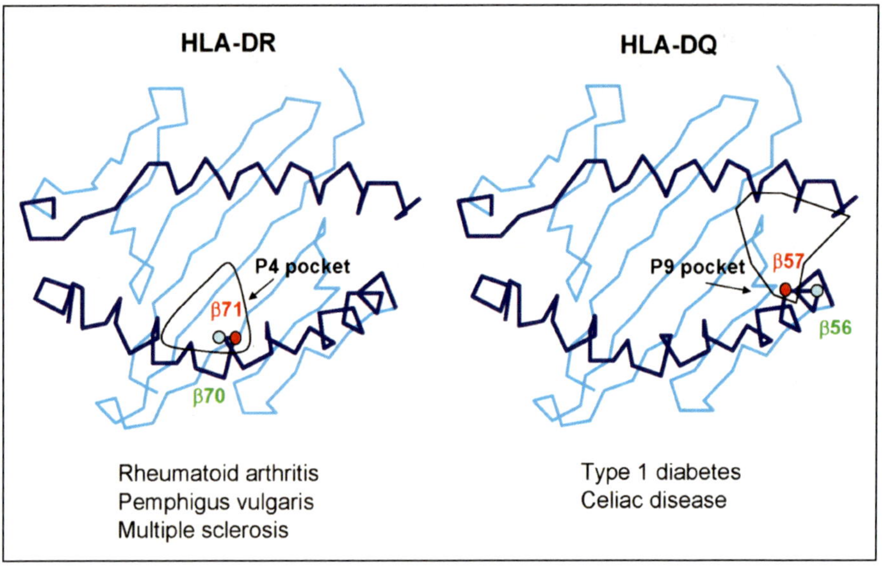

Figure 1. Key polymorphic MHC class II residues in DR and DQ associated human autoimmune diseases. The polymorphic DR β70 and β71 residues are important in DR associated autoimmune diseases and determine the shape and charge of the P4 pocket of the binding site. In the rheumatoid arthritis associated DR alleles (DRB1*0401, DRB1*0404 and DRB1*0101), β71 carries a positive charge (lysine or arginine). In contrast, both β70 and β71 are negatively charged in the pemphigus vulgaris (PV) associated DR allele (DRB1*0402). PV is an antibody-mediated autoimmune disease of the skin and the PV-associated DR4 subtype differs from a rheumatoid arthritis-associated DR4 subtype at only three positions in the binding site (DR β67, β70 and β71). In the multiple sclerosis associated DRB1*1501 molecule, β71 is a small, uncharged amino acid (alanine), resulting in a P4 pocket that is large and hydrophobic. The β57 polymorphism is critical in DQ associated autoimmune diseases. Susceptibility to type 1 diabetes is most closely associated with the DQB gene, and position β57 is not charged (an alanine) in the disease associated DQ8 and DQ2 molecules. In contrast, an aspartic acid residue is present at position β57 in the DQ molecules that either confer dominant protection from type 1 diabetes or are not associated with susceptibility to the disease. DQ2 and DQ8 also confer susceptibility to celiac disease, an inflammatory disease of the small intestine caused by dietary proteins, in particular wheat gliadins.

peptides are bound by a given MHC class II molecule.[3-6] Two modes of interaction permit high affinity binding of peptides: a sequence-independent mode based on formation of hydrogen bonds between the backbone of the peptide and conserved residues of the MHC class II binding site, and sequence-dependent interactions in which peptide side chains occupy defined pockets of the binding site.[1,2] Since peptides of different length can be bound by MHC molecules, the peptide residue that occupies the first pocket is referred to as the P1 anchor. Peptides are bound to MHC class II molecules in an extended conformation and five peptide side chains (P1, P4, P6, P7 and P9) in the core nine-amino acid segment can occupy pockets of the binding site.[2]

Structural Properties of HLA-DR Molecules Associated with Human Autoimmune Diseases

Structural and functional studies on DR molecules that confer susceptibility to rheumatoid arthritis (RA), pemphigus vulgaris (PV) and multiple sclerosis (MS) have identified features of the peptide binding site that are important for the binding of peptides from self-antigens. Particularly relevant are the polymorphic residues that shape the P4 pocket located in the center of the binding groove.

Susceptibility to rheumatoid arthritis is associated with the 'shared epitope', a segment of the DRβ chain helix (β67-74) that is very similar in sequence among disease-associated DR4 (DRB1*0401 and 0404) and DR1 (DRB1*0101) molecules.[7] In structural terms, this 'shared epitope' primarily defines the shape and charge of the P4 pocket.[8] The P4 pocket has a positive charge in the RA-associated DR1 and DR4 subtypes, due to the presence of a basic residue (lysine or arginine) at position β71 and the absence of an acidic residue at the other polymorphic residues that contribute to this pocket. In contrast, DR4 subtypes that do not confer susceptibility to RA carry a negative charge at positions β70 and β71 (DRB1*0402) or β74 (DRB1*0403, DRB1*0406, DRB1*0407) in the P4 pocket. Peptide binding studies have demonstrated that the RA-associated DR4 subtypes have a preference for negatively charged or small peptide side chains in the P4 pocket and that the β71 polymorphism is particularly important in determining binding specificity.[9]

Interestingly, susceptibility to pemphigus vulgaris is associated with a DR4 subtype (DRB1*0402) in which acidic residues are present at both β70 and β71 of the P4 pocket, resulting in a pocket with a negative charge.[10] PV is an autoimmune disease of the skin induced by autoantibodies against desmoglein-3, a keratinocyte surface protein, and these autoantibodies interfere with the interaction among keratinocytes and thus induce the formation of blisters in the skin and mucous membranes.[11] The PV-associated DR4 subtype is rare in the general population and differs from the RA-associated DRB1*0404 subtype only at three positions of the peptide binding site.[12] Two of these polymorphic residues (β70 and β71) are located in the P4 pocket and determine which peptides from the desmoglein-3 autoantigen can be presented to CD4 T cells. We have identified a peptide from human desmoglein-3 that is presented by the PV-associated DR4 subtype, but not other DR4 subtypes, to T cell clones isolated from patients with the disease. Presentation of this peptide was abrogated by mutation of residues β70 and β71, but not by mutation of β67, indicating that the polymorphic residues of the P4 pocket are critical. A second desmoglein-3 peptide that was also presented by the PV-associated DR4 molecule was identified using the same approach.[10] These data indicate that polymorphic MHC class II residues localized to one particular pocket of the DR binding site represent a key feature of MHC-linked susceptibility in a human autoimmune disease.

Susceptibility to multiple sclerosis (MS) is associated with the DR2 (DRB1*1501) haplotype. This MHC class II haplotype carries two functional DRβ chain genes (DRB1*1501 and DRB5*0101) and two different DR dimers can thus be formed by pairing with the nonpolymorphic DRα chain.[13] The structure of the DRB1*1501 molecule was determined with a bound peptide from human myelin basic protein (MBP) that is recognized by T cell clones isolated from patients with MS and normal donors.[14] Biochemical studies had demonstrated that two hydrophobic anchor residues (valine at P1 and phenylalanine at P4) were critical for high affinity binding.[15] A large, primarily hydrophobic P4 pocket was found to be a prominent feature of the DRB1*1501 peptide binding site. This pocket was occupied by a phenylalanine of the MBP peptide which made an important contribution to the binding of the MBP peptide to this MHC class II molecule. The presence of a small, uncharged residue (alanine) at the polymorphic DRβ71 position created the necessary room for the binding of a large hydrophobic side chain in the P4 pocket. The binding of aromatic side chains by the P4 pocket of DRB1*1501 is also facilitated by two aromatic residues of the P4 pocket (β26 Phe and β78 Tyr, of which β26 is polymorphic).[14] An alanine at β71 is relatively rare among DRB1 alleles since most alleles encode lysine, arginine or glutamic acid at this position.

These structural studies demonstrate that the polymorphic residues that shape the P4 pocket of the peptide binding site can be important determinants in DR associated human autoimmune diseases. Other polymorphic residues also contribute to the peptide binding specificities of these MHC class II molecules, but these key polymorphisms drastically change the repertoire of peptides that can be presented. The P4 pocket is the most polymorphic pocket of the DR binding site and the DR molecules associated with susceptibility to RA, PV and MS differ substantially in the shape and charge of the P4 pocket: the pocket carries a positive charge in the RA-associated DR1 and DR4 subtypes, a negative charge in the PV-associated DR subtype and is large and hydrophobic in the MS-associated DR2 (DRB1*1501) molecule.

Structure and Function of HLA-DQ Molecules That Confer Susceptibility to Type 1 Diabetes and Celiac Disease

Crystal Structure of HLA-DQ8 with a Bound Peptide from Human Insulin

The MHC region is the most important susceptibility locus for type 1 diabetes (*IDDM1*) and accounts for an estimated 42% to the familial clustering of the disease. By comparison, the contribution of other loci to familial clustering is relatively small, with an estimated 10% for *IDDM2* (insulin gene) and an even smaller fraction for other candidate loci.[16] Susceptibility is most closely associated with the DQB gene in the MHC class II region, based on linkage studies in families and association studies in patient and control groups.[17,18] The two alleles of the DQB gene that confer the highest risk for type 1 diabetes – DQB1*0201 and DQB1*0302 – encode the β chains of the DQ2 (DQA1*0501, DQB1*0201) and DQ8 (DQB1*0301, DQB1*0302) heterodimers. The risk for type 1 diabetes is greatly increased in individuals who are homozygous for these DQB genes and therefore express DQ8/DQ8 or DQ2/DQ2, and is even higher in subjects who are heterozygous and coexpress DQ8 and DQ2.[17,18] Analysis of MHC genes in different populations has demonstrated that these alleles of the DQB gene confer susceptibility in different ethnic groups, including Caucasians, Blacks and Chinese, providing further support for the hypothesis that the DQB gene rather than a closely linked gene is critical. A notable exception is Japan where the frequency of type 1 diabetes and these particular DQB alleles is relatively low, and where a different allele of DQB (DQB1*0401) confers susceptibility to the disease.[19,20]

These disease associations are highly specific since DQB alleles that encode proteins which differ at only one or a few polymorphic residues do not confer susceptibility to type 1 diabetes. Susceptibility to type 1 diabetes is strongly associated with the polymorphic DQ β57 residue. DQ molecules associated with susceptibility to type 1 diabetes carry a nonaspartic acid at this position (an alanine in DQ8 and DQ2), while an aspartic acid residue is present at β57 in DQ molecules that confer dominant protection from the disease (such as DQB1*0602) or are not associated with susceptibility to the disease.[17] The same polymorphic position is also critical in the NOD mouse model of the disease since β57 is a serine in I-A^{g7}, rather than an aspartic acid as in most murine I-A molecules.[21]

DQ8 was crystallized with a peptide from human insulin (B chain, res. 9-23) that represents a prominent T cell epitope for islet infiltrating CD4 T cells in NOD mice.[22,23] A T cell response to the insulin B (9-23) peptide has also been documented in patients with recent onset of type 1 diabetes and in prediabetics.[24] The insulin B (9-23) peptide binds with high affinity to DQ8 and the complex has a long half-life ($t_{1/2}$ >72 hours).[25] The crystal structure demonstrated particular features of DQ8 that allow presentation of this insulin peptide. Three side chains of the insulin peptide are buried in deep pockets of the DQ8 binding site, and two of these peptide side chains carry a negative charge (glutamic acid at P1 and P9). A tyrosine residue is bound in the P4 pocket, which is very deep and hydrophobic (Figs. 2 and 3).[23] The observation that acidic residues can be accommodated in two pockets of DQ8 has implications for the pathogenesis of type 1 diabetes and celiac disease, as discussed below.

Particularly important are the structural features of the P9 pocket of DQ8, which is in part shaped by residue β57 (Fig. 3). Both DQ8 and DQ2 carry an alanine at β57, rather than an aspartic acid residue which is present in alleles that do not confer susceptibility to type 1 diabetes. In MHC class II molecules with aspartic acid at this position, the P9 pocket is electrostatically neutral since the salt bridge between β57 aspartic acid and α76 arginine neutralizes the basic α76 residue, as shown in Figure 3C for the complex of DR1 and a influenza hemagglutinin peptide.[2] In contrast, the P9 pocket of DQ8 has a positive charge (blue color in Fig. 2), due to the absence of a negatively charged residue at β57. In the DQ8/insulin peptide complex, a salt bridge is instead formed between the glutamic acid side chain of the peptide and α76 arginine (Fig. 3B).[23] The formation of a salt bridge between the peptide and α76 accounts for the

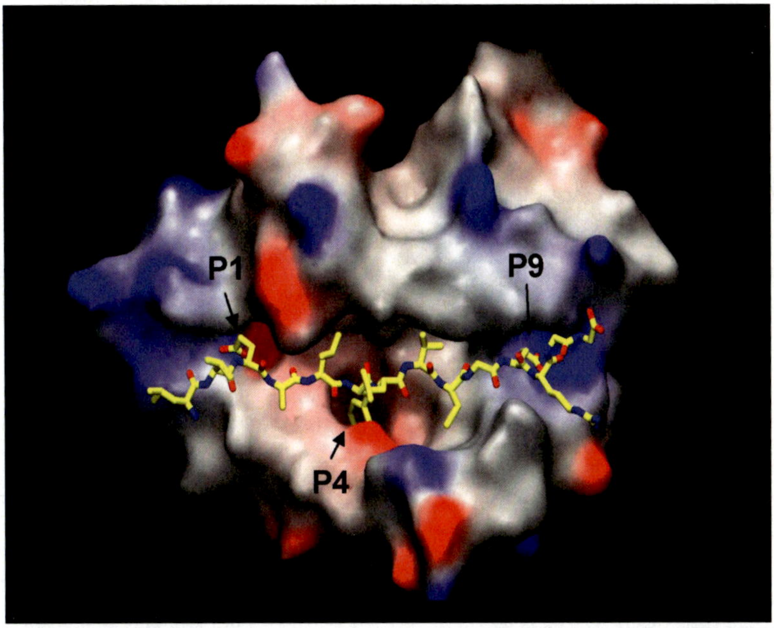

Figure 2. Crystal structure of the type 1 diabetes-associated DQ8 molecule with a bound peptide from human insulin. DQ8 was cocrystallized with the insulin B (9-23) peptide that is recognized by islet infiltrating T cells in NOD mice. An unusual feature of the structure is the presence of two acidic peptide side chains in pockets of the binding site (glutamic acid in both P1 and P9 pockets). The P9 pocket has a positive charge in DQ8 (blue color), due to the absence of a negative charge at β57. The P4 pocket of DQ8 is very deep and occupied by a tyrosine residue of the insulin peptide.

observed preference of the P9 pocket of DQ8 for negatively charged amino acids, and may contribute to the long half-life of the insulin peptide for DQ8. However, it is important to note that other residues can also be accommodated in the P9 pocket of DQ8, albeit with a reduced affinity.[25,26] The β57 polymorphism therefore has a drastic impact on the peptide binding specificity of DQ molecules: a preference for acidic peptide side chains is observed when β57 is a nonaspartic acid residue but such acidic side chains are strongly disfavored in the P9 pocket of MHC class II molecules with an aspartic acid at β57.

The crystal structure of I-A^{g7}, the MHC class II molecule that confers susceptibility to diabetes in NOD mice, has also been determined, allowing direct structural comparison of these diabetes-associated MHC molecules.[27,28] An important similarity between these structures is that the P9 pocket of both DQ8 and I-A^{g7} is basic. Peptide binding studies demonstrated that the P9 pocket of I-A^{g7} has a preference for negatively charged residues, as observed for DQ8.[29] In the I-A^{g7}/GAD peptide complex, a glutamic acid side chain occupies the P9 pocket and forms hydrogen bonds with α76 arginine and β57 serine (Fig. 3D).[27] Despite these important similarities, most of the polymorphic residues that shape the P9 pocket actually differ between DQ8 and I-A^{g7}, including residues β55-57 (Pro-Pro-Ala in DQ8 and Arg-His-Ser in I-A^{g7}, as shown in Figure 3B and 3D. The difference in the residues that shape the P9 pocket indicates that the alleles of DQB and I-Aβ that confer susceptibility to type 1 diabetes have evolved independently from their DQ and I-A ancestors, respectively, to converge with similar peptide-binding properties that confer some unknown advantage in immune protection that has the unfortunate side-effect of increasing the risk for type 1 diabetes.[23]

Due to the structural similarities, DQ8 and I-A^{g7} can present the same peptides.[25] The majority of peptides that were identified as T cell epitopes of insulin, GAD65 and HSP60 in

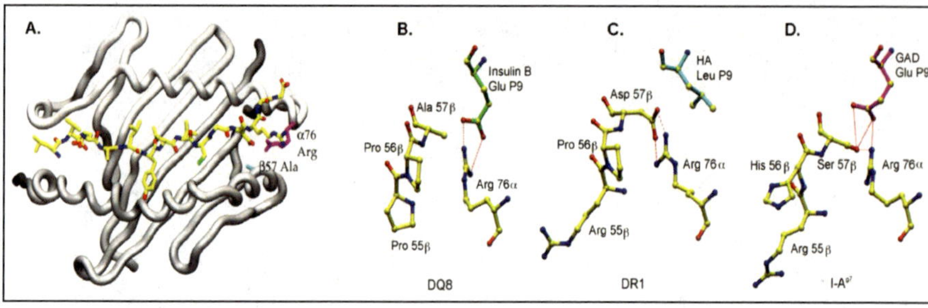

Figure 3. The β57 polymorphism determines the charge of the P9 pocket of the DQ8 peptide binding site. DQ β57 (blue color in Fig. 3A) is located on the helical segment of the DQ β chain and reaches into the P9 pocket of the binding site. Due the absence of a negative charge at this position, the positive charge of arginine 76 of the DQ α chain (α76 Arg, pink color) is not neutralized by formation of a salt bridge. As a result, the P9 pocket of DQ8 has a positive charge and a strong preference for acidic peptide side chains. In the DQ8 structure, a glutamic acid residue from the insulin peptide occupies this pocket and forms a salt bridge with α76 (Fig. 3B). β57 is also a nonaspartic acid residue in the MHC class II molecule (I-A^{g7}) expressed in NOD mice which develop spontaneous type 1 diabetes. Again, the P9 pocket carries a positive charge and has a strong preference for an acidic peptide side chain (glutamic acid in the structure of I-A^{g7} with a bound peptide from GAD65) (Fig. 3D). In contrast, a salt bridge is formed between β57 and α76 when an aspartic acid residue is located at β57. This results in a P9 pocket that is electrostatically neutral, as exemplified here by the structure of DR1 in which a hydrophobic residue of the bound influenza hemagglutinin peptide (leucine) occupies the P9 pocket (Fig. 3C). Reprinted from Nature Immunology with permission from the publisher.[23]

NOD mice also bind to DQ8. As discussed above, the P9 pocket of DQ8 and I-A^{g7} has a preference for negatively charged residues, and in addition, the P4 pocket of both molecules is large and hydrophobic. Differences are observed in the detailed architecture of the P1 pocket, which can accommodate a number of different amino acid side chains in both DQ8 and I-A^{g7}.[23,27,28]

The crystal structures demonstrate that β57, a key polymorphic residue, directly affects the interaction of these MHC class II molecules with peptides. The structural and functional similarities between DQ8 and I-A^{g7} suggest that similar antigen presentation events are involved in the development of type 1 diabetes in humans and NOD mice.

Presentation of Deamidated Gliadin Peptides by HLA-DQ8 and HLA-DQ2 in Celiac Disease

Susceptibility to celiac disease, a relatively common inflammatory disease of the small intestine, is associated with the same MHC class II molecules – DQ2 and DQ8 – that confer susceptibility to type 1 diabetes. The majority of patients with celiac disease express DQ2 (>90% in most ethnic groups) and/or DQ8. Celiac disease is one of the few HLA-associated diseases in which the critical antigen is known. The disease is caused by ingestion of cereal proteins, in particular wheat gliadins, and removal of these proteins from the diet results in clinical remission.[30] Celiac disease is much more prevalent in patients with type 1 diabetes (7.7-8.7% of biopsy confirmed cases) than in the general population (incidence of 0.2-0.5%). Antibodies to transglutaminase, a marker for celiac disease, are particularly common in type 1 diabetics who are homozygous for DQ2 (32.4% of antibody positive patients). The increased risk for celiac disease in patients with type 1 diabetes is, at least in part, due to the shared MHC class II genes.[31,32]

T cell clones specific for gliadins have been isolated from intestinal biopsies of patients with celiac disease, and these T cell clones are DQ2 or DQ8 restricted and proliferate in response to gliadins that have been proteolytically cleaved by pepsin or chymotrypsin. Patients with celiac

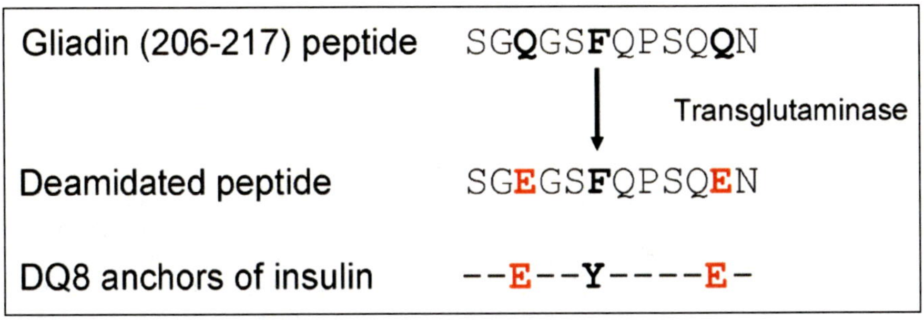

Figure 4. Enzymatic modification of a gliadin peptide creates a DQ8-restricted T cell epitope in celiac disease. Susceptibility to celiac disease, an inflammatory disease of the small intestine, is associated with DQ8 and DQ2. These MHC class II molecules present peptides from dietary proteins (gliadins) to gut-infiltrating T cells, and the T cell epitopes are created by deamidation of glutamine residues of gliadin by transglutaminase. This enzymatic modification converts glutamines to glutamic acid and thus creates the negatively charged anchor residues required for DQ8 and DQ2 binding. Modification of two glutamines in the gliadin (206-217) peptide results in a peptide that has very similar anchor residues to the insulin B (9-23) used for cocrystallization with DQ8: glutamic acid residues at P1 and P9, as well as an aromatic residue (tyrosine versus phenylalanine) at P4. These data thus explain how DQ8 confers susceptibility to two different autoimmune diseases - type 1 diabetes and celiac disease.

disease also develop antibodies to tissue transglutaminase, an enzyme in the intestinal mucosa that can deamidate glutamine residues to glutamic acid when limiting amounts of primary amines are present. Gliadins are very rich in glutamine and proline residues, and treatment of gliadin with transglutaminase dramatically increases the stimulatory capacity of the protein for DQ2 and DQ8 restricted T cell clones.[30,33]

A DQ8 restricted T cell epitope of gliadin was mapped to residues 206-217 within a natural pepsin fragment using T cell clones isolated from intestinal biopsies of two patients. Mass spec analysis of proteolytic gliadin fragments treated with transglutaminase demonstrated deamidation of glutamine 208 and 216. Synthetic peptides in which one or both of these residues were replaced by glutamic acid had a greatly increased stimulatory capacity for these DQ8 restricted T cell clones (Fig. 4).[34] The two glutamine/glutamic acid residues are spaced such that they could represent P1 and P9 anchors of the peptide, which would place phenylalanine 211 in the P4 pocket. When both glutamines are converted to glutamic acid, this gliadin peptide therefore has DQ8 anchors that are strikingly similar to the insulin B (9-23) peptide: glutamic acid at P1 and P9, and an aromatic residue (phenylalanine instead of tyrosine) at P4 (Figs. 2, 4).

Conversion of a single glutamine to glutamic acid (res. 65) is critical for the DQ2 restricted T cell response to gliadin. This gliadin segment (res. 57-75) contains two overlapping T cell epitopes, res. 57-68 and 62-75, centered around residue 65. For both peptides, conversion of glutamine 65 to glutamic acid greatly increases the stimulatory capacity for DQ2 restricted T cell clones isolated from the intestine as well as binding to DQ2. Binding of modified gliadin peptides to DQ8 and DQ2 is thus dependent on enzymatic modifications that create acidic peptide side chain(s).[35]

These studies thus provide a structural explanation for the association of susceptibility to two different autoimmune diseases with DQ8 and DQ2. The β57 polymorphism is critical in disease susceptibility since it permits binding of peptides with acidic side chains in the P9 pocket of the DQ8 binding site. The studies in celiac disease indicate that such epitopes can arise as the result of post-translational modifications. Recent studies have implicated enzymatic modifications of self-antigens in other autoimmune diseases, in particular rheumatoid arthritis. Enzymatic conversion of an arginine to citrulline by peptidyl arginine deiminase removes a positive charge from the arginine head group and thereby drastically alters the electrostatic properties of proteins or peptides. Autoantibodies to citrullinated proteins have been detected at early stages of rheumatoid arthritis, indicating that such post-translational modifications may be relevant in the disease process.[36,37]

Disease-Associated MHC Class II Molecules and Thymic Repertoire Selection

The structural and functional studies described above demonstrate that polymorphic residues that are critical in MHC-linked susceptibility to autoimmune diseases determine the shape and charge of key pockets of the peptide binding site. Alleles that confer susceptibility differ from nonassociated alleles at only one or a few positions in the binding site, implying a high degree of specificity. Peptide binding experiments have demonstrated that disease-associated MHC molecules bind peptides from candidate autoantigens, but other peptides from the same autoantigens can be bound by MHC molecules that do not confer susceptibility to the disease. The high degree of specificity implied by the genetic data could, however, be explained by a two-stage model in which the disease-associated MHC polymorphisms determine the outcome of two critical antigen presentation events: presentation of peptides in the thymus that promote positive selection of potentially pathogenic T cell populations, followed later by presentation of peptides from autoantigens to the same T cells in the target organ and draining lymph nodes.

Recent work in the NOD mouse model of type 1 diabetes has provided experimental support for this hypothesis.[38,39] These studies were based on peptide ligands that have been identified for a series of islet-specific T cell clones reactive with an islet secretory granule antigen.[40,41] These clones were isolated by two research groups from islets of prediabetic NOD mice or spleen/lymph nodes of diabetic NOD mice and were shown to cause diabetes following transfer to NOD *scid/scid* mice.[41,42] The BDC-2.5 T cell receptor (TCR) has also been used to generate TCR transgenic mice which develop spontaneous diabetes.[43] The native autoantigen is not known, but analysis of combinatorial peptide libraries has provided a series of peptide mimetics that stimulate these T cell clones/hybridomas at low peptide concentrations. Surprisingly, six of seven independent clones/hybridomas were stimulated by the same peptide mimetics, indicating that the majority of these clones have the same antigen specificity.[40,41]

Since conventional assays that rely on effector T cell functions are not particularly suitable for analysis of the thymic T cell repertoire, we examined the T cell repertoire using tetrameric forms of MHC class II/peptide complexes.[38] A series of I-A^{g7} tetramers were generated by a peptide exchange procedure in which a covalently linked, low affinity CLIP peptide was exchanged with different peptides following proteolytic cleavage of the linker. No CD4 T cell populations could be identified for two GAD65 peptides, but tetramers with a peptide mimetic recognized by the BDC-2.5 and other islet-specific T cell clones labeled a distinct $CD4^+$ T cell population in the thymus of young NOD mice. Tetramer-positive cells were identified in the immature $CD4^+CD8^{lo}$ population that arises during positive selection, and in larger numbers in the more mature $CD4^+CD8^-$ population. The T cell population was already present in the thymus of 2-week old NOD mice before the typical onset of insulitis. An expanded population of these T cells was also observed in the thymus of B10 mice congenic for *H-2*^{g7}, indicating that the NOD MHC genes were sufficient for positive selection of this T cell population on a different genetic background.

The frequency of these cells ($1{:}10^3$ to $1{:}2x10^3$) is several orders of magnitude higher than the average precursor frequency estimated for T cells with a given MHC/peptide specificity in the naïve T cell pool ($1{:}10^6$ to $1{:}10^7$). Tetramer labeling was specific, based on a number of criteria: (1) Discrete cell populations were not detected in the thymus of NOD mice with a panel of control tetramers; (2) The tetramer-labeled cell population could be significantly enriched with anti-PE microbeads, while no enrichment of cells labeled with control tetramers was observed; (3) The cell population was present in the thymus of NOD and B10.*H-2*^{g7}, but not B10 control mice; (4) Staining was greatly reduced by a single amino acid substitution in the peptide known to affect activation of T cell clones/hybridomas reactive with the islet autoantigen; (5) Two mimic peptides known to stimulate the same islet-specific T cell clones labeled this thymic T cell population, even though these peptides only shared sequence identity at four positions within the nine-amino acid core.[38] Similar findings were reported by Stratmann et al who generated an I-A^{g7} tetramer with a covalently linked BDC mimic peptide.[39] T cell hybridomas isolated based on tetramer labeling responded to the mimic peptide and islets in the presence of antigen presenting cells, indicating that the T cells identified with this tetramer were islet-reactive.[39] Based on these data we propose a model in which I-A^{g7} confers susceptibility to type 1 diabetes by biasing positive selection in the thymus and later presenting peptides from islet autoantigens to such T cells in the periphery.

These findings have important implications for thymic T cell repertoire development, in particular in terms of MHC-linked susceptibility to autoimmunity. The surprisingly high frequency of CD4 T cells identified with I-A^{g7}/BDC tetramers demonstrates that the T cell repertoire in NOD mice can be highly biased, apparently because positive selection of this population is efficient while negative selection is either inefficient or largely absent. An important role of thymic repertoire selection in susceptibility to autoimmunity could explain the exquisite allele specificity observed for disease-associated versus nonassociated MHC class II alleles. A key aspect of MHC-associated susceptibility to type 1 diabetes is the presence of a nonaspartic acid residue at position 57 of both DQ and I-A β chains.[17,21] Based on these data, we propose that MHC class II molecules which confer susceptibility to type 1 diabetes act at two distinct sites: initially in the thymus by promoting efficient positive selection of potentially pathogenic T cell populations and later in pancreatic lymph nodes and islets by presenting islet-derived peptides that induce differentiation of these T cells into effector cells that initiate and propagate the inflammatory process. The stringent structural requirements for peptide presentation implied by the genetic data could thus be explained by the requirement for presentation of different peptides in the thymus and the periphery to the same T cell population. This two-stage model (Fig. 5) of MHC-linked susceptibility could thus account for the observation that particular structural properties of I-A^{g7} and DQ8 are tied to disease susceptibility. In most other DQ and I-A molecules, the aspartic acid residue present at β57 forms a salt bridge with arginine α76, but this salt-bridge is not formed in DQ8 and I-A^{g7}. Arginine α76 is instead available to form a salt bridge with acidic peptide side chains bound in the P9 pocket.[23] The β57 polymorphism may thus permit presentation of positively selecting peptides (with an acidic residue at P9) and simultaneously prevent binding of peptides that could induce negative selection of relevant T cell populations (peptides with side chains that cannot be accommodated in the P9 pocket). Experiments in transgenic NOD mice support this hypothesis since mice that coexpressed a mutant I-A^{g7} β chain with substitutions of residues β56 and 57 of the P9 pocket were protected from the disease.[44] A substantial level of positive selection may also occur for other T cell populations that are relevant in the disease process in NOD mice.

Several other lines of evidence indicate that thymic repertoire selection is critical in the development of type 1 diabetes. In humans, susceptibility to the disease is influenced by the promoter region of the insulin gene (*IDDM2* locus) and protective alleles are associated with higher levels of insulin mRNA in the thymus.[45,46] In NOD mice, a defect in thymic negative selection has been reported. Kishimoto and Sprent demonstrated that negative selection in NOD mice was impaired for a population of semi-mature thymocytes in the medulla with a $CD4^{+}CD8^{-}HSA^{Hi}$ phenotype.[47] Reduced levels of apoptosis were observed for this cell population in vitro following stimulation with anti-CD3 or anti-CD3 plus anti-CD28 or in vivo following injection of the superantigen staphylococcus enterotoxin B (SEB). This defect in apoptosis was not observed in NOR, B6.*H-2^{g7}* or (B6.*H-2^{g7}*xNOD)F_1 mice.[47] Lesage et al demonstrated a T cell intrinsic defect in thymic negative selection in NOD mice based on a transgenic model in which a membrane-bound form of hen egg lysozyme (HEL) was expressed in islets, along with a HEL-specific TCR. Negative selection of HEL specific T cells was defective on the NOD but not the B10 background, and experiments in bone marrow chimeras demonstrated that the defect was T cell intrinsic.[48]

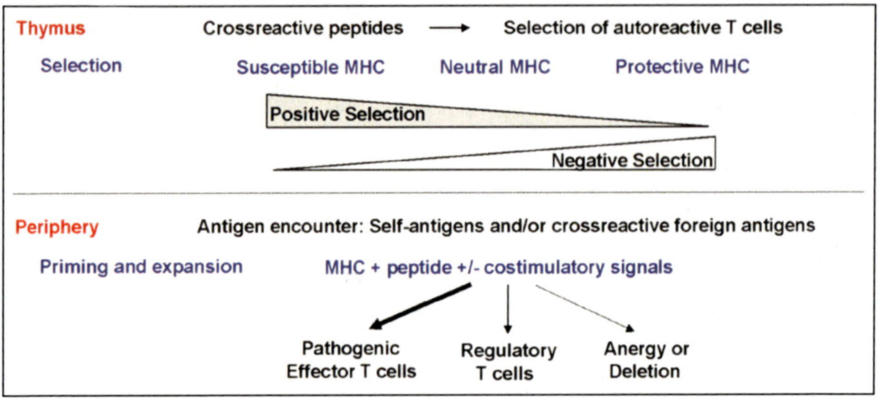

Figure 5. Disease-associated MHC class II molecules may influence susceptibility to autoimmunity by shaping the T cell repertoire in the thymus. Recent studies in the NOD mouse model have demonstrated thymic expansion of an islet-specific CD4 T cell population due to efficient positive selection. Two antigen presentation events may therefore be relevant in MHC-linked susceptibility to autoimmunity: presentation of thymic self-peptides that promote positive selection of a potentially pathogenic T cell population, followed later by presentation of peptides from the target organ to this T cell population and differentiation of these T cells into effector cells. Protective MHC class II molecules may either induce thymic deletion of potentially pathogenic T cell populations and/or induce the generation of regulatory T cells.

A failure of negative selection has also been implicated for the immunodominant T cell epitope of myelin proteolipid protein (PLP, res. 139-151) in SJL mice. Immunization with this peptide induces a severe, chronic form of experimental autoimmune encephalomyelitis (EAE). Only an alternatively spliced form that did not include the exon encoding the PLP (139-151) epitope was detected in the thymus, while both splicing variants were expressed in the target organ. This failure of negative selection is evidenced by the fact that PLP (139-151) specific T cells can be readily detected in nonimmunized mice in a T cell proliferation assay.[49,50] It is possible that the same mechanism is responsible for the observation that T cells recognized by I-A^{g7}/BDC tetramers are not deleted in the thymus. MHC class II molecules that confer susceptibility to an autoimmune disease may thus set the stage for disease development by permitting the emergence of potentially pathogenic T cell populations from the thymus.

Acknowledgements

I would like to thank my colleagues and collaborators for their major contributions to work discussed here, in particular Drs. Kon Ho Lee and Don C. Wiley, as well as Drs. Mei-Huei Jang, Nilufer Seth, Laurent Gauthier, Bei Yu and Dorothee Hausmann. I would also like to thank Drs. Don Wiley and Kon Ho Lee for providing (Figs. 2 and 3). This work was supported by grants from the NIH (PO1 AI45757, RO1 NS044914), the Juvenile Diabetes Research Foundation International, a Career Development Award from the American Diabetes Association (ADA) and the National Multiple Sclerosis Society.

References

1. Brown JH, Jardetzky TS, Gorga JC et al. Three-dimensional structure of the human class II histocompatibility antigen HLA-DR1. Nature 1993; 364:33-39.
2. Stern LJ, Brown JH, Jardetzky TS et al. Crystal structure of the human class II MHC protein HLA-DR1 complexed with an influenza virus peptide. Nature 1994; 368:215-221.
3. Hunt DF, Michel H, Dickinson TA et al. Peptides presented to the immune system by the murine class II major histocompatibility complex molecule I-Ad. Science 1992; 256:1817-1820.

4. Chicz RM, Urban RG, Gorga JC et al. Specificity and promiscuity among naturally processed peptides bound to HLA-DR alleles. J Exp Med 1993; 178:27-47.
5. Lanzavecchia A, Reid PA, Watts C. Irreversible association of peptides with class II MHC molecules in living cells. Nature 1992; 357:249-252.
6. Jensen PE. Long-lived complexes between peptide and class II major histocompatibility complex are formed at low pH with no requirement for pH neutralization. J Exp Med 1992; 176:793-798.
7. Gregersen PK, Silver J, Winchester RJ. The shared epitope hypothesis. An approach to understanding the molecular genetics of susceptibility to rheumatoid arthritis. Arthritis Rheum 1987; 30:1205-1213.
8. Dessen A, Lawrence CM, Cupo S et al. X-ray crystal structure of HLA-DR4 (DRA*0101, DRB1*0401) complexed with a peptide from human collagen II. Immunity 1997; 7:473-481.
9. Hammer J, Gallazzi F, Bono E et al. Peptide binding specificity of HLA-DR4 molecules: Correlation with rheumatoid arthritis association. J Exp Med 1995; 181:1847-1855.
10. Wucherpfennig KW, Yu B, Bhol K et al. Structural basis for major histocompatibility complex (MHC)-linked susceptibility to autoimmunity: Charged residues of a single MHC binding pocket confer selective presentation of self-peptides in pemphigus vulgaris. Proc Natl Acad Sci USA 1995; 92:11935-11939.
11. Amagai M, Klaus-Kovtun V, Stanley JR. Autoantibodies against a novel epithelial cadherin in pemphigus vulgaris, a disease of cell adhesion. Cell 1991; 67:869-877.
12. Scharf SJ, Friedmann A, Brautbar C et al. HLA class II allelic variation and susceptibility to pemphigus vulgaris. Proc Natl Acad Sci USA 1988; 85:3504-3508.
13. Sone T, Tsukamoto K, Hirayama K et al. Two distinct class II molecules encoded by the genes within HLA-DR subregion of HLA-Dw2 and Dw12 can act as stimulating and restriction molecules. J Immunol 1985; 135:1288-1298.
14. Smith KJ, Pyrdol J, Gauthier L et al. Crystal structure of HLA-DR2 (DRA*0101, DRB1*1501) complexed with a peptide from human myelin basic protein. J Exp Med 1998; 188:1511-1520.
15. Wucherpfennig KW, Sette A, Southwood S et al. Structural requirements for binding of an immunodominant myelin basic protein peptide to DR2 isotypes and for its recognition by human T cell clones. J Exp Med 1994; 179:279-290.
16. Davies JL, Kawaguchi Y, Bennett ST et al. A genome-wide search for human type 1 diabetes susceptibility genes. Nature 1994; 371:130-136.
17. Todd JA, Bell JI, McDevitt HO. HLA-DQ beta gene contributes to susceptibility and resistance to insulin-dependent diabetes mellitus. Nature 1987; 329:599-604.
18. Noble JA, Valdes AM, Cook M et al. The role of HLA class II genes in insulin-dependent diabetes mellitus: Molecular analysis of 180 Caucasian, multiplex families. Am J Hum Genet 1996; 59:1134-1148.
19. Nepom GT, Erlich H. MHC class-II molecules and autoimmunity. Annu Rev Immunol 1991; 9:493-525.
20. Awata T, Kuzuya T, Matsuda A et al. Genetic analysis of HLA class II alleles and susceptibility to type 1 (insulin-dependent) diabetes mellitus in Japanese subjects [published erratum appears in Diabetologia 1992 Sep;35(9):906]. Diabetologia 1992; 35:419-424.
21. Acha-Orbea H, McDevitt HO. The first external domain of the nonobese diabetic mouse class II I-A beta chain is unique. Proc Natl Acad Sci USA 1987; 84:2435-2439.
22. Wegmann DR, Norbury-Glaser M, Daniel D. Insulin-specific T cells are a predominant component of islet infiltrates in prediabetic NOD mice. Eur J Immunol 1994; 24:1853-1857.
23. Lee KH, Wucherpfennig KW, Wiley DC. Structure of a human insulin peptide-HLA-DQ8 complex and susceptibility to type 1 diabetes. Nat Immunol 2001; 2:501-507.
24. Alleva DG, Crowe PD, Jin L et al. A disease-associated cellular immune response in type 1 diabetics to an immunodominant epitope of insulin. J Clin Invest 2001; 107:173-180.
25. Yu B, Gauthier L, Hausmann DH et al. Binding of conserved islet peptides by human and murine MHC class II molecules associated with susceptibility to type I diabetes. Eur J Immunol 2000; 30:2497-2506.
26. Kwok WW, Domeier ME, Johnson ML et al. HLA-DQB1 codon 57 is critical for peptide binding and recognition. J Exp Med 1996; 183:1253-1258.
27. Corper AL, Stratmann T, Apostolopoulos V et al. A structural framework for deciphering the link between I-Ag7 and autoimmune diabetes. Science 2000; 288:505-511.
28. Latek RR, Suri A, Petzold SJ et al. Structural basis of peptide binding and presentation by the type I diabetes-associated MHC class II molecule of NOD mice. Immunity 2000; 12:699-710.
29. Hausmann DH, Yu B, Hausmann S et al. pH-dependent peptide binding properties of the type I diabetes-associated I-Ag7 molecule: Rapid release of CLIP at an endosomal pH. J Exp Med 1999; 189:1723-1734.

30. Sollid LM. Molecular basis of celiac disease. Annu Rev Immunol 2000; 18:53-81.
31. Gillett PM, Gillett HR, Israel DM et al. High prevalence of celiac disease in patients with type 1 diabetes detected by antibodies to endomysium and tissue transglutaminase. Can J Gastroenterol 2001; 15:297-301.
32. Bao F, Yu L, Babu S et al. One third of HLA DQ2 homozygous patients with type 1 diabetes express celiac disease-associated transglutaminase autoantibodies. J Autoimmun 1999; 13:143-148.
33. Molberg O, McAdam SN, Korner R et al. Tissue transglutaminase selectively modifies gliadin peptides that are recognized by gut-derived T cells in celiac disease. Nat Med 1998; 4:713-717.
34. van de Wal Y, Kooy YM, van Veelen PA et al. Small intestinal T cells of celiac disease patients recognize a natural pepsin fragment of gliadin. Proc Natl Acad Sci USA 1998; 95:10050-10054.
35. Arentz-Hansen H, Korner R, Molberg O et al. The intestinal T cell response to alpha-gliadin in adult celiac disease is focused on a single deamidated glutamine targeted by tissue transglutaminase. J Exp Med 2000; 191:603-612.
36. Schellekens GA, de Jong BA, van den Hoogen FH et al. Citrulline is an essential constituent of antigenic determinants recognized by rheumatoid arthritis-specific autoantibodies. J Clin Invest 1998; 101:273-281.
37. Masson-Bessiere C, Sebbag M, Girbal-Neuhauser E et al. The major synovial targets of the rheumatoid arthritis-specific antifilaggrin autoantibodies are deiminated forms of the alpha- and beta-chains of fibrin. J Immunol 2001; 166:4177-4184.
38. Jang MH, Seth NP, Wucherpfennig KW. Ex vivo analysis of thymic CD4 T cells in nonobese diabetic mice with tetramers generated from I-A(g7)/class II-associated invariant chain peptide precursors. J Immunol 2003; 171:4175-4186.
39. Stratmann T, Martin-Orozco N, Mallet-Designe V et al. Susceptible MHC alleles, not background genes, select an autoimmune T cell reactivity. J Clin Invest 2003; 112:902-914.
40. Judkowski V, Pinilla C, Schroder K et al. Identification of MHC class II-restricted peptide ligands, including a glutamic acid decarboxylase 65 sequence, that stimulate diabetogenic T cells from transgenic BDC2.5 nonobese diabetic mice. J Immunol 2001; 166:908-917.
41. Yoshida K, Martin T, Yamamoto K et al. Evidence for shared recognition of a peptide ligand by a diverse panel of nonobese diabetic mice-derived, islet-specific, diabetogenic T cell clones. Int Immunol 2002; 14:1439-1447.
42. Haskins K, Portas M, Bergman B et al. Pancreatic islet-specific T-cell clones from nonobese diabetic mice. Proc Natl Acad Sci USA 1989; 86:8000-8004.
43. Katz JD, Wang B, Haskins K et al. Following a diabetogenic T cell from genesis through pathogenesis. Cell 1993; 74:1089-1100.
44. Singer SM, Tisch R, Yang XD et al. Prevention of diabetes in NOD mice by a mutated I-Ab transgene. Diabetes 1998; 47:1570-1577.
45. Vafiadis P, Bennett ST, Todd JA et al. Insulin expression in human thymus is modulated by INS VNTR alleles at the IDDM2 locus. Nat Genet 1997; 15:289-292.
46. Pugliese A, Zeller M, Fernandez Jr A et al. The insulin gene is transcribed in the human thymus and transcription levels correlated with allelic variation at the INS VNTR-IDDM2 susceptibility locus for type 1 diabetes. Nat Genet 1997; 15:293-297.
47. Kishimoto H, Sprent J. A defect in central tolerance in NOD mice. Nat Immunol 2001; 2:1025-1031.
48. Lesage S, Hartley SB, Akkaraju S et al. Failure to censor forbidden clones of CD4 T cells in autoimmune diabetes. J Exp Med 2002; 196:1175-1188.
49. Klein L, Klugmann M, Nave KA et al. Shaping of the autoreactive T-cell repertoire by a splice variant of self protein expressed in thymic epithelial cells. Nat Med 2000; 6:56-61.
50. Anderson AC, Nicholson LB, Legge KL et al. High frequency of autoreactive myelin proteolipid protein-specific T cells in the periphery of naive mice: Mechanisms of selection of the self-reactive repertoire. J Exp Med 2000; 191:761-770.

CHAPTER 2

Genomic Variation and Autoimmune Disease

Silke Schmidt and Lisa F. Barcellos

Abstract

Genetic epidemiology is the study of the relationship between genomic and phenotypic variation with a goal to uncover the genetic basis of monogenic or complex disorders. A variety of study designs are available, and the importance of choosing an approach that is appropriate for the goals of the study cannot be over-emphasized. In addition to study design, important issues include selection of genetic marker type and number of markers to be tested, as well as the use of genotyping technology. In this chapter, we review these important features of genetic epidemiology studies with particular emphasis on applications to autoimmune conditions.

Introduction

Throughout this chapter, we assume that a qualitative (binary) phenotype is being investigated, i.e., all of the individuals enrolled for the study are classified as affected, unaffected, or unknown. Analysis strategies for quantitative traits are reviewed elsewhere.[1] We give an overview of study design considerations and statistical analysis methods, first for linkage, then for association analysis. Next, we discuss genotyping methods, focusing on the most common type of genomic variation, the single-nucleotide polymorphisms (SNPs) that have been made available to the research community as part of the Human Genome Project. We then review example linkage and association studies for autoimmune disorders. We end this chapter with a brief overview of new genome-wide screening approaches, including the use of DNA pooling for increased cost efficiency.

Study Design and Methods of Linkage Analysis

If the goal of the study is to identify regions in the human genome likely to harbor susceptibility genes for the phenotype of interest, a data set suitable for linkage analysis should be collected. Here, no assumptions are made a priori about the involvement of any particular gene or genomic region in the disease process. At minimum, an informative data set would be composed of families with at least two sampled affected, biologically related individuals (e.g., families with at least one affected sibling pair), but much more information per family is contributed by extended pedigrees with more distantly related sampled individuals from two or more generations. Linkage analysis evaluates whether the joint inheritance pattern of disease phenotype and marker genotype in the collected pedigrees suggests that the underlying disease and marker locus are physically located close to one another ("linked") on the same chromosome. The biological basis of linkage between two loci is meiosis, the cell division that creates haploid gametes (sperm and ova) from diploid mother cells to ensure that the fusion of two gametes upon fertilization creates another diploid individual. During meiosis, homologous chromosomes pair up and exchange genetic material by crossing-over of an individual's maternal and paternal chromosome strands, thus creating a mosaic of "recombinant" segments with

Immunogenetics of Autoimmune Disease, edited by Jorge Oksenberg and David Brassat.

differing parental origin. The key observation for linkage analysis is the fact that recombination between any two loci on the same chromosome is more likely to occur the further apart the loci are, since greater distance provides more physical opportunity for recombination to occur. Therefore, the distance between two loci can be measured by the frequency with which new combinations of grandparental alleles are observed in the offspring resulting from the fusion of two haploid gametes (recombination frequency).

When only one generation of affected individuals is sampled and cosegregation of disease phenotype and marker genotype cannot be directly observed, the extent of linkage can be measured by evaluating marker allele sharing among affected relative pairs. This approach is based on the intuitive idea that pairs of relatives who share the same phenotype (e.g., both are affected) are expected to show above-average sharing of alleles at marker loci that are physically close to the disease locus causing the shared phenotype.[2] The most commonly used statistical methods for both types of linkage analysis are briefly reviewed below.

Model-Based Lod Score Analysis

A likelihood approach to model-based pedigree analysis has traditionally been applied to localize genes for Mendelian disorders, which are relatively rare in the general population and typically due to defects in a single gene with a large effect on disease risk. However, with some modifications, the same approach can be applied to the analysis of complex diseases including autoimmune disorders. For the analysis of a single marker, the pedigree likelihood is a function of the recombination fraction θ, which measures the proportion of new combinations of grandparental disease and marker alleles in the offspring generation due to recombination in the parental meiosis. Since only disease phenotypes, rather than genotypes, are observed, it is necessary to assume a specific genetic model for the relationship of disease phenotype and genotype in order to make inferences about the recombination fraction between the underlying loci. The components of a genetic model include allele frequency at disease and marker loci, mode of inheritance (dominant, recessive, additive, multiplicative), and probabilities of being affected given all possible genotypes at the unknown disease locus (penetrances). Using the assumed model parameters, the algorithm that computes the pedigree likelihood infers probabilities of underlying disease genotypes given observed phenotypes, which are then scored as recombinant or nonrecombinant with the observed marker genotypes. A likelihood ratio test comparing the pedigree likelihood under linkage ($\theta<1/2$) with the one under no linkage ($\theta=1/2$) is computed and the lod score is defined as the $\log_{10}$ of this likelihood ratio. A lod score of 3.0 or greater means that the observed pedigree data are at least $10^3=1000$ times more likely under linkage than under no linkage. This has traditionally been considered as statistically significant evidence for linkage, although this stringent threshold is rarely exceeded in the genetic analysis of complex disorders. Model-based lod score analysis for complex traits is typically carried out by (i) not letting unaffected individuals contribute information about their underlying disease genotype ("affecteds-only analysis", see[3] for details) and (ii) introducing a heterogeneity parameter, which allows for an estimated proportion of pedigrees not to be linked to the marker locus under study.[4] The analysis of multiple markers simultaneously (multipoint linkage analysis) is a straightforward, albeit computationally demanding extension of the single-point analysis described above and requires genetic maps (order and distances between markers) as an additional input parameter. Several freely available software packages implement model-based (parametric) lod score analysis, including VITESSE,[5] FASTLINK,[6] GENEHUNTER[7] and ALLEGRO.[8]

Model-Free Lod Score Analysis

While model-based linkage analysis essentially scores parental meioses as recombinant or nonrecombinant using observed or inferred genotypes at marker and disease locus, model-free approaches simply assess the evidence for excess marker allele sharing in pairs of sampled relatives who share the same disease phenotype. If the shared phenotype is due to shared genotypes at a putative disease locus, genotypes of nearby markers are expected to exhibit allele sharing

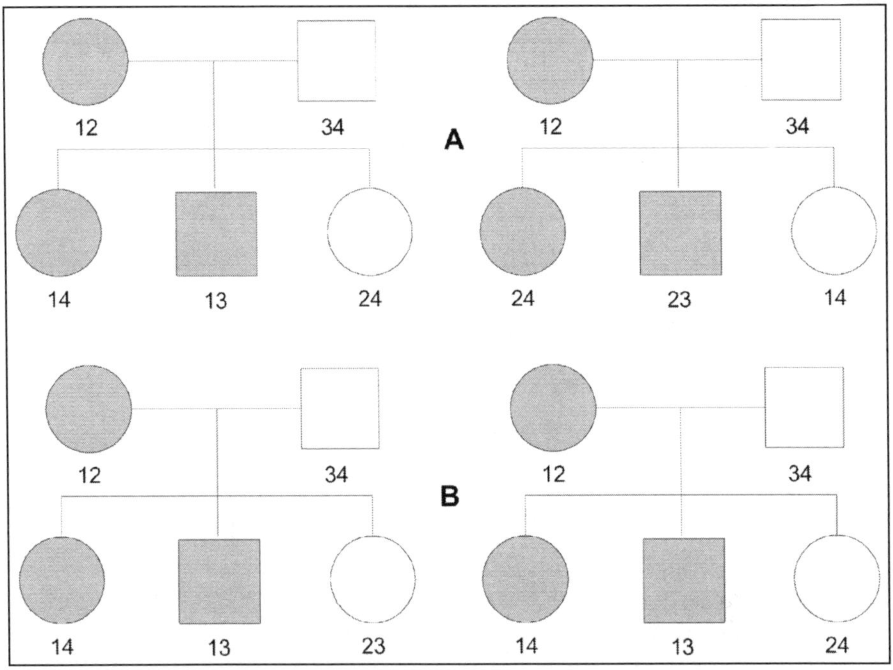

Figure 1. Comparison of linkage and association for a marker with four alleles. Squares denote males, circles denote females. Shaded symbols denote affected individuals. Marker genotypes are shown below symbols. Panel A: Presence of linkage but not association. Linkage is a property of loci, and different alleles at the same marker locus may cosegregate with the disease phenotype in different pedigrees. Panel B: Presence of linkage and association (linkage disequilibrium). Association is a property of alleles. Thus, the same marker allele is preferentially transmitted to affected offspring in different pedigrees.

above and beyond the background sharing determined by the biological relationship between these relatives. Thus, the estimation of allele sharing probabilities does not require explicit assumptions about genotype-phenotype relationships and is less "model-based" than the traditional lod score analysis. Likelihood-based methods for single-point and multipoint allele-sharing analysis among affected relative pairs have been implemented in several software packages, including GENEHUNTER-PLUS,[9] MERLIN[10] and ALLEGRO.[8] They primarily differ in the complexity of pedigrees they can handle and in computational speed. The likelihood-ratio statistics implemented in these programs are typically also log10-transformed and reported as (nonparametric) lod scores. The most common approach to linkage studies using affected relative pairs utilizes sibships with two or more affected individuals.

Study Design for Association Analysis

If the goal of the study is to test specific candidate regions identified in prior genome-wide linkage studies, or to test particular genes considered to be plausible susceptibility candidates based on biological or functional relevance, a study design for evaluating allelic association may be preferred. While linkage analysis examines intra-familial coinheritance of two or more *loci*, family-based association analysis assesses whether particular *alleles* are preferentially transmitted to affected rather than unaffected individuals across a collection of pedigrees. Therefore, linkage, but *not* association, exists when the same marker locus cosegregates with the disease phenotype in multiple pedigrees, but different alleles at this locus are transmitted with the putative disease allele in different pedigrees (Fig. 1, panel A). Linkage *and* association exist when the *same* marker allele is coinherited with the putative disease allele in different pedigrees, and the two alleles are then said to be in linkage disequilibrium (LD) in the population (Fig. 1, panel B). LD is generated when the susceptibility allele is first generated by mutation, at which point it exists only on the one particular ancestral haplotype of alleles at polymorphic loci surrounding it on the same chromosome. In present-day chromosomes, LD is a population-specific measure of the extent to which this originally very tight association has been broken up over time. In a randomly mating population, the decay of LD is primarily determined by the recombination frequency between the disease locus and adjacent loci, but is also strongly influenced by stochastic factors. LD can only persist over many generations when marker and disease loci are so tightly linked that their alleles almost never recombine. Therefore, the detection of LD between a putative disease allele and a measured marker allele provides a much greater resolution of the most likely location of the susceptibility locus than the detection of linkage. As a rule of thumb, LD in outbred populations may at best persist over physical distances of 50-100 kb, with highly variable local patterns across the human genome, whereas linkage is commonly observed for loci as far apart as 20 Mb. LD in inbred or isolated populations is maintained over much larger physical distances, for example, up to several Mb.[11] Greater statistical power to detect disease loci is often reported for association compared to linkage analysis.[12] An intuitive explanation is that linkage analysis only evaluates recombination information provided by the observed meioses within the collected pedigrees, whereas LD takes into account information from the unobserved meioses presumably connecting these pedigrees historically, given a genetically homogeneous population, although those pedigree structures are unknown to the investigator.[13]

It is important to note that alleles can be associated for reasons other than linkage, i.e., close physical proximity. For example, subgroups of a population with different marker allele frequencies may exist. If one subgroup happens to have a higher disease prevalence than another and affected individuals are thus sampled primarily from this subgroup, whereas unaffected individuals are sampled primarily from the other subgroup, marker allele frequencies may appear to be different in affected and unaffected individuals. However, this type of allelic association may exist even when marker and disease locus are physically located on two entirely different chromosomes and are thus completely unlinked.

A family-based association analysis may be performed on pedigrees with at least two sampled first-degree relatives, of which at least one is affected with the disease of interest. Alternatively, the investigator may collect a series of unrelated patients (cases), which is compared to a suitably matched collection of unrelated individuals without the disease of interest (controls). Family-based analysis can extract information about allelic association when the second sampled relative is either a parent, regardless of affection status, or an unaffected sibling. When methods that appropriately test for association in the presence of linkage are used[14] the same families that contribute information about linkage can also be included in a family-based association analysis. Spouses and offspring of an affected family member may also contribute information about allelic transmission.[15]

The main advantage of family-based over case-control association analysis is that it protects from the detection of spurious allelic association due to reasons other than linkage, since family-based controls are always genetically matched to the cases. The above example of different marker allele and disease frequencies in population subgroups illustrated the concept of allelic association that is *not* due to linkage and thus not helpful for mapping and identifying disease susceptibility genes. It is an example of the well-known confounding problem of epidemiologic case-control studies more generally. In this situation, the unknown subgroup membership of cases and controls, which is associated with both marker and disease allele frequency, is the confounder that causes false-positive evidence for marker-disease association. When such subgroups are defined by ethnicity and the investigator carefully documents each individual's ethnicity as part of the basic study information, confounding can be controlled either by matching cases and controls on ethnicity at the study design stage or by performing ethnicity-specific comparisons at the analysis stage. Therefore, the detection of false-positive association in a case-control study is only a potential problem if there is concern that subgroups cannot be correctly identified and that cases and controls may thus remain imperfectly matched on genetic background ("population stratification"). This concern received considerable attention in the genetic-epidemiologic literature after early reports of obvious false-positive associations in admixed populations[16] and has been a major driving force for the development of family-based tests of association. However, the issue has recently been debated in a more balanced fashion, suggesting that the early examples probably represented a worst-case scenario easily avoided with a reasonably well-designed epidemiologic study.[17,18] Empirical examples and analytical calculations demonstrated that subgroup differences in disease prevalence and marker allele frequencies had to be quite extreme to produce false-positive evidence for association, making it unlikely that such extreme differences would be unknown to the study investigator. Furthermore, several approaches have been proposed to assess, on the basis of genetic marker data for the actually sampled cases and controls, whether they are reasonably well matched on genetic background and how to correct for the presence of genome-wide marker allele frequency differences when they are not.[19-21] These ideas have become known as "genomic control" approaches and have further alleviated the concern about unknown population stratification in genetic case-control studies.

The question remains, however, whether a family-based or case-control study design should be chosen by the investigator. As mentioned above, the answer to this question is highly dependent on the specific goals of the study. In the absence of population stratification, case-control studies have been shown to be substantially more powerful than family-based studies for detecting main effects of disease-associated alleles.[22] On the other hand, family-based studies can be more powerful for the examination of gene-gene (GxG) and gene-environment (GxE) interaction,[23,24] particularly for genes with rare allele frequency. One of the most versatile family-based designs is the ascertainment of patients and their parents (case-parent triad), which was shown to provide good statistical power for estimating GxG and GxE interaction.[25] It also allows for the examination of parent-of-origin effects (e.g., imprinting) and the effect of maternal genotypes on the offspring's risk of disease.[26] Such effects may be of particular interest for conditions like birth defects and childhood disorders. For estimating main genetic effects, the "controls" in a case-parent triad design are the nontransmitted alleles at the marker locus. While GxE interaction is estimable from case-parent triad data, main environmental effects cannot be estimated due to the lack of such an implicit control.

The case-parent design may not be a feasible option for studies of late-onset disorders, since most parents of affected individuals are typically deceased by the time the study is conducted. The ascertainment of unaffected siblings of patients has been proposed as an alternative, but this design generally has lower power than case-parent triad or unrelated case-control studies for detecting main genetic effects. It may also suffer from overmatching of siblings with respect to some environmental factors, which negatively impacts the estimation of GxE interaction.[24] For late-onset disorders, phenotypic misclassification of unaffected siblings may present a problem and further restrict the pool of eligible sibling controls to include only those unaffected at an older age than the proband's age at onset.

Family-Based Association Analysis Methods

As mentioned above, the primary motivation for the development of family-based association analysis methods was the concern about false-positive evidence for association from case-control studies in populations with incompletely matched genetic background. One of the first approaches was the transmission/disequilibrium test (TDT), which is based on a matched-pairs comparison (McNemar test) of alleles transmitted and nontransmitted from heterozygous parents to affected offspring.[27] Various extensions of the TDT for nuclear families soon followed, allowing for more than one affected offspring, multiple marker alleles, missing parents, and the presence of one or more unaffected siblings. A widely used and very general family-based association test is the pedigree disequilibrium test (PDT),[14] which was the first test of association that can be applied in extended pedigrees and is valid even in the presence of linkage. When applied to nuclear families composed of affected offspring and their parents, it is similar to the original TDT. When applied to discordant sibships (at least one affected and one unaffected sibling), it is a slight modification of the sibship disequilibrium test (SDT).[28] Its strength is the combination of association evidence contributed by multiple parent-offspring triads and/or discordant sibships in extended pedigrees. A version that simultaneously scores the transmission of two alleles to affected offspring and can be more powerful under dominant and recessive modes of inheritance is also available (geno-PDT).[29] However, both versions of the PDT can only evaluate a single locus at a time and require genotypes from both parents to evaluate allelic transmission to affected offspring, i.e., the PDT cannot analyze incomplete triads composed of one genotyped parent and affected offspring.

An alternative to the PDT that incorporates information from incomplete parent-offspring triads and can analyze the transmission of haplotypes (combination of alleles at multiple loci in close physical proximity) in addition to single loci is the family-based association test implemented in the program FBAT.[30] The challenge posed by the analysis of more than one marker locus simultaneously is the presence of "unknown phase", which refers to a lack of knowledge about the cooccurrence of alleles on a single chromosome for individuals heterozygous at more than one locus. Recently, the original FBAT program was extended to accommodate missing phase information for haplotype analysis.[31] A disadvantage of the FBAT method is that it decomposes extended families into several nuclear families and employs only a variance correction to account for the relatedness of these nuclear families. A likelihood-based approach for haplotype analysis in extended pedigrees has been implemented in the PDTPHASE module of the UNPHASED package.[32]

Population-Based Association Analysis Methods

If cases and controls share the same genetic background and controls represent the source population that gave rise to the cases, case-control analysis of genetic markers is in principle quite similar to standard epidemiologic analyses, which have traditionally evaluated the association between environmental exposures and disease status. The primary decisions that have to be made by the investigator are (i) how to control for the effects of confounding variables, such as age and sex, and (ii) which inheritance model should be assumed for the unknown disease locus. Effects of confounding variables can be controlled at the design stage, by using individually or frequency-matched ascertainment of controls. Alternatively, a stratified analysis that examines genetic effects separately in strata defined by the confounders, or a logistic regression model that includes confounders as model covariates may be chosen. Regarding the inheritance model, it is very difficult to make general recommendations. If there were some prior evidence that the unknown disease locus may act in a dominant or recessive fashion, it would be reasonable to test that particular model in a case-control analysis. Suppose the geno-PDT gave evidence for over-transmission of a homozygous marker genotype to affected offspring, suggesting a recessive model for the disease gene whose allele may be in LD with the respective marker allele. The investigator may then choose to code only that homozygous genotype as "exposed" in a logistic regression model for unrelated cases and controls and use the other two genotypes as the reference (unexposed) group. In the absence of any prior information, the additive model has been suggested as a fairly robust test in the sense that it does not incur severe loss of statistical power when the true model is either dominant or recessive.[33] For a biallelic marker, this model may be coded by counting the number of times the minor allele at an SNP marker occurs in the three possible genotypes, i.e., the model covariate would take on values 0, 1, and 2 for genotypes 1/1, 1/2, 2/2, respectively, if "2" denotes the minor allele.

Several methods are available for testing the association of marker haplotypes with disease risk in a logistic regression model. One of the most comprehensive approaches has been implemented in the "haplo.stats"program, which requires the availability of either the S-plus (Insightful Corporation, Inc.) or R package for statistical analysis (http://www.r-project.org).[34,35] This program uses the EM algorithm[36] for likelihood-based analyses to account for the unknown phase of individuals that are heterozygous at more than one marker locus. As a regression model, it provides the ability to adjust for case-control differences in confounding variables or nongenetic risk factors for the disease under study, and it also implements test of haplotype-environment interactions.

Genetic Markers and Detection Methods

Being able to distinguish between genotypes that are relevant to a particular phenotype of interest is a major goal in studies of human disease. Advances in both molecular biology and genotyping technology have led to the development of many types of molecular markers. Microsatellites, or short tandemly repeated sequence motifs, were the first marker type to take full advantage of PCR technology. They are highly polymorphic, abundant and fairly evenly distributed throughout most areas of human genome. The construction of genetic maps in humans and several animals, and the majority of linkage studies and positional cloning of human disease genes during the past 10-15 years have been accomplished using microsatellite markers.[37] However, the recent completion of a draft sequence of the human genome[38] and resulting identification of many single nucleotide polymorphisms (SNPs) has markedly changed the scope and complexity of studies to identify disease genes. A genome wide SNP map has expanded from an initial draft containing 4000 in 1999, to a current version with over 6 million validated SNPs (see dbSNP at www.ncbi.nlm.nih.gov/ SNP). The main advantages of SNPs for complex disease gene mapping include their low mutation rate, abundant numbers throughout the human genome, ease of typing (i.e., not prone to the 'slippage' seen with microsatellite repeats) and high potential for an automated high throughput analysis (discussed below). It is estimated that SNPs occur on average once every 300-500 base pairs, and that the number of SNPs within the human genome (defined by a minor allele frequency of $\geq 1\%$ in at least one population) is likely to be at least 15 million.[39]

Utilizing dense screening panels of SNP markers, the genome has recently been characterized as a series of regions with high levels of LD or 'blocks' separated by short discrete segments of very low LD,[40,41] and the categorization of these blocks is in progress. Block patterns have been observed within the major histocompatibility complex (MHC) on ch. 6p21[42-44] in the immunoglobulin cluster on 5q31[40,45] and throughout several other chromosomes.[46,47] It is anticipated that a complete understanding of these patterns across the genome will greatly facilitate efforts to map disease complex disease genes by significantly reducing the number of genetic markers needed to detect disease associations.[48] To this end, the National Institutes of Health recently funded the Haplotype Mapping (or 'HapMap') project, an international effort (International HapMap Consortium) to create a genome-wide catalogue of common haplotype blocks in several different human populations.[49-51] The overall goal of this Consortium is to provide publicly available tools (http:// www.hapmap.org) that will allow the indirect association approach to be applied readily to any candidate region suggested by family-based linkage studies or biologically relevant candidate gene in the genome. Ultimately, this approach could be utilized for whole genome disease gene scans[51] (discussed below).

The extraordinary increase in genetic information and molecular markers for genetic mapping resulting from the Human Genome Project and HapMap efforts has been paralleled by significant progress in biotechnology. SNP identification and detection technologies have evolved from labor intensive, time consuming, and costly processes to some of the most highly automated, robust, and relatively inexpensive methods. The nearly completed and publicly available human genome sequence provides an invaluable reference against which all other sequencing data can be compared.[38,52] Today, SNP discovery for any given project is therefore only limited by available funding. While DNA sequencing is the gold standard of SNP discovery, historically it has been labor intensive and quite expensive. A number of other methods have been developed for local, targeted, SNP discovery including denaturing high performance liquid chromatography, and are reviewed elsewhere.[53]

The number of SNP genotyping methods has also grown significantly in recent years and many robust approaches are currently available. The ideal technology must be easily and reliably developed from DNA sequence information, robust, cost efficient, flexible and automated for ease of genotyping and data analysis.[53] Over the last decade, several methodologies have been described and utilized for sequence specific detection that employ hybridization, primer extension, ligation, or even combinations of these techniques. Although a variety of enzymatic and detection technologies have resulted in a number of robust SNP genotyping approaches and platforms, including several with very high throughput capabilities,[54-57] no single available method is ideally suited for all applications; for example, some platforms can readily identify SNP genotypes, but not variation due to insertion/deletion polymorphisms. New approaches must be developed to lower the cost and increase the speed of detection for SNP and other types of genetic variants.

Genetic Studies of Autoimmune Disorders

Independent genome-wide linkage searches of several autoimmune disorders have been performed and reported elsewhere.[58-67] A large number of candidate regions containing loci that collectively contribute to disease predisposition have been identified, including the MHC region. Linkage results from autoimmune disorders have demonstrated complex patterns as compared with traditional linkage studies of monogenic diseases. A greater number of linked loci with lower significance levels have been reported, and support a complex genetic etiology. For example, in type 1 diabetes (T1D) to date, three chromosomal regions have been identified definitively, six appear suggestive, and more than ten are implicated provisionally.[64,68,69] Several studies have provided strong evidence for overlap between different diseases of candidate regions and/or genes. Becker et al[70] recently compared linkage results from 23 human and experimental immune-mediated diseases. Clustering of susceptibility loci was detected, suggesting that in some cases, part of the pathophysiology of clinically distinct autoimmune disorders may be controlled by a common set of genes.[71,72] Other investigations also support this notion, including a recent genome scan of rheumatoid arthritis (RA) in which several identified regions had been previously implicated in studies of multiple sclerosis (MS), systemic lupus erythematosus (SLE) or inflammatory bowel disease (IBD).[59] Similar results have also been obtained in studies of experimental models of autoimmune disease.[73-77] Recent meta-analyses of many of these datasets have been performed separately for each autoimmune disease[60,68,78-81] and together in some cases[81] using both nonparametric pooled analyses of raw data and nonparametric ranking methods of p-values.

Further support for the presence of common autoimmune susceptibility genes comes from family studies. Familial clustering of multiple autoimmune diseases has been previously reported[82-90] and is more common than the coexistence of more than one disease within an individual. In a recent report, Broadley et al[85] investigated the prevalence of autoimmune disease in first-degree relatives of probands with MS using a case-control method. Their results showed a significant excess of autoimmune disease within these families, whereas the frequency of other chronic (nonautoimmune) diseases was not increased. Both Heinzlef et al[86] and Broadley et al[85] noted a higher prevalence of autoimmune thyroid disease (ATD) in MS families, which may suggest a relationship between the two conditions, although the specific mechanisms are not known. An increased prevalence of psoriasis previously reported by Midgard et al[91] was also observed by Broadley and colleagues.[85] Studies of associations between MS and other common autoimmune conditions such as T1D or IBD have provided suggestive, but also conflicting results.[85,88,89,92] Overall, the available data collectively support the notion that not only is the same autoimmune disease more prevalent in pedigrees of individuals affected with a given disorder, but other autoimmune conditions are increased as well. However, while a number of shared genotypes may genetically predispose to autoimmunity, the specific phenotype in individual family members could be determined by disease specific genes or environmental factors that may or may not be mutually exclusive.[93]

Clinical or phenotypic heterogeneity almost certainly contributes to the disparity observed between linkage screens in autoimmune disorders and other complex diseases where different loci may be contributing to particular disease phenotypes. For example, in recent genome screens of multiple affected SLE families stratified by distinct phenotypic features such as the presence of renal disease, hemolytic anemia, vitiligo, thrombocytopenia, RA and other clinical manifestations, additional prominent regions of linkage were identified[94-100] and await confirmation. Concordance in MS families for early and late clinical manifestations,[101-103] and in RA families for seropositivity and presence of nodules[104] has also been observed, further indicating that genes are likely to influence disease severity or other aspects of the clinical phenotype. In future screens, a strategy for genome-wide association studies that explicitly addresses heterogeneity will be ideal. In addition to predisposing genetic components within a subgroup of a particular disease, variables such as age of disease onset, gender, or other clinical manifestations can also be used for stratification, while at the same time maintaining use of large sample numbers for increased statistical power.

Candidate gene investigations are still very reasonable strategies for gene discovery in autoimmune disease. This approach takes advantage of both the biological understanding of the disease phenotype and the increased statistical efficiency of association-based methods of analysis, provided that the datasets are adequately powered. A candidate gene approach can be viewed as an important first step in exploring potential causal pathways between genetic variants and complex disorders.[105] Genes for study are selected based on functional relevance or location within a candidate region identified through linkage analyses. Associations with MHC region genes and specific HLA class II alleles have been confirmed for many autoimmune diseases including MS,[106] RA,[107] SLE,[108] T1D,[64] ATD,[109] IBD,[110] and others. For many of these conditions, strong evidence for the involvement of nonMHC genes has also been demonstrated, including *CARD15* in IBD,[111] *NOS2A* in MS,[112] and *PDCD1* in SLE and RA.[113,114] Perhaps the most compelling candidate gene for susceptibility to autoimmunity is the *CTLA4* locus on ch.2q33 which encodes a costimulatory molecule expressed on the surface of activated T cells.[115] Investigations have shown, with increasing evidence, that *CTLA4* variants are associated with autoimmune endocrinopathies such as T1D and ATD (Graves' disease and autoimmune hypothyroidism) as well as autoimmune Addison's disease and SLE.[77,116-119] Functional studies have shown that an associated *CTLA4* haplotype appears to correlate with lower mRNA levels of a soluble form of CTLA-4;[119] however other different alterations of soluble CTLA-4 have been reported.[120] Further efforts are needed to determine how variation within the *CTLA4* locus influences the development of autoimmunity.

New Approaches to Genome Wide Screening to Detect Disease Associations

Due to the increasing availability of SNPs in the human genome and decreasing costs of high-throughput SNP genotyping technologies, it may soon become feasible to conduct genome-wide association studies at sufficiently high marker density, thus "by-passing" linkage studies as a means to identify candidate regions for more detailed association analysis. However, since LD decays much faster than linkage, a substantially larger number of markers is necessary to detect LD of marker and susceptibility alleles, and estimates of the exact number depend on the population under study, the variability of LD across genomic regions, marker and disease allele frequencies, and the strength of the genetic effect. LD is much more a function of the specific genetic history of a population than linkage, which can be examined with essentially the same set of markers in different populations. It has been estimated that at least on the order of 300,000 and 1,000,000 SNPs would be required for genome-wide LD analysis in nonAfrican and African populations, respectively.[39,41,121] It is not yet clear how to best deal with the substantial multiple testing problem posed by the analysis of such a large number of markers,[122] and current genotyping costs are still too high to make genome-wide association studies a feasible alternative to linkage-based screens.

The use of DNA pooling has been proposed as one approach to significantly reduce the time and expense of a genome screen for association.[22,123-126] Pooling allows allele frequencies in groups of individuals to be measured and compared using far fewer PCR amplifications for marker assays than are used for individual genotyping. Although both careful quantitation of DNA samples and construction of pools are necessary when using pooled amplifications, this is performed just once for an entire screen and constitutes a small fraction of the actual typing effort. In general, a two or three stage approach is optimal whereby initial screens can be conducted using DNA pooling, and then only those sites yielding positive results are confirmed using individual genotyping.[123,126] Since the number of true loci is likely to be small in comparison with the number of candidate loci, many nonassociated regions could be excluded from further study by initially screening with pooled analyses. Several different methods for determining microsatellite marker allele frequencies and detecting disease associations have been published,[125,127-134] and the Genetic Analysis of Multiple Sclerosis in Europeans or 'GAMES' initiative recently completed the first-ever genome-wide association screen across multiple populations for any complex trait using large panels of PCR-based microsatellite markers and pooled DNA samples. This extraordinary effort was described as a series of papers in the October 2003 issue of Journal of Neuroimmunology (see ref 135). Microsatellite markers, however, can pose technical challenges even when used for individual sample genotyping due to both stutter artifacts and preferential amplification, which can vary significantly between markers.[123,136] Each marker behaves differently and needs to be carefully characterized initially, using individual genotyping to identify number of alleles and potential PCR related artifacts. Though it can be a time-consuming process, the use of mathematical methods for correction of these artifacts has also been suggested in order to obtain more accurate microsatellite frequencies.[136-138] DNA pooling strategies to screen the genome employing SNP markers are expected to be more successful, and several SNP genotyping approaches have recently been extended successfully to pooled DNA samples.[126,139]

Summary

In summary, there are many design and analysis options for mapping susceptibility genes for complex disorders. The choice between different study designs is largely determined by the characteristics of the disease under study and available resources. For example, the typical age at onset of the disease has a strong impact on whether a design using parental, sibling, or unrelated controls is appropriate; the diagnostic methods and budgetary resources may determine whether it is feasible to collect family members that could live in geographically distant regions or whether a population-based case-control design is more efficient. Statistical analysis methods and genotyping technologies continue to evolve, and genotyping costs are certain to decrease further over the next few years, making it likely that whole-genome association studies using a high-density SNP map will become feasible in the very near future. To make optimal use of the increasing availability of genomic resources, the investigator's choice of study design and analysis methods will likely become one of the most important determinants of the success in mapping complex disease genes.

References

1. Blangero J, Williams JT, Almasy L. Quantitative trait locus mapping using human pedigrees. Hum Biol 2000; 72(1):35-62.
2. Penrose LS. The general purpose sibpair linkage test. Ann Eugen 1953; 18(2):120-124.
3. Terwilliger JD, Ott J. Handbook of Human Genetic Linkage. Baltimore: Johns Hopkins University Press, 1994.
4. Ott J. The number of families required to detect or exclude linkage heterogeneity. Am J Hum Genet 1986; 39(2):159-165.
5. O'Connell JR, Weeks DE. The VITESSE algorithm for rapid exact multilocus linkage analysis via genotype set-recoding and fuzzy inheritance. Nat Genet 1995; 11(4):402-408.
6. Schaffer AA, Gupta SK, Shriram K et al. Avoiding recomputation in linkage analysis. Hum Hered 1994; 44(4):225-237.

7. Kruglyak L, Daly MJ, Reeve-Daly MP et al. Parametric and nonparametric linkage analysis: A unified multipoint approach. Am J Hum Genet 1996; 58(6):1347-1363.
8. Gudbjartsson DF, Jonasson K, Frigge ML et al. Allegro, a new computer program for multipoint linkage analysis. Nat Genet 2000; 25(1):12-13.
9. Kong A, Cox NJ. Allele-sharing models: LOD scores and accurate linkage tests. Am J Hum Genet 1997; 61(5):1179-1188.
10. Abecasis GR, Cherny SS, Cookson WO et al. Merlin—rapid analysis of dense genetic maps using sparse gene flow trees. Nat Genet 2002; 30(1):97-101.
11. Varilo T, Savukoski M, Norio R et al. The age of human mutation: Genealogical and linkage disequilibrium analysis of the CLN5 mutation in the finnish population. Am J Hum Genet 1996; 58(3):506-512.
12. Risch N, Merikangas K. The future of genetic studies of complex human diseases. Science 1996; 273(5281):1516-1517.
13. Terwilliger JD, Goring HH. Gene mapping in the 20th and 21st centuries: Statistical methods, data analysis, and experimental design. Hum Biol 2000; 72(1):63-132.
14. Martin ER, Monks SA, Warren LL et al. A test for linkage and association in general pedigrees: The pedigree disequilibrium test. Am J Hum Genet 2000; 67(1):146-154.
15. Lee WC. Genetic association studies of adult-onset diseases using the case-spouse and case-offspring designs. Am J Epidemiol 2003; 158(11):1023-1032.
16. Knowler WC, Williams RC, Pettitt DJ et al. Gm3;5,13,14 and type 2 diabetes mellitus: An association in American Indians with genetic admixture. Am J Hum Genet 1988; 43(4):520-526.
17. Wacholder S, Rothman N, Caporaso N. Population stratification in epidemiologic studies of common genetic variants and cancer: Quantification of bias. J Natl Cancer Inst 2000; 92(14):1151-1158.
18. Wacholder S, Rothman N, Caporaso N. Counterpoint: Bias from population stratification is not a major threat to the validity of conclusions from epidemiological studies of common polymorphisms and cancer. Cancer Epidemiol Biomarkers Prev 2002; 11(6):513-520.
19. Devlin B, Roeder K. Genomic control for association studies. Biometrics 1999; 55(4):997-1004.
20. Pritchard JK, Stephens M, Rosenberg NA et al. Association mapping in structured populations. Am J Hum Genet 2000; 67(1):170-181.
21. Reich DE, Goldstein DB. Detecting association in a case-control study while correcting for population stratification. Genet Epidemiol 2001; 20(1):4-16.
22. Risch N, Teng J. The relative power of family-based and case-control designs for linkage disequilibrium studies of complex human diseases I. DNA pooling. Genome Res 1998; 8(12):1273-1288.
23. Gauderman WJ. Sample size requirements for association studies of gene-gene interaction. Am J Epidemiol 2002; 155(5):478-484.
24. Gauderman WJ. Sample size requirements for matched case-control studies of gene-environment interaction. Stat Med 2002; 21(1):35-50.
25. Schaid DJ. Case-parents design for gene-environment interaction. Genet Epidemiol 1999; 16(3):261-273.
26. Weinberg CR, Wilcox AJ, Lie RT. A log-linear approach to case-parent-triad data: Assessing effects of disease genes that act either directly or through maternal effects and that may be subject to parental imprinting. Am J Hum Genet 1998; 62(4):969-978.
27. Spielman RS, McGinnis RE, Ewens WJ. Transmission test for linkage disequilibrium: The insulin gene region and insulin-dependent diabetes mellitus (IDDM). Am J Hum Genet 1993; 52(3):506-516.
28. Horvath S, Laird NM. A discordant-sibship test for disequilibrium and linkage: No need for parental data. Am J Hum Genet 1998; 63(6):1886-1897.
29. Martin ER, Bass MP, Gilbert JR et al. Genotype-based association test for general pedigrees: The genotype-PDT. Genet Epidemiol 2003; 25(3):203-213.
30. Rabinowitz D, Laird N. A unified approach to adjusting association tests for population admixture with arbitrary pedigree structure and arbitrary missing marker information. Hum Hered 2000; 50(4):211-223.
31. Horvath S, Xu X, Lake SL et al. Family-based tests for associating haplotypes with general phenotype data: Application to asthma genetics. Genet Epidemiol 2004; 26(1):61-69.
32. Dudbridge F. Pedigree disequilibrium tests for multilocus haplotypes. Genet Epidemiol 2003; 25(2):115-121.
33. Schaid DJ. General score tests for associations of genetic markers with disease using cases and their parents. Genet Epidemiol 1996; 13(5):423-449.
34. Schaid DJ, Rowland CM, Tines DE et al. Score tests for association between traits and haplotypes when linkage phase is ambiguous. Am J Hum Genet 2002; 70(2):425-434.

35. Lake SL, Lyon H, Tantisira K et al. Estimation and tests of haplotype-environment interaction when linkage phase is ambiguous. Hum Hered 2003; 55(1):56-65.
36. Dempster AP, Laird NM, Rubin DB. Maximum likelihood from incomplete data via the EM algorithm (with discussion). J R Stat Soc B 1977; B39:1-38.
37. Litt M, Luty JA. A hypervariable microsatellite revealed by in vitro amplification of a dinucleotide repeat within the cardiac muscle actin gene. Am J Hum Genet 1989; 44(3):397-401.
38. Lander ES, Linton LM, Birren B et al. Initial sequencing and analysis of the human genome. Nature 2001; 409(6822):860-921.
39. Botstein D, Risch N. Discovering genotypes underlying human phenotypes: Past successes for mendelian disease, future approaches for complex disease. Nat Genet 2003; 33(Suppl):228-237.
40. Daly MJ, Rioux JD, Schaffner SF et al. High-resolution haplotype structure in the human genome. Nat Genet 2001; 29(2):229-232.
41. Gabriel SB, Schaffner SF, Nguyen H et al. The structure of haplotype blocks in the human genome. Science 2002; 296(5576):2225-2229.
42. Jeffreys AJ, Kauppi L, Neumann R. Intensely punctate meiotic recombination in the class II region of the major histocompatibility complex. Nat Genet 2001; 29(2):217-222.
43. Walsh EC, Mather KA, Schaffner SF et al. An integrated haplotype map of the human major histocompatibility complex. Am J Hum Genet 2003; 73(3):580-590.
44. Stenzel A, Lu T, Koch WA et al. Patterns of linkage disequilibrium in the MHC region on human chromosome 6p. Hum Genet 2004; 114(4):377-385.
45. Anderson EC, Slatkin M. Population-genetic basis of haplotype blocks in the 5q31 region. Am J Hum Genet 2004; 74(1):40-49.
46. Patil N, Berno AJ, Hinds DA et al. Blocks of limited haplotype diversity revealed by high-resolution scanning of human chromosome 21. Science 2001; 294(5547):1719-1723.
47. Dawson E, Abecasis GR, Bumpstead S et al. A first-generation linkage disequilibrium map of human chromosome 22. Nature 2002; 418(6897):544-548.
48. Cardon LR, Abecasis GR. Using haplotype blocks to map human complex trait loci. Trends Genet 2003; 19(3):135-140.
49. Couzin J. Human genome. HapMap launched with pledges of $100 million. Science 2002; 298(5595):941-942.
50. Couzin J. Genomics. New mapping project splits the community. Science 2002; 296(5572):1391-1393.
51. The International HapMap project. Nature 2003; 426(6968):789-796.
52. Venter JC, Adams MD, Myers EW et al. The sequence of the human genome. Science 2001; 291(5507):1304-1351.
53. Kwok PY, Chen X. Detection of single nucleotide polymorphisms. Curr Issues Mol Biol 2003; 5(2):43-60.
54. Oliphant A, Barker DL, Stuelpnagel JR et al. BeadArray technology: Enabling an accurate, cost-effective approach to high-throughput genotyping. Biotechniques. 2002; (Suppl):56-58, 60-51.
55. Kennedy GC, Matsuzaki H, Dong S et al. Large-scale genotyping of complex DNA. Nat Biotechnol 2003; 21(10):1233-1237.
56. Matsuzaki H, Loi H, Dong S et al. Parallel genotyping of over 10,000 SNPs using a one-primer assay on a high-density oligonucleotide array. Genome Res 2004; 14(3):414-425.
57. Fakhrai-Rad H, Zheng J, Willis TD et al. SNP discovery in pooled samples with mismatch repair detection. Genome Res 2004; 14(7):1404-1412.
58. Barmada MM, Brant SR, Nicolae DL et al. A genome scan in 260 inflammatory bowel disease-affected relative pairs. Inflamm Bowel Dis 2004; 10(1):15-22.
59. Jawaheer D, Seldin MF, Amos CI et al. A genomewide screen in multiplex rheumatoid arthritis families suggests genetic overlap with other autoimmune diseases. Am J Hum Genet 2001; 68(4):927-936.
60. Jawaheer D, Seldin MF, Amos CI et al. Screening the genome for rheumatoid arthritis susceptibility genes: A replication study and combined analysis of 512 multicase families. Arthritis Rheum 2003; 48(4):906-916.
61. Gaffney PM, Kearns GM, Shark KB et al. A genome-wide search for susceptibility genes in human systemic lupus erythematosus sib-pair families. Proc Natl Acad Sci USA 1998; 95(25):14875-14879.
62. Gaffney PM, Ortmann WA, Selby SA et al. Genome screening in human systemic lupus erythematosus: Results from a second minnesota cohort and combined analyses of 187 sib-pair families. Am J Hum Genet 2000; 66(2):547-556.
63. Tomer Y. Genetic dissection of familial autoimmune thyroid diseases using whole genome screening. Autoimmun Rev 2002; 1(4):198-204.
64. Hirschhorn JN. Genetic epidemiology of type 1 diabetes. Pediatr Diabetes 2003; 4(2):87-100.

65. Coraddu F, Sawcer S, Feakes R et al. HLA typing in the united kingdom multiple sclerosis genome screen. Neurogenetics 1998; 2(1):24-33.
66. Coraddu F, Sawcer S, D'Alfonso S et al. A genome screen for multiple sclerosis in sardinian multiplex families. Eur J Hum Genet 2001; 9(8):621-626.
67. Haines JL, Ter-Minassian M, Bazyk A et al. A complete genomic screen for multiple sclerosis underscores a role for the major histocompatability complex. The Multiple Sclerosis Genetics Group [see comments]. Nat Genet 1996; 13(4):469-471.
68. Cox NJ, Wapelhorst B, Morrison VA et al. Seven regions of the genome show evidence of linkage to type 1 diabetes in a consensus analysis of 767 multiplex families. Am J Hum Genet 2001; 69(4):820-830.
69. Onengut-Gumuscu S, Concannon P. Mapping genes for autoimmunity in humans: Type 1 diabetes as a model. Immunol Rev 2002; 190:182-194.
70. Becker KG, Simon RM, Bailey-Wilson JE et al. Clustering of nonmajor histocompatibility complex susceptibility candidate loci in human autoimmune diseases. Proc Natl Acad Sci USA 1998; 95(17):9979-9984.
71. Becker KG. The common genetic hypothesis of autoimmune/inflammatory disease. Curr Opin Allergy Clin Immunol 2001; 1(5):399-405.
72. Becker KG. The common variants/multiple disease hypothesis of common complex genetic disorders. Med Hypotheses 2004; 62(2):309-317.
73. Bergsteinsdottir K, Yang HT, Pettersson U et al. Evidence for common autoimmune disease genes controlling onset, severity, and chronicity based on experimental models for multiple sclerosis and rheumatoid arthritis. J Immunol 2000; 164(3):1564-1568.
74. Vyse TJ, Todd JA. Genetic analysis of autoimmune disease. Cell 1996; 85(3):311-318.
75. Merriman TR, Cordell HJ, Eaves IA et al. Suggestive evidence for association of human chromosome 18q12-q21 and its orthologue on rat and mouse chromosome 18 with several autoimmune diseases. Diabetes 2001; 50(1):184-194.
76. Morahan G, Morel L. Genetics of autoimmune diseases in humans and in animal models. Curr Opin Immunol 2002; 14(6):803-811.
77. Raman K, Mohan C. Genetic underpinnings of autoimmunity—lessons from studies in arthritis, diabetes, lupus and multiple sclerosis. Curr Opin Immunol 2003; 15(6):651-659.
78. A meta-analysis of whole genome linkage screens in multiple sclerosis. J Neuroimmunol 2003; 143(1-2):39-46.
79. A meta-analysis of genomic screens in multiple sclerosis. The transatlantic multiple sclerosis genetics cooperative. Mult Scler 2001; 7(1):3-11.
80. van Heel DA, Fisher SA, Kirby A et al. Inflammatory bowel disease susceptibility loci defined by genome scan meta-analysis of 1952 affected relative pairs. Hum Mol Genet 2004; 13(7):763-770.
81. Wise LH, Lanchbury JS, Lewis CM. Meta-analysis of genome searches. Ann Hum Genet 1999; 63(Pt 3):263-272.
82. Ginn LR, Lin JP, Plotz PH et al. Familial autoimmunity in pedigrees of idiopathic inflammatory myopathy patients suggests common genetic risk factors for many autoimmune diseases. Arthritis Rheum 1998; 41(3):400-405.
83. Lin JP, Cash JM, Doyle SZ et al. Familial clustering of rheumatoid arthritis with other autoimmune diseases. Hum Genet 1998; 103(4):475-482.
84. Firooz A, Mazhar A, Ahmed AR. Prevalence of autoimmune diseases in the family members of patients with pemphigus vulgaris. J Am Acad Dermatol 1994; 31(3 Pt 1):434-437.
85. Broadley SA, Deans J, Sawcer SJ et al. Autoimmune disease in first-degree relatives of patients with multiple sclerosis. A UK survey. Brain 2000; 123(Pt 6):1102-1111.
86. Heinzlef O, Alamowitch S, Sazdovitch V et al. Autoimmune diseases in families of French patients with multiple sclerosis. Acta Neurol Scand 2000; 101(1):36-40.
87. McCombe PA, Chalk JB, Pender MP. Familial occurrence of multiple sclerosis with thyroid disease and systemic lupus erythematosus. J Neurol Sci 1990; 97(2-3):163-171.
88. Minuk GY, Lewkonia RM. Possible familial association of multiple sclerosis and inflammatory bowel disease. N Engl J Med 1986; 314(9):586.
89. Sadovnick AD, Paty DW, Yannakoulias G. Concurrence of multiple sclerosis and inflammatory bowel disease. N Engl J Med 1989; 321(11):762-763.
90. Henderson RD, Bain CJ, Pender MP. The occurrence of autoimmune diseases in patients with multiple sclerosis and their families. J Clin Neurosci 2000; 7(5):434-437.
91. Midgard R, Gronning M, Riise T et al. Multiple sclerosis and chronic inflammatory diseases. A case-control study. Acta Neurol Scand 1996; 93(5):322-328.
92. Marrosu MG, Cocco E, Lai M et al. Patients with multiple sclerosis and risk of type 1 diabetes mellitus in Sardinia, Italy: A cohort study. Lancet 2002; 359(9316):1461-1465.

93. Bias WB, Reveille JD, Beaty TH et al. Evidence that autoimmunity in man is a Mendelian dominant trait. Am J Hum Genet 1986; 39(5):584-602.
94. Namjou B, Nath SK, Kilpatrick J et al. Stratification of pedigrees multiplex for systemic lupus erythematosus and for self-reported rheumatoid arthritis detects a systemic lupus erythematosus susceptibility gene (SLER1) at 5p15.3. Arthritis Rheum 2002; 46(11):2937-2945.
95. Namjou B, Nath SK, Kilpatrick J et al. Genome scan stratified by the presence of anti-double -stranded DNA (dsDNA) autoantibody in pedigrees multiplex for systemic lupus erythematosus (SLE) establishes linkages at 19p13.2 (SLED1) and 18q21.1 (SLED2). Genes Immun 2002; 3(Suppl 1):S35-41.
96. Nath SK, Kelly JA, Namjou B et al. Evidence for a susceptibility gene, SLEV1, on chromosome 17p13 in families with vitiligo-related systemic lupus erythematosus. Am J Hum Genet 2001; 69(6):1401-1406.
97. Nath SK, Kelly JA, Reid J et al. SLEB3 in systemic lupus erythematosus (SLE) is strongly related to SLE families ascertained through neuropsychiatric manifestations. Hum Genet 2002; 111(1):54-58.
98. Kelly JA, Thompson K, Kilpatrick J et al. Evidence for a susceptibility gene (SLEH1) on chromosome 11q14 for systemic lupus erythematosus (SLE) families with hemolytic anemia. Proc Natl Acad Sci USA 2002; 99(18):11766-11771.
99. Scofield RH, Bruner GR, Kelly JA et al. Thrombocytopenia identifies a severe familial phenotype of systemic lupus erythematosus and reveals genetic linkages at 1q22 and 11p13. Blood 2003; 101(3):992-997.
100. Quintero-Del-Rio AI, Kelly JA, Kilpatrick J et al. The genetics of systemic lupus erythematosus stratified by renal disease: Linkage at 10q22.3 (SLEN1), 2q34-35 (SLEN2), and 11p15.6 (SLEN3). Genes Immun 2002; 3(Suppl 1):S57-62.
101. Brassat D, Azais-Vuillemin C, Yaouanq J et al. Familial factors influence disability in MS multiplex families. French Multiple Sclerosis Genetics Group. Neurology 1999; 52(8):1632-1636.
102. Barcellos LF, Oksenberg JR, Green AJ et al. Genetic basis for clinical expression in multiple sclerosis. Brain 2002; 125(Pt 1):150-158.
103. Kantarci OH, de Andrade M, Weinshenker BG. Identifying disease modifying genes in multiple sclerosis. J Neuroimmunol 2002; 123(1-2):144-159.
104. Jawaheer D, Lum RF, Amos CI et al. Clustering of disease features within 512 multicase rheumatoid arthritis families. Arthritis Rheum 2004; 50(3):736-741.
105. Tabor HK, Risch NJ, Myers RM. Opinion: Candidate-gene approaches for studying complex genetic traits: Practical considerations. Nat Rev Genet 2002; 3(5):391-397.
106. Barcellos LF, Oksenberg JR, Begovich AB et al. HLA-DR2 dose effect on susceptibility to multiple sclerosis and influence on disease course. Am J Hum Genet 2003; 72(3):710-716.
107. Jawaheer D, Li W, Graham RR et al. Dissecting the genetic complexity of the association between human leukocyte antigens and rheumatoid arthritis. Am J Hum Genet 2002; 71(3):585-594.
108. Graham RR, Ortmann WA, Langefeld CD et al. Visualizing human leukocyte antigen class II risk haplotypes in human systemic lupus erythematosus. Am J Hum Genet 2002; 71(3):543-553.
109. Simmonds MJ, Gough SC. Unravelling the genetic complexity of autoimmune thyroid disease: HLA, CTLA-4 and beyond. Clin Exp Immunol 2004; 136(1):1-10.
110. Duerr RH. The genetics of inflammatory bowel disease. Gastroenterol Clin North Am 2002; 31(1):63-76.
111. Bonen DK, Cho JH. The genetics of inflammatory bowel disease. Gastroenterology 2003; 124(2):521-536.
112. Barcellos LF, Begovich AB, Reynolds RL et al. Linkage and association with the NOS2A locus on chromosome 17q11 in multiple sclerosis. Ann Neurol 2004; 55(6):793-800.
113. Prokunina L, Castillejo-Lopez C, Oberg F et al. A regulatory polymorphism in PDCD1 is associated with susceptibility to systemic lupus erythematosus in humans. Nat Genet 2002; 32(4):666-669.
114. Prokunina L, Padyukov L, Bennet A et al. Association of the PD-1.3A allele of the PDCD1 gene in patients with rheumatoid arthritis negative for rheumatoid factor and the shared epitope. Arthritis Rheum 2004; 50(6):1770-1773.
115. Brunet JF, Denizot F, Luciani MF et al. A new member of the immunoglobulin superfamily—CTLA-4. Nature 1987; 328(6127):267-270.
116. Vaidya B, Pearce S. The emerging role of the CTLA-4 gene in autoimmune endocrinopathies. Eur J Endocrinol 2004; 150(5):619-626.
117. Chistiakov DA, Turakulov RI. CTLA-4 and its role in autoimmune thyroid disease. J Mol Endocrinol 2003; 31(1):21-36.
118. Kristiansen OP, Larsen ZM, Pociot F. CTLA-4 in autoimmune diseases—a general susceptibility gene to autoimmunity? Genes Immun 2000; 1(3):170-184.

119. Ueda H, Howson JM, Esposito L et al. Association of the T-cell regulatory gene CTLA4 with susceptibility to autoimmune disease. Nature 2003; 423(6939):506-511.
120. Oaks MK, Hallett KM. Cutting edge: A soluble form of CTLA-4 in patients with autoimmune thyroid disease. J Immunol 2000; 164(10):5015-5018.
121. Kruglyak L. Prospects for whole-genome linkage disequilibrium mapping of common disease genes. Nat Genet 1999; 22(2):139-144.
122. Wille A, Hoh J, Ott J. Sum statistics for the joint detection of multiple disease loci in case-control association studies with SNP markers. Genet Epidemiol 2003; 25(4):350-359.
123. Barcellos LF, Klitz W, Field LL et al. Association mapping of disease loci, by use of a pooled DNA genomic screen. Am J Hum Genet 1997; 61(3):734-747.
124. Kirov G, Williams N, Sham P et al. Pooled genotyping of microsatellite markers in parent-offspring trios. Genome Res 2000; 10(1):105-115.
125. Mohlke KL, Erdos MR, Scott LJ et al. High-throughput screening for evidence of association by using mass spectrometry genotyping on DNA pools. Proc Natl Acad Sci USA 2002; 99(26):16928-16933.
126. Sham P, Bader JS, Craig I et al. DNA Pooling: A tool for large-scale association studies. Nat Rev Genet 2002; 3(11):862-871.
127. Bansal A, van den Boom D, Kammerer S et al. Association testing by DNA pooling: An effective initial screen. Proc Natl Acad Sci USA 2002; 99(26):16871-16874.
128. Chen J, Germer S, Higuchi R et al. Kinetic polymerase chain reaction on pooled DNA: A high-throughput, high-efficiency alternative in genetic epidemiological studies. Cancer Epidemiol Biomarkers Prev 2002; 11(1):131-136.
129. Germer S, Holland MJ, Higuchi R. High-throughput SNP allele-frequency determination in pooled DNA samples by kinetic PCR. Genome Res 2000; 10(2):258-266.
130. Daniels J, Holmans P, Williams N et al. A simple method for analyzing microsatellite allele image patterns generated from DNA pools and its application to allelic association studies. Am J Hum Genet 1998; 62(5):1189-1197.
131. Daniels J, McGuffin P, Owen MJ et al. Molecular genetic studies of cognitive ability. Hum Biol 1998; 70(2):281-296.
132. Collins HE, Li H, Inda SE et al. A simple and accurate method for determination of microsatellite total allele content differences between DNA pools. Hum Genet 2000; 106(2):218-226.
133. Plomin R, Hill L, Craig IW et al. A genome-wide scan of 1842 DNA markers for allelic associations with general cognitive ability: A five-stage design using DNA pooling and extreme selected groups. Behav Genet 2001; 31(6):497-509.
134. Williams NM, Spurlock G, Norton N et al. Mutation screening and LD mapping in the VCFS deleted region of chromosome 22q11 in schizophrenia using a novel DNA pooling approach. Mol Psychiatry 2002; 7(10):1092-1100.
135. Barcellos LF, Thomson G. Genetic analysis of multiple sclerosis in Europeans. J Neuroimmunol 2003; 143(1-2):1-6.
136. Setakis E. Statistical analysis of the GAMES studies. J Neuroimmunol 2003; 143(1-2):47-52.
137. Perlin MW, Lancia G, Ng SK. Toward fully automated genotyping: Genotyping microsatellite markers by deconvolution. Am J Hum Genet 1995; 57(5):1199-1210.
138. LeDuc C, Miller P, Lichter J et al. Batched analysis of genotypes. PCR Methods Appl 1995; 4(6):331-336.
139. Norton N, Williams NM, Williams HJ et al. Universal, robust, highly quantitative SNP allele frequency measurement in DNA pools. Hum Genet 2002; 110(5):471-478.

Chapter 3

Endocrine Diseases:

Type I Diabetes Mellitus

Regine Bergholdt, Michael F. McDermott and Flemming Pociot

Introduction

Type 1 diabetes (T1D) [MIM 222100] is the third most prevalent chronic disease of childhood, affecting up to 0.4% of individuals in some populations by age 30 years, with an overall lifetime risk of nearly 1%.[1,2] T1D is caused by absolute insulin deficiency due to destruction of the pancreatic β-cells. The majority of T1D cases are believed to develop as a result of immune-mediated destruction of the β-cells, leaving a small proportion of idiopathic cases in which immune markers cannot be detected, which are caused by other pathogenetic mechanisms such as rare genetic syndromes, β-cell lytic virus infections, or environmental factors.[3] T1D is associated with an increased risk of premature death due to acute complications and chronic disabling and life-threatening manifestations, including eye disease and blindness, renal failure, neuropathy and cardiovascular disease.[4]

The etiology of T1D is unknown, but it is recognized that both genetic and environmental determinants are important in defining disease risk. Family studies, including twin studies, have shown that T1D clusters in families,[5] but does not segregate with a known mode of inheritance. The incidence and prevalence of T1D have increased, and also the age at onset in some populations has decreased over the last decades.[6-8] These data, coupled with the incomplete concordance for the phenotype in monozygotic twins (30%-70%),[9,10] and differences in incidence between genetically comparable populations,[2] suggest that the penetrance of T1D alleles is strongly influenced by environmental factors. T1D is clustered in families with an overall genetic risk ratio (λ_S) of approximately 15.[11] At least one locus that contributes strongly to T1D occurring in several family members resides within the major histocompatibility complex (MHC) on chromosome 6p21. However, HLA genes (*IDDM1*) of the MHC region alone cannot explain the familial incidence of T1D. In the general population, individuals who carry the high-risk haplotypic combination of *HLA-DRB1*04-DQB1*0302/DRB1*03-DQB1*0201* have ~5% absolute risk of T1D. However, within affected sib-pair families, this genotype has ~20% risk.[12,13] Secondly, a number of nonHLA loci have been identified which have small yet significant effect on T1D risk – see below. Finally, the observed risk of T1D in first- and second-degree relatives declines in a pattern consistent with multiplicative effects of multiple loci.[14]

The HLA Region in T1D Susceptibility

The MHC represents the most intensively studied 4 Mb in the human genome. Associations between autoimmune disease and alleles of genes in this region are among the most consistent findings in human genetics. Genetic, functional, structural and animal model studies all suggest that HLA genes are the major genetic component of the MHC region in T1D susceptibility. The association between HLA and susceptibility to T1D was made in the early 1970s[15,16] and

Immunogenetics of Autoimmune Disease, edited by Jorge Oksenberg and David Brassat.

Table 1. T1D HLA-DQ/DR susceptible and protective haplotypes[11,17,24]

Genotype *DQA1-DQB1-DRB1*	
Susceptible haplotypes	
Haplotype 1	Haplotype 2
0501-0201-03	*0301-0302-0401*
0301-0302-0401	*0301-0302-0401*
0501-0201-03	*0301-0302-0405*
0301-0302-0401	*0401-0402-0801*
0301-0302-0401	*03-03-0901*
0501-0201-03	*03-03-0901*
0501-0201-03	*0501-0201-03*
0301-0302-0401	*0201-0201-0701*
Protective haplotypes	
0301-0301-0403	
0501-0301-1101	
0103-0603-1301	
0102-0602-1501	

Haplotypes and -combinations are ranked according to the degree of susceptibility, with the most susceptible at top. The protective haplotypes may confer dominant protection, as in the case of *0102-0602-1501* in presence of the susceptible *0301-0302-0401* haplotype.

has been consistently reproduced since then. Studies have suggested that HLA class II genes (*DRB1* and *-DQB1*) are the primary determinants of *IDDM1*,[17-24] (Table 1) However, due to the strong linkage disequilibrium (LD) between these loci it has been very difficult to study the effect of individual *HLA-DQ* or *-DR* genes. The frequency of HLA class II susceptibility alleles correlates well with the population incidence of T1D,[22] and studies suggest that the HLA (*IDDM1*) may account for nearly 40% of the observed familial clustering of T1D, with a locus-specific genetic risk ratio (λ_S) of approximately 3.[14] The contribution of the *IDDM1* region is easily detectable in genome-wide linkage analysis, as indicated by a LOD score of 116 in a recent combined analysis of more than 1400 T1D affected sib-pair (ASP) families.[25] The influence of this region on genetic susceptibility to T1D is complex, with epistasis between *DQB1* and *DRB1*, as demonstrated by disease association of particular *DQB1-DRB1* haplotypes, trans or genotype effects involving *DQA1*, *DQB1* and *DRB1* as well as yet unidentified genes that modify class II risk. Therefore, the risk conferred by a class II genotype may differ from that predicted from the two haplotypes expressed. The hierarchy of susceptibility effects for HLA class II haplotypes range across a 200-fold risk gradient, and within the high-risk *DRB1*04* group in the presence of *DQB1*0302*, there is a 20 fold difference in susceptibility effect.[11,24] There is evidence that the degree of risk conferred by different combinations of class II alleles is determined by the predicted structure and function of peptide-binding pockets of the *DRB1* molecule.[26] The peptide-binding ability of the class II molecule is dependent on certain amino acids of the *HLA-DQB1* and *DRB1* chains.[26-31] In particular, protective alleles contain aspartic acid (Asp) at residue 57 of the *HLA-DQB1* molecule, whereas the predisposing alleles encode alanine, valine or serine residues at the same position.[32] However, this important and confirmed effect of residue 57 in peptide binding of HLA class II molecules[33,34] cannot account for all the complexity of HLA and T1D associations (e.g., Asp57 is not associated with T1D in the Japanese population, where other residues seem of importance[35,36]). Animal studies have provided evidence that the predisposing MHC class II molecules mediate disease, at least in part, by presenting β-cell derived peptides to diabetogenic T cells. Regarding the MHC class II associated protection effect the data are less clear, although a recent study suggested that the structure of the *DQ*0602* molecule may facilitate presentation of an expanded peptide repertoire during thymic maturation critical for the dominant effect observed.[31]

Although the classical HLA genes represent good candidates, given their immunological roles, LD surrounding these genes has made it difficult to rule out effects from neighboring genes, many with immune function, in influencing disease susceptibility. A role for MHC complex genes other than class II genes was initially suggested by Thomsen et al[37] and Pociot et al[38] by studying *HLA-DR3/4* heterozygous individuals, and by Robinson et al[39] using a family study design, which to some degree eliminated the LD effects involving *HLA-DQ/DR* loci; however, in all these studies the number of subjects/families was small.

An association with *HLA-DPB1* alleles has been observed in several studies.[13,26,40-43] Taken together, these studies support an effect for three *DPB1* alleles, *DPB1*0202, DPB1*0301,* and *DPB1*0402,* on T1D susceptibility. *DPB*'0202* and *DPB1*0301* are positively and *DPB1*0402* negatively associated. Whether the *DPB1* locus is causally involved or merely a marker for T1D susceptibility, these studies suggest that *DPB1* genotyping can increase the predictive power of HLA genetics for T1D susceptibility. Additional susceptibility loci in the class II region include the antigen-processing genes (*TAP1, TAP2, LMP2,* and *LMP7*), although current evidence suggests that these are not directly involved in T1D.[44-46] The tumor necrosis factor and lymphotoxin genes (*TNF* and *LT*) have been extensively studied[38,47-49] and shown some evidence for association independent of *DRB1* and *DQB1*. Furthermore, another class of MHC genes, MHC Class I chain-related genes (MIC) has been identified, The *MICA* gene is located between the *TNFA* and the *HLA-B* genes,[50] and contains an exon 5 tri-nucleotide repeat polymorphism that has been demonstrated to be independently associated with T1D in several populations.[51-55] Many additional *MICA* gene polymorphisms have been identified and it may be that other variants, e.g., leading to amino acid substitutions in the extracellular domain of the *MICA* molecule, are better candidates for the observed T1D association than the most frequently investigated exon 5 repeat polymorphism (exon 5 encodes part of the intracellular part of the *MICA* molecule). The strongest evidence for susceptibility genes in the class I region, however, comes from recent systematic assessment of microsatellite markers spanning this region.[56-62]

Despite intensive efforts in the analysis of classical HLA genes no definitively causal variants have been identified in T1D. Studies of classical HLA genes have often implicated more than one allele at a single locus as influencing T1D susceptibility. Another observation from MHC studies in T1D is that an extended haplotype, rather than a single variant, is associated with disease. This suggests that one should consider all genes of the MHC region, rather than focusing only on the classical HLA loci.

NonHLA Genes in T1D Susceptibility

HLA-encoded susceptibility to T1D accounts for approximately half of the observed familial clustering of the disease leaving the rest to other (nonHLA) genes and environmental factors. Genome-wide scans have been intensively used in the search for genetic determinants for T1D. The first scans for linkage to T1D, using fewer than 100 affected sib-pair families, identified chromosome 6p21 (*IDDM1*) as the major T1D risk locus.[63,64] Subsequent studies identified other putative T1D loci on several chromosomes.[25,65-68] However, despite the fact that there was strong statistical evidence supporting linkage for some of these regions in the initial reports, most regions have not been clearly established in multiple populations.[11] A major barrier to T1D gene identification, given the likely small locus-specific contribution (low λ_S) for nonHLA genes, is the limited number of available affected sib-pair families with T1D.

Very recently a joint analysis of data from previous T1D genome-wide scans,[67,68] as well as genome scanning of new families was performed.[25] This effort has been achieved under the auspices of the Type 1 Diabetes Genetics Consortium (T1DGC) (http://www.t1dgc.org). T1DGC assembled families and merged data from three large genome scans and added new data from 254 families not previously scanned. This family collection provided ~95% power to detect a locus with locus-specific $\lambda_S > 1.3$ and $P=10^{-4}$. The increased sample size allowed the

Table 2. Genomic loci likely to confer susceptibility in T1D

Chromosome	Closest Marker	LOD
2q31-q33	*D2S2167*	3.34
3p13-p14	*D3S1261*	1.52
6p21	*TNFA*	116.3
9q33-q34	*D9S260*	2.2
10p14-q11	*D10S1426*	3.21
11p15	*D11S922*	1.87
12q14-q12	*D12S375*	1.66
16p12-q11.1	*D16S3131*	1.88
16q22-q24	*D16S504*	2.64
19p13.3-p13.2	*INSR*	1.92

Adapted from reference 25.

exclusion of over 80% of the human genome for locus-specific, but population independent, effects of $\lambda_S \geq 1.3$. This represents one of the largest genome scans ever performed in a multifactorial disease. Some *IDDM* loci were confirmed, whereas other previously suggested *IDDM* loci, were excluded. In addition to continued support for T1D susceptibility related to the MHC (*IDDM1*), nine regions were identified that supported nonHLA-linked susceptibility;[25] these are listed in Table 2 and described below.

2q31-q33

This region includes the *IDDM12* locus, which been attributed to SNPs in the 3′ UTR of the cytotoxic T-lymphocyte-associated protein 4 gene (*CTLA4*) gene;[69] however, the modest λ_S value predicted for the associated SNPs at *CTLA4* seem unlikely to account fully for the magnitude of the observed evidence for linkage. The *CTLA4* region on chromosome 2q33 has been linked with susceptibility to several autoimmune diseases; the encoded molecule is a costimulatory receptor, involved in, and conferring an inhibitory effect on T-cell activation. There are two known isoforms of CTLA-4 in humans: a full-length transmembrane form expressed transiently on activated T cells, and a soluble form generated by alternative splicing of the transmembrane domain and expressed mainly in inactivated T cells.

Several *CTLA4* gene variants have been identified. These include polymorphisms in the 5′ flanking and promoter region, one coding SNP, an *A49G* variant leading to a threonine to alanine replacement in the signal peptide and polymorphisms in the 3′UTR. Many of these variations have been associated with autoimmune diseases as T1D, systemic lupus erythematosus, celiac disease, Graves disease and autoimmune hypothyroid disease, and may be a common susceptibility factor in autoimmunity in general.[70] The most comprehensive SNP and LD mapping analysis of this locus[69] identified the *G6230A* SNP as the predominant marker for T1D risk although the presence of causative SNP(s) in the 5′ end of the gene was not ruled out. The *G6230A* SNP was reported to correlate with higher mRNA level of soluble CTLA-4 in unstimulated T-cells from individuals heterozygous for the T1D protective haplotype (*A49, A6230*) compared to the predisposing haplotype (*G49, G6230*).[69] The observation was limited to the soluble form and no allelic differences were reported for the full-length CTLA-4 isoform. This observation is not easily compatible with the observation in other autoimmune diseases, where higher levels of soluble CTLA-4 were found in patients vs. controls, and the fact that blockage of the CD28/CTLA-4 pathway by CTLA-4-immunoglobulin seems to be a promising treatment in autoimmune diseases.[70] Thus, further studies are needed to clarify the functional role of *CTLA4* in T1D pathogenesis. Based on the functional data observed in[69] and other studies[70] no clear molecular model to explain the increased risk for autoimmunity has yet emerged and additional studies are warranted.

11p15

This region, also referred to as *IDDM2*, includes the insulin gene, *INS*, expressed specifically in the β-cell and thymus. Insulin is an early detectable auto antigen in T1D; a minisatellite, VNTR (variable number of tandem repeats), arising from tandem repetition of 14-15 basepairs in the 5′ regulatory region of the *INS* gene, most probably represents the primary locus for *IDDM2*. The class I alleles of the *INS VNTR*, which confers genetic risk to T1D, lead to lower insulin expression in the thymus as well as higher insulin expression in the β-cell compared to the dominant protective class III alleles. This may attenuate the development of central tolerance to insulin, at the same time as providing high antigen expression in the β-cell.[71] Certain class III alleles, which silence thymic *INS* expression, however, also confer genetic predisposition to T1D.[72] Furthermore there is evidence for interaction between the *INS* and *HLA* loci in conferring susceptibility to T1D.[68]

6q21

This region corresponds to *IDDM15*, for which strong support for linkage to T1D has been observed previously.[66,68,73] *IDDM15* appears as one of the major nonHLA susceptibility loci also in the T1DGC combined genome scan.[25] Due to its proximity to the MHC the influence of this locus on T1D susceptibility is only properly appreciated when the HLA effect is taken into account.[68,73] To further define the effects of this locus, increased information content in the HLA region and in the region surrounding *IDDM15*, will be useful. No obvious candidate gene has yet been identified, and the closest microsatellite marker was *D6S283*.[25] This locus is partially overlapping with the region associated with some cases of neonatal transitoric diabetes.[73]

16p12-q11.1

Support for a T1D susceptibility locus on chromosome 16p12-q11.1 has been observed independently in both the combined UK and US families,[67] as well as in the Scandinavian families,[68] and remains strong in the recent combined genome scan,[25] (Table 2). A recent analysis of four rheumatoid arthritis (RA) genome scans[74] also reported evidence for linkage at chromosome 16p-cen. Since RA, anti-thyroid autoimmune disease and T1D cluster in families more often than expected by chance,[75] evidence for linkage for any one of these autoimmune diseases could be informative for others. No candidate gene has yet emerged from studies of this region on chromosome 16.

16q22-q24

An additional region on chromosome 16, 16q22-q24 was identified from the combined genome scan,[25] (Table 2), but no candidate genes have been proposed. This region has not been identified before in T1D genome scans. However, it was mapped as a susceptibility locus for several other autoimmune diseases, including psoriasis,[76] asthma[77] and celiac disease,[78] supporting the probable existence of common genetic factors underlying autoimmunity, and hence, giving additional support to this locus.

10p14-q13

This region includes the *IDDM10* locus, and linkage of T1D to this region is well supported by the recent combined T1DGC genome scan,[25] as well as past studies.[65,67] However, other than association analyses of the functional candidate gene *GAD2*, which suggest that this gene is not a T1D susceptibility locus,[79-81] there have been relatively few follow-up studies and no other genes have been reported as candidates for *IDDM10*.

19p13.3-p13.2

This region was also suggested from the recent combined genome scan.[25] The region is of interest as the linkage peak corresponds exactly to the insulin receptor gene, *INSR*. The interleukin 12 receptor β-1 gene (*IL12RB1*) is located in the proximity of the *INSR* gene; this gene is also of potential interest in T1D, since the *IL12B* gene, encoding a subunit of the IL-12 molecule (the ligand of the IL-12 receptor), has been suggested as a candidate gene in T1D, although data are contrasting.[82,83] However, fine mapping remains to be performed, and no polymorphism or gene has been demonstrated to account for the T1D linkage in this region.

In addition, three regions, **3p13-p14, 9q33-q34** and **12q14-q12**, have been suggested as linked to T1D in the combined genome scan[25] (Table 2), and none of them corresponds to previously identified *IDDM* loci. Regarding these regions, no candidate genes has yet been proposed, however fine mapping will be important in defining the effects of this region on susceptibility to T1D.

Additional Candidate Genes

In addition to linkage analysis, association studies of variants in selected candidate genes, with a likely functional significance, have also been valuable in determining potentially important T1D genes. Some of the most validated, interesting and recently identified, are listed below.

Vitamin D Receptor

There is increasing evidence of the key role of vitamin D levels in T1D susceptibility.[84] Vitamin D has important immunomodulatory properties[85] and depletion or relative resistance may play a part in the etiology of both T1D and T2D, possibly through effects on insulin secretion.[86] It has been shown that allelic variations in the vitamin D receptor (*VDR*) gene is a significant determinant of the amount of VDR mRNA and VDR protein expressed,[87] and may also affect plasma concentrations of 1,25$(OH)_2D_3$, and response to oral vitamin D.[88] An association between *VDR* polymorphisms and T1D has been reported in several populations,[89-95] although not necessarily with the same VDR polymorphisms. However, no associations were found with T1D susceptibility in the Finnish population,[96] and furthermore no convincing evidence of association was found between a total of 98 *VDR* SNPs, including the four commonly studied SNPs (*FokI, BsmI, ApaI*, and *TaqI VDR* SNPs) and T1D in a very large family collection from UK, Finland, Norway, Romania and US.[97] The phenotypic consequences of genetic heterogeneity are likely to be very different in populations exposed to varying amounts of UV-light; furthermore, evidence from animal experiments and human observational studies suggests that some dietary micronutrients, in particular vitamin D, may protect against the development of T1D.[98] Further work remains to be done on this gene-environment interaction in T1D susceptibility.

EIF2AK3

Interestingly, the Scandinavian T1D genome scan[68] identified a region on chromosome 2p12, marker *D2S113*, near the gene for eukaryotic translation-initiation factor-2 α kinase-3 (*EIF2AK3*), in which disease-causing mutations have been identified in patients with Wolcott-Rallison syndrome (neonatal insulin-dependent diabetes and epiphyseal dysplasia).[99] On that basis additional markers were selected to cover the *EIF2AK3* region, and evidence of linkage at this locus increased to a LOD score of 2.6 in HLA-DR3/4 positive ASPs.[68] Also, an association between the region around the *EIF2AK3* locus and T1D susceptibility has been found in South Indian subjects.[100] Although common *EIF2AK3* mutations were excluded in T1D patients in this population, excess transmission of the common alleles of two polymorphic markers (*D2S1786* and *15INDEL*, located within the gene) downstream of *EIF2AK3*, either singly (*D2S1786*, $P=0.01$ and *15INDEL*, $P=0.02$) or as a combination ($P<0.001$), were found in 234 families with a T1D proband. There was also a clear paternal effect for the *15INDEL* marker ($P=0.005$) on disease susceptibility. The presence of the common allele of both markers was found in decreased frequency in the subjects with normal glucose tolerance compared to probands with T1D (both $P\leq 0.0001$). Recently, functional implications (influences on kinase activity) of variants in the *EIF2AK3* gene in Wolcott-Rallison patients, was evaluated.[101]

PTPN22

The lymphoid-specific phosphatase, LYP, encoded by the *PTPN22* gene, is a powerful inhibitor of T-cell activation, acting by dephosphorylating T-cell receptor-associated kinases. LYP is a 110 kDa protein tyrosine phosphatase, expressed in lymphocytes, that inhibits T-cell activation by physically associating through its proline-rich N-terminal motif, with the SH3 domain of the Csk kinase.[102] This suppresses the Src kinase family members, Lck[103] and Fyn, that mediate signaling via T-cell receptors. *PTPN22* is therefore a candidate gene for all autoimmune diseases mediated by T-cells. A SNP (rs2476601) in *PTPN22*, C1858T, in codon 620 results in an amino acid substitution from arginine (Arg) to tryptophan (Trp). The allele encoding Trp demonstrated strong association to T1D, originally in case-control designs in two ethnically different populations.[104] In addition, the functional consequence of this amino acid substitution has been studied, and only the LYP with the Arg620 was found to form a complex with the negative regulatory Csk kinase, whereas the LYP molecule with the Trp620 did not.[104] The *PTPN22* gene maps to chromosome 1p13, a region which has been weakly linked to rheumatoid arthritis,[105] as well as to systemic lupus erythematosus,[106] however not to T1D, suggesting that this gene also may be important in systemic autoimmune diseases. Another recent report has demonstrated association of the rs2476601 SNP in *PTPN22* to rheumatoid arthritis in two independent samples,[107] as well as the inability of the LYP variant, carrying the Trp allele, to bind Csk and thereby down-regulate T-cell activation.[107] Familial clustering of several autoimmune diseases is well documented, and *PTPN22* may be a link in a shared etiology or common factors contributing to general immune dysregulation. Association of the minor Trp encoding allele of rs2476601 in *PTPN22* has additionally been shown to be associated with human systemic lupus erythematosus.[108] Knockout mice deficient for *PTPN22* show selective dysregulation in the effector/memory T-cell system.[109] Replication of the association of rs2476601 to T1D was recently published in two reports; a large T1D family as well as a large case-control cohort was used in one report,[110] and in addition evidence for association to Grave's disease, another autoimmune disease, was demonstrated. In a second report association was confirmed in a large cohort of US T1D multiplex families.[111] Another recent report also demonstrated association to Grave's disease as well as Addison's disease.[112] In the recent study by T1DGC, linkage of T1D on 1p11-p12 (*D1S206*) is weakly supported ($P = 1.4 \times 10^{-2}$); however, *PTPN22* is contained within the LOD-1 support interval.[25] Taken together these recent reports strongly support the *PTPN22* gene having an important role in T1D, with a genetic variant probably having important functional consequences on T1D pathogenesis.

SUMO4

Two independent groups have recently identified another new T1D candidate gene, *SUMO4*, a novel member of a family of small ubiqutin-like modifiers with an effect on inhibitor kappa B alpha (IκBα) action.[113,114] The gene is located in the *IDDM5* region on chromosome 6q25, already identified in several genome scans.[64,66,115] The *SUMO4* gene, which consists of only one exon, is located in intron 6 of another potential T1D candidate gene, *TAB2* (TAK1-binding protein 2, mediating TAK1 activation in the IL-1 signaling pathway). Both genes are involved in nuclear factor-kappa B (NF-κB) activation, playing a role in apoptosis of pancreatic β-cells. The *SUMO* (small ubiquitin-like modifier) gene family consists of *SUMO1* to *SUMO4*, showing substantial homology to each other, as well as high conservation among species.

The *SUMO4* gene was identified as a result of fine mapping the *IDDM5* region,[116] and several SNPs in a 200 kb region demonstrated T1D association. The *SUMO4* gene was cloned and strong T1D association was demonstrated in several populations. A missense mutation, at codon 55 substituting methionine (Met) with valine (Val), was identified and functional studies support this SNP as important in T1D pathogenesis. *SUMO4* conjugates to IκBα and negatively regulates NFκB transcriptional activity, whereas the substitution to Val at codon 55 resulted in 5.5 times greater NFκB transcriptional activity, as well as approximately 2 times greater expression of a NFκB dependent gene, *IL12B*.[116] Another group,[117,118] simultaneously identified the same gene and the same SNP; however, it was the Met encoding allele of the Met55Val substitution of *SUMO4*, which was most strongly associated with T1D in this report. Furthermore, the Met variant was shown to be associated with higher levels of activated heat shock factor transcription factors when compared to the Val variant, a factor that may be directly involved in T1D pathogenesis through abnormal heat shock protein expression in pancreatic β-cells. Heat shock proteins are 'molecular chaperons' involved in assembly of proteins and processing and presentation of antigens.[119,120] However, Bohren et al[118] observed no differences in expression levels of NF-κB among the two variants, as opposed to the findings in the report from Guo et al.[116] These studies support *SUMO4* as an important gene involved in regulatory immunogenetic networks and hence in T1D pathogenesis. However, more studies are clearly needed in order to clarify the discrepancies regarding this association, as well as the functional consequences of the SNP, to establish whether this is indeed a novel T1D susceptibility gene.

Conclusion

T1D is a multifactorial disease of which the pathogenetic molecular mechanisms are still not fully understood. However, recent progress within the genetics of T1D, e.g., with the establishment of T1DGC, are likely to facilitate future studies within this complex field.

Among the different T1D genome scans there has been a pronounced lack of reproducibility of identified linked regions.[63-68] The recently completed combined genome scan of UK, US and Scandinavian T1D families, including more than 1400 multiplex families, is an example of a concerted action of increasing sample size and thereby power to the levels necessary for convincing identification of T1D loci of only modest effects.[25] In this large sample, strong evidence for the HLA region was observed, whereas, only moderate support for T1D linkage was obtained for additional loci (Table 2). The identified regions, or a large proportion of them, are, however, likely to harbor T1D susceptibility genes due to the power of the study. Systematic fine mapping of these regions are needed to characterize variation(s) of the gene or genes responsible for the observed linkage signal in the different regions. This should be followed by functional characterization of the biological effect of the identified genetic variants. Systematic fine mapping is laborious and complex, one linkage peak covers many genes (up to 1000) and may be composed of several susceptibility loci, as already known from animal models.[32,121] Furthermore, a linkage signal may be observed due to the chance clustering of several disease loci, each with relatively weak locus-specific effects.[25] Such complexity probably also, at least partly, explains some of the difficulties in obtaining reproducible association results. Also contributing to the complexity of the genetics of T1D is the interaction between different loci, and probably also gene-environment interactions. Interactions between susceptibility loci for T1D have been demonstrated in several studies.[25,64,65,68,122] Gene-gene interaction is likely to be a very important factor in genetic predisposition, and further identification of such interactions will help in understanding the molecular basis of T1D. A recent approach used high throughput chip-based mass spectrometry in the 6p21 region as a method to screen for differences in SNP allele frequencies, among pooled DNA from individuals with several multifactorial diseases as well as controls.[123] This method seems of value in prioritizing genes and SNPs in large linkage regions. In line with this method, the use of knowledge regarding differences in gene expression, under different conditions or in different tissues, may also be useful in mapping genes. Such genes, which are responsible for the variation in human gene expression, are likely to have an impact on phenotype.[124] In addition, novel analytical approaches, e.g., neural network-based methods, have proven valuable in T1D.[125] Association studies of genes with a plausible biological mechanism in T1D, is still a valuable method, as seen from the additional T1D candidate genes mentioned in this review as well as several other studies. Increasingly, the focus is moving to genome-wide association studies, using SNPs; this approach is now technically possible and will probably be more broadly applied in the near future. The so called HapMap project, a haplotype-based map of informative SNPs covering the entire genome (www.hapmap.org) will add tremendously to this effort. Genome-wide association studies may be more powerful than linkage studies in identifying loci of interest in multifactorial diseases.

Future collaborative efforts, in combination with new tools and increased sample size should increase the chances of identifying T1D susceptibility loci and unravelling the molecular basis of T1D.

References

1. Mølbak AG, Christau B, Marner B et al. Incidence of insulin-dependent diabetes mellitus in age groups over 30 years in Denmark. Diabet Med 1994; 11(7):650-655.
2. Karvonen M, Viik-Kajander M, Moltchanova E et al. Incidence of childhood type 1 diabetes worldwide. Diabetes Care 2000; 23(10):1516-1526.
3. Alberti K, Zimmet P. Definition, diagnosis and classification of diabetes mellitus and its complications. Part 1: Diagnosis and classification of diabetes mellitus provisional report of a WHO consultation. Diabet Med 1998; 15(7):539-553.
4. Borch-Johnsen K. The prognosis of insulin-dependent diabetes mellitus. An epidemiological approach. Dan Med Bull 1989; 36(4):336-348.
5. Hirschhorn J. Genetic epidemiology of type 1 diabetes. Ped Diab 2003; 4(2):87-100.
6. Hyttinen V, Kaprio J, Kinnunen L et al. Genetic liability of type 1 diabetes and the onset age among 22,650 young Finnish twin pairs: A nationwide follow-up study. Diabetes 2003; 52(4):1052-1055.
7. Svensson J, Carstensen B, Molbak A et al. Increased risk of childhood type 1 diabetes in children born after 1985. Diabetes Care 2002; 25(12):2197-2201.
8. Onkamo P, Karvonen M, Tuomilehto J. Worldwide increase in incidence of Type I diabetes—the analysis of the data on published incidence trends. Diabetolog 1999; 42(12):1395-1403.
9. Kyvik K, Green A, Beck-Nielsen H. Concordance rates of insulin dependent diabetes mellitus: A population based study of young Danish twins. BMJ (Clinical research ed.) 1995; 311(7010):913-917.
10. Redondo M, Yu L, Hawa M et al. Heterogeneity of type I diabetes: Analysis of monozygotic twins in Great Britain and the United States. Diabetolog 2001; 44(3):354-362.
11. Pociot F, McDermott MF. Genetics of Type 1 diabetes mellitus. Genes Immun 2002; 3(5):235-249.
12. Noble J, Valdes A, Cook M et al. The role of HLA class-II genes in Insulin-dependent diabetes mellitus - Molecular analysis of 180 caucasian, multiplex families. Am J Hum Genet 1996; 59(5):1134-1148.
13. Valdes A, Noble J, Clerget-Darpoux F et al. Modeling of HLA class II susceptibility to Type I diabetes reveals an effect associated with DPB1. Genet Epidem 2001; 21(3):212-223.
14. Rich S. Mapping genes in diabetes. Genetic epidemiological perspective. Diabetes 1990; 39(11):1315-1319.
15. Singal D, Blajchman M. Histocompatibility (HL-A) antigens, lymphocytotoxic antibodies and tissue antibodies in patients with diabetes mellitus. Diabetes 1973; 22(6):429-432.
16. Nerup J, Platz P, Andersen O et al. HL-A antigens and diabetes mellitus. Lancet 1974; 2(7885):864-866.
17. Koeleman B, Lie B, Undlien D et al. Genotype effects and epistasis in type 1 diabetes and HLA-DQ trans dimer associations with disease. Genes Immun 2004; 5(5):381-388.
18. She JX. Susceptibility to type I diabetes: HLA-DQ and DR revisited. Immunol Tod 1996; 17(7):323-329.
19. Thorsby E. Invited anniversary review: HLA associated diseases. Human Immun 1997; 53(1):1-11.
20. Dorman J, Bunker C. HLA-DQ locus of the human leukocyte antigen complex and type 1 diabetes mellitus: A HuGE review. Epidemiol Rev 2000; 22(2):218-227.
21. Undlien DE, Lie BA, Thorsby E. HLA complex genes in type 1 diabetes and other autoimmune diseases. Which genes are involved? Trends Genet 2001; 17(2):93-100.
22. Ronningen K, Keiding N, Green A et al. Correlations between the incidence of childhood-onset type I diabetes in Europe and HLA genotypes. Diabetolog 2001; 44(Suppl 3):B51-B59.
23. Cucca F, Todd J. HLA susceptibility to type 1 diabetes: Methods and mechanisms. In: Browning M, McMichaels A, eds. HLA and MHC: Genes, molecules and function. Oxford: BIOS Scientific Publishers Ltd, 1996:383-406.
24. Lambert A, Gillespie K, Thomson G et al. Absolute risk of childhood-onset type 1 diabetes defined by human leukocyte antigen class II genotype: A population-based study in the United Kingdom. J Clin. Endocrinol Metab 2004; 89(8):4037-4043.

25. Type 1 Diabetes Genetics Consortium. Type 1 Diabetes: Evidence for susceptibility loci from four genome-wide scans in 1435 multiplex families. Diabetes 2005; In press.
26. Cucca F, Lampis R, Congia M et al. A correlation between the relative predisposition of MHC class II alleles to type 1 diabetes and the structure of their proteins. Hum Mol Gen 2001; 10(19):2025-2037.
27. Lee K, Wucherpfennig K, Wiley D. Structure of a human insulin peptide-HLA-DQ8 complex and susceptibility to type I diabetes. Nat Immunol 2001; 2(6):501-507.
28. Latek R, Suri A, Petzold S et al. Structural basis of peptide binding and presentation by the type I diabetes-associated MHC class II molecule of NOD mice. Immunity 2000; 12(6):699-710.
29. Stratmann T, Apostolopoulos V, Mallet-Designe V et al. The I-Ag7 MHC class II molecule linked to murine diabetes is a promiscuous peptide binder. J Immunol 2000; 165(6):3214-3225.
30. Chao C, Sytwu H, Chen E et al. The role of MHC class II molecules in susceptibility to type I diabetes: Identification of peptide epitopes and characterization of the T cell repertoire. PNAS US 1999; 96(16):9299-9304.
31. Siebold C, Hansen B, Wyer J et al. Crystal structure of HLA-DQ0602 that protects against type 1 diabetes and confers strong susceptibility to narcolepsy. PNAS US 2004; 101(7):1999-2004.
32. Todd JA, Wicker LS. Genetic protection from the inflammatory disease type 1 diabetes in humans and animal models. Immunity 2001; 15(3):387-395.
33. Corper A, Stratmann T, Apostolopoulos V et al. A structural framework for deciphering the link between I-Ag7 and autoimmune diabetes. Science 2000; 288(5465):505-511.
34. Kwok W, Domeier M, Johnson M et al. HLA-DQB1 codon 57 is critical for peptide binding and recognition. J Exp Med 1996; 183(3):1253-1258.
35. Awata T, Kuzuya T, Matsuda A et al. High frequency of aspartic acid at position 57 of HLA-DQ beta-chain in Japanese IDDM patients and nondiabetic subjects. Diabetes 1990; 39(2):266-269.
36. Yamagata K, Hanafusa T, Nakajima H et al. HLA-DP and susceptibility to insulin-dependent diabetes mellitus in Japanese. Tissue Antigens 1991; 38(3):107-110.
37. Thomsen M, Molvig J, Zerbib A et al. The susceptibility to insulin-dependent diabetes mellitus is associated with C4 allotypes independently of the association with HLA-DQ alleles in HLA-DR3,4 heterozygotes. Immunogenetics 1988; 28(5):320-327.
38. Pociot F, Molvig J, Wogensen L et al. A tumour necrosis factor beta gene polymorphism in relation to monokine secretion and insulin-dependent diabetes mellitus. Scand J Immunol 1991; 33(1):37-49.
39. Robinson W, Barbosa J, Rich S et al. Homozygous parent affected sib pair method for detecting disease predisposing variants: Application to insulin dependent diabetes mellitus. Genet Epidem 1993; 10(5):273-288.
40. Erlich H, Rotter J, Chang J et al. Association of HLA-DPB1*0301 with IDDM in Mexican-Americans. Diabetes 1996; 45(5):610-614.
41. Noble J, Valdes A, Thomson G et al. The HLA class II locus DPB1 can influence susceptibility to type 1 diabetes. Diabetes 2000; 49(1):121-125.
42. Lie B, Akselsen H, Joner G et al. HLA associations in insulin-dependent diabetes mellitus: No independent association to particular DP genes. Human Immun 1997; 55(2):170-175.
43. Cruz T, Valdes A, Santiago A et al. DPB1 alleles are associated with type 1 diabetes susceptibility in multiple ethnic groups. Diabetes 2004; 53(8):2158-2163.
44. Caillat-Zucman S, Daniel S, Djilali-Saiah I et al. Family study of linkage disequilibrium between TAP2 transporter and HLA class II genes. Absence of TAP2 contribution to association with insulin-dependent diabetes mellitus. Human Immun 1995; 44(2):80-87.
45. van Endert P, Liblau R, Patel S et al. Major histocompatibility complex-encoded antigen processing gene polymorphism in IDDM. Diabetes 1994; 43(1):110-117.
46. Undlien D, Akselsen H, Joner G et al. No independent associations of LMP2 and LMP7 polymorphisms with susceptibility to develop IDDM. Diabetes 1997; 46(2):307-312.
47. Bidwell J, Keen L, Gallagher G et al. Cytokine gene polymorphism in human disease: On-line databases, supplement 1. Genes Immun 2001; 2(2):61-70.
48. Bidwell J, Keen L, Gallagher G et al. Cytokine gene polymorphism in human disease: On-line databases. Genes Immun 1999; 1(1):3-19.
49. Pociot F, Wilson AG, Nerup J et al. No independent association between a tumor necrosis factor-alpha promotor region polymorphism and insulin-dependent diabetes mellitus. Eur J Immun 1993; 23(11):3050-3053.
50. MHC Sequencing Consortium. Complete sequence and gene map of a human major histocompatibility complex. Nature 1999; 401(6756):921-923.
51. Gambelunghe G, Ghaderi M, Cosentino A et al. Association of MHC Class I chain-related A (MIC-A) gene polymorphism with Type I diabetes. Diabetolog 2000; 43(4):507-514.

52. Bilbao J, Martin-Pagola A, Calvo B et al. Contribution of MIC-A polymorphism to type 1 diabetes mellitus in basques. Ann NY Acad Sci 2002; 958(1):321-324.
53. Sanjeevi CB, Kanungo A, Berzina L et al. MHC class I chain-related gene A alleles distinguish malnutrition-modulated diabetes, insulin-dependent diabetes, and noninsulin- dependent diabetes mellitus patients from Eastern India. Ann NY Acad Sci 2002; 958(1):341-344.
54. Tica V, Nikitina-Zake L, Donadi E et al. MIC-A Genotypes 4/5.1 and 9/9 are positively associated with type 1 diabetes mellitus in brazilian population. Ann NY Acad Sci 2003; 1005(1):310-313.
55. Gupta M, Nikitina-Zake L, Zarghami M et al. Association between the transmembrane region polymorphism of MHC class I chain related gene-A and type 1 diabetes mellitus in Sweden. Human Immun 2003; 64(5):553-561.
56. Moghaddam P, Zwinderman A, de Knijff P et al. TNFa microsatellite polymorphism modulates the risk of IDDM in Caucasians with the high-risk genotype HLA DQA1*0501-DQB1*0201/DQA1*0301-DQB1*0302. Belgian Diabetes Registry. Diabetes 1997; 46(9):1514-1515.
57. Nejentsev S, Reijonen H, Adojaan B et al. The effect of HLA-B allele on the IDDM risk defined by DRB1*04 subtypes and DQB1*0302. Diabetes 1997; 46(11):1888-1892.
58. Lie B, Todd J, Pociot F et al. The predisposition to type 1 diabetes linked to the human leukocyte antigen complex includes at least one nonclass II gene. Am J Hum Genet 1999; 64(3):793-800.
59. Nejentsev S, Gombos Z, Laine A et al. Nonclass II HLA gene associated with type 1 diabetes maps to the 240-kb region near HLA-B. Diabetes 2000; 49(12):2217-2221.
60. Herr M, Dudbridge F, Zavattari P et al. Evaluation of fine mapping strategies for a multifactorial disease locus: Systematic linkage and association analysis of IDDM1 in the HLA region on chromosome 6p21. Hum Mol Gen 2000; 9(9):1291-1301.
61. Cordell H, Clayton D. A unified stepwise regression procedure for evaluating the relative effects of polymorphisms within a gene using case/control or family data: Application to HLA in type 1 diabetes. Am J Hum Genet 2002; 70(1):124-141.
62. Zavattari P, Lampis R, Motzo C et al. Conditional linkage disequilibrium analysis of a complex disease superlocus, IDDM1 in the HLA region, reveals the presence of independent modifying gene effects influencing the type 1 diabetes risk encoded by the major HLA-DQB1, -DRB1 disease loci. Hum Mol Gen 2001; 10(8):881-889.
63. Hashimoto L, Habita C, Beressi JP et al. Genetic mapping of a susceptibility locus for insulin-dependent diabetes mellitus on chromosome 11q. Nature 1994; 371(6493):161-164.
64. Davies JL, Kawaguchi Y, Bennett ST et al. A genome-wide search for human type-1 diabetes susceptibility genes. Nature 1994; 371(6493):130-136.
65. Mein CA, Esposito L, Dunn MG et al. A search for type 1 diabetes susceptibility genes in families from the United Kingdom. Nature Genet 1998; 19(3):297-300.
66. Concannon P, Gogolin-Ewens KJ, Hinds DA et al. A second-generation screen of the human genome for susceptibility to insulin-dependent diabetes mellitus. Nature Genet 1998; 19(3):292-296.
67. Cox NJ, Wapelhorst B, Morrison VA et al. Seven regions of the genome show evidence of linkage to type 1 diabetes in a consensus analysis of 767 multiplex families. Am J Hum Genet 2001; 69(4):820-830.
68. Nerup J, Pociot F, European Consortium for IDDM genome studies. A genomewide scan for Type 1-diabetes susceptibility in Scandinavian families: Identification of new loci with evidence of interactions. Am J Hum Genet 2001; 69(6):1301-1313.
69. Ueda H, Howson JMM, Esposito L et al. Association of the T-cell regulatory gene CTLA4 with susceptibility to autoimmune disease. Nature 2003; 423(6939):506-511.
70. Pociot F. CTLA-4 in Autoimmune Disease. In: Pociot F, ed. Georgetown, Texas, USA: Landes Bioscience, 2004.
71. Pugliese A, Zeller M, Fernandez A et al. The insulin gene is transcribed in the human thymus and transcription levels correlate with allelic variation at the ins vntr-iddm2 susceptibility locus for type-1 diabetes. Nature Genet 1997; 15(3):293-297.
72. Vafiadis P, Ounissi-Benkalha H, Palumbo M et al. Class III alleles of the variable number of tandem repeat insulin polymorphism associated with silencing of thymic insulin predispose to type 1 diabetes. J Clin Endocrinol Metab 2001; 86(8):3705-3710.
73. Delepine M, Pociot F, Habita C et al. Evidence of a nonMHC susceptibility locus in type I diabetes linked to HLA on chromosome 6. Am J Hum Genet 1997; 60(1):174-187.
74. Fisher S, Lanchbury J, Lewis C. Meta-analysis of four rheumatoid arthritis genome-wide linkage studies: Confirmation of a susceptibility locus on chromosome 16. Arthritis Rheum 2003; 48(5):1200-1206.
75. Tait K, Marshall T, Berman J et al. Clustering of autoimmune disease in parents of siblings from the Type 1 diabetes Warren repository. Diabet Med 2004; 21(4):358-362.

76. Nair R, Henseler T, Jenisch S et al. Evidence for two psoriasis susceptibility loci (HLA and 17q) and two novel candidate regions (16q and 20p) by genome-wide scan. Hum Mol Gen 1997; 6(8):1349-1356.
77. Ober C, Tsalenko A, Parry R et al. A second-generation genomewide screen for asthma-susceptibility alleles in a founder population. Am J Hum Genet 2000; 67(5):1154-1162.
78. King A, Yiannakou J, Brett P et al. A genome-wide family-based linkage study of coeliac disease. Ann Hum Gen 2000; 64(Pt 6):479-490.
79. Rambrand T, Pociot F, Ronningen K et al. Genetic markers for glutamic acid decarboxylase do not predict insulin-dependent diabetes mellitus in pairs of affected siblings. The Danish Study Group of Diabetes in Childhood. Hum Genet 1997; 99(2):177-185.
80. Wapelhorst B, Bell G, Risch N et al. Linkage and association studies in insulin-dependent diabetes with a new dinucleotide repeat polymorphism at the GAD65 locus. Autoimmun 1995; 21(2):127-130.
81. Johnson G, Payne F, Nutland S et al. A comprehensive, statistically powered analysis of GAD2 in type 1 diabetes. Diabetes 2002; 51(9):2866-2870.
82. Morahan G, Huang DX, Ymer SI et al. Linkage disequilibrium of a type 1 diabetes susceptibility locus with a regulatory IL12B allele. Nature Genet 2001; 27(2):218-221.
83. Bergholdt R, Ghandil P, Johannesen J et al. Genetic and functional evaluation of an interleukin-12 polymorphism (IDDM18) in families with type 1 diabetes. J Med Genet 2004; 41(4):e39.
84. Hypponen E, Laara E, Reunanen A et al. Intake of vitamin D and risk of type 1 diabetes: A birth-cohort study. Lancet 2001; 358(9292):1500-1503.
85. Lemire J. Immunomodulatory role of 1,25-dihydroxyvitamin D3. J Cell Biochem 1992; 49(1):26-31.
86. Hitman G, Mannan N, McDermott M et al. Vitamin D receptor gene polymorphisms influence insulin secretion in Bangladeshi Asians. Diabetes 1998; 47(4):688-690.
87. Ogunkolade B, Boucher B, Prahl J et al. Vitamin D receptor (VDR) mRNA and VDR protein levels in relation to vitamin D status, insulin secretory capacity, and VDR genotype in Bangladeshi Asians. Diabetes 2002; 51(7):2294-2300.
88. Zmuda J, Cauley J, Ferrell R. Molecular epidemiology of vitamin D receptor gene variants. Epidemiol Rev 2000; 22(2):203-217.
89. McDermott M, Ramachandran A, Ogunkolade B et al. Allelic variation in the vitamin D receptor influences susceptibility to IDDM in Indian Asians. Diabetolog 1997; 40(8):971-975.
90. Pani M, Knapp M, Donner H et al. Vitamin D receptor allele combinations influence genetic susceptibility to type 1 diabetes in Germans. Diabetes 2000; 49(3):504-507.
91. Chang T, Lei H, Yeh J et al. Vitamin D receptor gene polymorphisms influence susceptibility to type 1 diabetes mellitus in the Taiwanese population. Clin Endocrinol 2000; 52(5):575-580.
92. Fassbender W, Goertz B, Steinhauer B et al. VDR gene polymorphisms are overrepresented in german patients with type 1 diabetes compared to healthy controls without effect on biochemical parameters of bone metabolism. Hormone Met 2002; 34(6):330-337.
93. Guja C, Marshall S, Welsh K et al. The study of CTLA-4 and vitamin D receptor polymorphisms in the Romanian type 1 diabetes population. J Cell Mol Med 2002; 6(1):75-81.
94. Koeleman B, Valdigem G, Eerligh P et al. Seasonality of birth in patients with type 1 diabetes. Lancet 2002; 359(9313):1246-7, (author reply 1247-8).
95. Audi L, Marti G, Esteban C et al. VDR gene polymorphism at exon 2 start codon (FokI) may have influenced Type 1 diabetes mellitus susceptibility in two Spanish populations. Diabet Med 2004; 21(4):393-394.
96. Turpeinen H, Hermann R, Vaara S et al. Vitamin D receptor polymorphisms: No association with type 1 diabetes in the Finnish population. Eur J Endocrinol 2003; 149(6):591-596.
97. Nejentsev S, Cooper J, Godfrey L et al. Analysis of the vitamin D receptor gene sequence variants in type 1 diabetes. Diabetes 2004; 53(10):2709-2712.
98. Hypponen E. Micronutrients and the risk of type 1 diabetes: Vitamin D, vitamin E, and nicotinamide. Nutr Rev 2004; 62(9):340-347.
99. Delepine M, Nicolino M, Barrett T et al. EIF2AK3, encoding translation initiation factor 2-α kinase 3, is mutated in patients with Wolcott-Rallison syndrome. Nature Genet 2000; 25(4):406-409.
100. Allotey R, Mohan V, McDermott M et al. The EIF2AK3 gene region and type I diabetes in subjects from South India. Genes Immun 2004; 5(8):648-652.
101. Senee V, Vattem KM, Delepine M et al. Wolcott-Rallison Syndrome: Clinical, genetic, and functional study of EIF2AK3 mutations and suggestion of genetic heterogeneity. Diabetes 2004; 53(7):1876-1883.
102. Cloutier J, Veillette A. Association of inhibitory tyrosine protein kinase p50csk with protein tyrosine phosphatase PEP in T cells and other hemopoietic cells. EMBO J 1996; 15(18):4909-4918.

103. Bergman M, Mustelin T, Oetken C et al. The human p50csk tyrosine kinase phosphorylates p56lck at Tyr-505 and down regulates its catalytic activity. EMBO J 1992; 11(8):2919-2924.
104. Bottini N. A functional variant of lymphoid tyrosine phosphatase is associated with type I diabetes. Nature Genet 2004; 36(4):337-338.
105. Jawaheer D, Seldin M, Amos C et al. Screening the genome for rheumatoid arthritis susceptibility genes: A replication study and combined analysis of 512 multicase families. Arthritis Rheum 2003; 48(4):906-916.
106. Gaffney P, Kearns G, Shark K et al. A genome-wide search for susceptibility genes in human systemic lupus erythematosus sib-pair families. PNAS US 1998; 95(25):14875-14879.
107. Begovich A, Carlton V, Honigberg L et al. A missense single-nucleotide polymorphism in a gene encoding a protein tyrosine phosphatase (PTPN22) is associated with rheumatoid arthritis. Am J Hum Genet 2004; 75(2):330-337.
108. Kyogoku C, Langefeld C, Ortmann W et al. Genetic association of the R620W polymorphism of protein tyrosine phosphatase PTPN22 with human SLE. Am J Hum Genet 2004; 75(3):504-507.
109. Hasegawa K, Martin F, Huang G et al. PEST domain-enriched tyrosine phosphatase (PEP) regulation of effector/memory T cells. Science 2004; 303(5658):685-689.
110. Smyth D, Cooper J, Collins J et al. Replication of an association between the lymphoid tyrosine phosphatase locus (LYP/PTPN22) with type 1 diabetes, and evidence for its role as a general autoimmunity locus. Diabetes 2004; 53(11):3020-3023.
111. Onengut-Gumuscu S, Ewens KG, Spielman RS et al. A functional polymorphism (1858C/T) in the PTPN22 gene is linked and associated with type I diabetes in multiplex families. Genes Immun 2004; 5(8):678-680.
112. Velaga M, Wilson V, Jennings C et al. The codon 620 tryptophan allele of the lymphoid tyrosine phosphatase (LYP) gene is a major determinant of Graves' disease. J Clin Endocrinol Metab 2004; 89(11):5862-5865.
113. Desterro J, Rodriguez M, Hay R. SUMO-1 modification of IkappaBalpha inhibits NF-kappaB activation. Mol Cell 1998; 2(2):233-239.
114. Karin M. How NF-kappaB is activated: The role of the IkappaB kinase (IKK) complex. Oncogene 1999; 18(49):6867-6874.
115. Luo D, Buzzetti R, Rotter J et al. Confirmation of three susceptibility genes to insulin-dependent diabetes mellitus: IDDM4, IDDM5 and IDDM8. Hum Mol Gen 1996; 5(5):693-698.
116. Guo D, Li M, Zhang Y et al. A functional variant of SUMO4, a new I kappa B alpha modifier, is associated with type 1 diabetes. Nature Genet 2004; 36(8):837-841.
117. Owerbach D, Pina L, Gabbay K. A 212-kb region on chromosome 6q25 containing the TAB2 gene is associated with susceptibility to type 1 diabetes. Diabetes 2004; 53(7):1890-1893.
118. Bohren K, Nadkarni V, Song J et al. A M55V polymorphism in a novel SUMO gene (SUMO-4) differentially activates heat shock transcription factors and is associated with susceptibility to type I diabetes mellitus. J Biol Chem 2004; 279(26):27233-27238.
119. Birk O, Elias D, Weiss A et al. NOD mouse diabetes: The ubiquitous mouse hsp60 is a beta-cell target antigen of autoimmune T cells. J Autoimmun 1996; 9(2):159-166.
120. Jones D, Coulson A, Duff G. Sequence homologies between hsp60 and autoantigens. Immunol Tod 1993; 14(3):115-118.
121. Nguyen C, Limaye N, Wakeland E. Susceptibility genes in the pathogenesis of murine lupus. Arthritis Res 2002; 4(Suppl 3):S255-S263.
122. Cordell H, Todd J, Bennett S et al. Two-locus maximum lod score analysis of a multifactorial trait: Joint consideration of IDDM2 and IDDM4 with IDDM1 in type 1 diabetes. Am J Hum Genet 1995; 57(4):920-934.
123. Herbon N, Werner M, Braig C et al. High-resolution SNP scan of chromosome 6p21 in pooled samples from patients with complex diseases. Genomics 2003; 81(5):510-518.
124. Morley M, Molony C, Weber T et al. Genetic analysis of genome-wide variation in human gene expression. Nature 2004; 430(7001):743-747.
125. Pociot F, Karlsen AE, Pedersen CB et al. Novel analytical methods applied to type 1 diabetes genome scan data. Am J Hum Genet 2004; 74(4):647-660.

CHAPTER 4

Endocrine Diseases:
Graves' and Hashimoto's Diseases

Yoshiyuki Ban and Yaron Tomer

Abstract

The autoimmune thyroid diseases (AITD) are complex diseases which are caused by an interaction between susceptibility genes and environmental triggers. Genetic susceptibility in combination with external factors (e.g., dietary iodine) are believed to initiate the autoimmune response to thyroid antigens. Abundant epidemiological data, including family and twin studies, point to a strong genetic influence on the development of AITD. Various techniques have been employed to identify the genes contributing to the etiology of AITD, including candidate gene analysis and whole genome screening. These studies have enabled the identification of several loci (genetic regions) that are linked with AITD, and in some of these loci putative AITD susceptibility genes have been identified. Some of these genes/loci are unique to Graves' disease (GD) and Hashimoto's thyroiditis (HT) and some are common to both diseases, indicating that there is a shared genetic susceptibility to GD and HT. The putative GD and HT susceptibility genes include both immune modifying genes (e.g., HLA, CTLA-4) and thyroid specific genes (e.g., TSHR, Tg). Most likely these loci interact and their interactions may influence disease phenotype and severity.

Introduction

The autoimmune thyroid diseases (AITD) include a number of conditions which have in common cellular and humoral immune responses targeted at the thyroid gland. The AITD include Graves' disease (GD) and Hashimoto's thyroiditis (HT), both of which involve infiltration of the thyroid by T and B cells reactive with thyroid antigens, production of thyroid autoantibodies, with the resultant clinical manifestations (hyperthyroidism in GD and hypothyroidism in HT) (reviewed in refs. 1,2). While the etiology of the immune response to the thyroid remains unknown, there is solid evidence for a major genetic influence on the development of AITD (reviewed in refs. 3,4). Therefore, the current paradigm is that AITD are complex diseases in which susceptibility genes and environmental triggers act in concert to initiate the autoimmune response to the thyroid. In this review we focus on the genes already found to contribute to AITD. While proof that a gene causes AITD requires functional studies, the genes we will discuss are strong candidates, and their functions are now being investigated. We will not discuss in detail the genetic regions linked with AITD in which no candidate gene has yet been identified.

Genetic Epidemiology of AITD

The familial occurrence of AITD has been reported by investigators for many years. Early studies showing familial aggregation of AITD were mostly observational, based on careful family histories from patients.[5,6] Later, in the 1960s Hall and Stanbury[7] showed that 33% of

Immunogenetics of Autoimmune Disease, edited by Jorge Oksenberg and David Brassat.

Table 1. Some HLA association studies in GD performed in Caucasians

Country	No. of Patients	HLA Allele	Relative Risk/p-Value	Reference
Belgium	194	DRB1*0301	2.53	27
Canada	175	B8	3.1	18
		DR3	5.7	
Denmark	86	B8	2.80	17
		Dw3	3.94	
Germany	253	DR3	2.52	31
Hungary	256	B8	3.48	173
		DR3	4.8	
Sweden	78	B8	4.4	32
		DR3	3.9	
U.K.	127	B8	2.77	35
		DR3	2.13	
U.K.	101	DR3	1.10	174
U.S.A.	65	DR3	3.38	21
U.S.A.	92	DRB1*03	2.6	175
		DRB1*08	3.2	
U.K.	120	DQA1*0501	3.8	24
U.K.	228	DRB1*0304	2.7	23
		DQB1*0301	1.9	
		DQA1*0501	3.2	
U.S.A.	94	DQA1*0501	3.71	25

siblings of patients with GD or HT developed AITD themselves. Additionally, they found that 56% of siblings of AITD patients had thyroid antibodies (TAbs).[7] A recent survey by our own group revealed that 41/114 (36%) of GD patients with ophthalmopathy reported a family history of AITD and 36/114 (32%) had a first degree relative with AITD.[8]

The sibling risk ratio (λs), which is the ratio of the prevalence of the disease in siblings of affected individuals compared to the prevalence of the disease in the general population,[9] serves as a good estimate of disease heritability, with λs >5 considered significant. The λs in AITD has been estimated to be between 5.9[3] and >10 in AITD,[8,10,28] supporting a strong genetic influence on the development of AITD.

Several large twin studies have been reported from Denmark showing a higher concordance of AITD in monozygotic (MZ) twins when compared to dizygotic (DZ) twins. For GD the concordance was 35% in MZ twins and 3% in DZ twins.[11,12] A recent GD twin study from California confirmed the Danish twin study results.[13] Twin studies in HT have shown concordance rates of 55% and 0% in MZ and DZ twins, respectively.[14] The concordance rates for TAbs were also reported to be higher in MZ twins compared to DZ twins. In a recent study from the UK the concordance rates for thyroglobulin antibodies (Tg- Ab) were 59% and 23% for MZ and DZ twins, respectively.[15] The concordance rates for thyroid peroxidase antibodies (TPO-Ab) were 47% and 29% for MZ and DZ twins, respectively.[15] Thus, the twin data confirm with remarkable clarity the presence of a substantial inherited susceptibility to AITD.

Susceptibility Genes in AITD Immune Related Genes

The Human Leukocyte Antigen (HLA) Gene (Table 1)

The major histocompatibility complex (MHC) region, encoding the HLA glycoproteins, consists of a complex of genes located on chromosome 6p21.[16] Since the HLA region is highly polymorphic and contains many immune response genes it was the first candidate genetic region to be studied for association and linkage with AITD. GD was initially found to be associated with HLA-B8 in Caucasians.[17,18] Subsequently, it was found that GD was more strongly associated with HLA-DR3, which is now known to be in linkage disequilibrium with HLA-B8 (reviewed in ref. 19). The frequency of DR3 in GD patients was generally 40-55% and in the general population ~15-30% giving a RR for people with HLA- DR3 of up to 4.0.[18,20-22] A recent family-based study from the UK using the transmission disequilibrium test (TDT) confirmed the results of the case control studies.[23] Among Caucasians, HLA-DQA1*0501 was also shown to be associated with GD (RR = 3.8),[24-26] bu studies have suggested that the primary susceptibility allele in GD is indeed HLA-DR3 (HLA-DRB1*03).[27] We have recently shown that specific DR sequence variants are associated with GD.[29] The pattern of transmission of HLA alleles from parents to offspring was also studied. A recent study suggested a preferential transmission of HLA susceptibility alleles from fathers to affected offspring, whereas maternal susceptibility alleles were not transmitted more frequently than expected.[30] This may suggest parental imprinting in the transmission of HLA susceptibility alleles to affected offspring.

The role of HLA polymorphisms on the clinical expression of GD has also been explored. Some groups reported an association between the likelihood of relapse of GD and HLA-DR3 but most other investigators were unable to confirm this observation.[31-33] Studies of HLA associations in Graves' ophthalmopathy (GO) have produced conflicting results with some workers reporting increased frequency of HLA-DR3 in patients with GO, and others reporting no difference in the distribution of HLA-DR alleles between GD patients with and without ophthalmopathy.[17,18,34,35] These results were not surprising in view of our recent segregation analysis which showed no genetic influences on the development of GO.[8] Likewise, no difference in the DR3 frequency was found in GD patients with and without pretibial myxedema.[18] Some workers have suggested that local factors such as orbital pressure play an important role in the development of GO and pretibial myxedema.[36]

Data on HLA haplotypes in HT have been less definitive than in GD. Initial studies failed to demonstrate an association between goitrous HT and HLA A- B- or C- antigens.[37] Later studies showed an association of goitrous HT with HLA- DR5 (RR=3.1)[38] and of atrophic HT with DR3 (RR=5.1).[39] Associations of HT with HLA-DR3 in Caucasians has been confirmed in subsequent studies,[40,41] and further supported by studies of transgenic mice.[42] An association between HT and HLA-DQw7 (DQB1*0301) has also been reported in Caucasians.[43,44]

Linkage studies of HLA in AITD have been largely negative.[45-47] Only one recent study from the UK showed weak evidence for linkage between GD and the HLA region,[48] and an additional study reported linkage only when conditioning on DR3.[49] It is difficult to explain why the HLA genes show consistent association with GD but no evidence for linkage. The lack of linkage means that HLA-DR3, as measured, does not cause the familial segregation of GD, while the relatively strong association showed that HLA-DR3 conferred a generalized increase in risk for GD in the general population. Indeed, we were able to show that HLA was associated with GD in both sporadic GD patients and probands from GD families, giving similar RRs (unpublished data).

The Cytotoxic T Lymphocyte Antigen-4 (CTLA-4) Immune Regulatory Cluster on Chromosome 2q33 (Table 2)

Costimulatory molecules are critical to the activation of T cells by antigen presenting cells (APCs). APCs activate T cells by presenting to the T cell receptor an antigenic peptide bound to an HLA class II protein on the cell surface. However, a second signal is also required for T cell activation and these costimulatory signals may be provided by the APCs themselves or other local cells.[50] The costimulatory signals are provided by a variety of proteins which are expressed on APCs (e.g., B7-1, B7-2, B7h, CD40) and interact with receptors (CD28, CTLA-4, and CD40L) on the surface of CD4+ T-lymphocytes during antigen presentation.[50] Whereas, the binding of B7 to CD28 on T cells costimulates T cell activation, the presence of CTLA-4,

Table 2. Some CTLA-4 association studies in autoimmune thyroid diseases in Caucasians and non-Caucasian population

CTLA-4 Polymorphism	Country	Ethnic Group	Dis.	No.	RR*/P Value	Ref.
CTLA-4(AT)	USA	Caucasians	GD	133	2.82	53
CTLA-4(AT)	UK	Caucasians	GD	112	2.12.2	56
			HT	44		
CTLA-4(AT)	Hong-Kong	Chinese	GD	94	p= 0.037	54
CTLA-4(AT)	Japan	Japanese	GD+HT	349	1.8	131
Thr/Ala $(A/G)_{49}$	Germany	Caucasians	GD	305	2.0	55
Thr/Ala $(A/G)_{49}$	UK	Caucasians	GD	94	p= 0.003	76
Thr/Ala $(A/G)_{49}$	UK	Caucasians	GD	379	1.6	61
Thr/Ala $(A/G)_{49}$	UK	Caucasians	GD	484	p< 0.0001	75
Thr/Ala $(A/G)_{49}$	USA	Caucasians	GD	85	1.6	8
Thr/Ala $(A/G)_{49}$	Germany	Caucasians	HT	73	p< 0.04	63
Thr/Ala $(A/G)_{49}$	Italy	Caucasians	HT	126	NS*	64
Thr/Ala $(A/G)_{49}$	UK	Caucasians	HT	158	1.57	58
Thr/Ala $(A/G)_{49}$	Slovenia	Caucasians	TAb's	67	p< 0.005	71
Thr/Ala $(A/G)_{49}$	Japan	Japanese	GD	153	2.64	60
Thr/Ala $(A/G)_{49}$	Korea	Korean	GD	97	1.6NS	73
			HT	110		

*RR: relative risk; NS: not significant

which has a higher affinity for B7, down regulates T-cell activation by competing for the binding of B7 to CD28. A new member of this family of costimulatory molecules, 'inducible costimulator' (ICOS) was identified by Hutloff et al.[51] Unlike the constitutively expressed CD28, ICOS is induced on the T-cell surface and does not upregulate the production of interleukin (IL)-2, but induces the synthesis of IL-4.[52] Interestingly, CD28, CTLA-4 and ICOS form a gene cluster in a 300 kb region on chromosome 2q33. Thus, associations of autoimmune diseases with this region may represent the effects of any of these 3 genes alone or in combination due to linkage disequilibrium.

Recently, there have been several reports demonstrating an association between the CTLA-4 gene and AITDs.[53-57] The initial studies found an association between a microsatellite marker located at the 3' untranslated region (3'UTR) of the CTLA-4 gene and GD, giving a RR of 2.1 to 2.8.[53,56] Later, two SNPs were also identified in the CTLA-4 gene: (1) at position 49 in the CTLA-4 leader peptide (A/G_{49}) resulting in an alanine/threonine polymorphism; and (2) in the promoter of CTLA-4 at position -318 (C/T_{-318}). Case-control studies from several groups, including our own, have shown an association between the alanine (G) polymorphism and GD with a RR of ~2.0.[8,55,58-60] The association of CTLA-4 and GD has also been confirmed in a family based study using TDT analysis.[61] In contrast, association studies using the C/T_{-318} SNP of CTLA-4 have been less consistent with some showing association[59] and others not.[62] CTLA-4 has been reported to be associated with HT in Caucasians.[56,58,63] There have been two reports of no association of HT with CTLA-4, most likely due to lack of power.[59,64]

Since CTLA-4 is a non specific costimulatory molecule it is expected to confer susceptibility to AITD and autoimmunity in general and not specifically to GD.[65] Indeed, CTLA-4 was reported to be associated and linked with all forms of AITD (GD, HT, and TAbs, see below), and with many autoimmune diseases such as Type 1 diabetes mellitus (T1DM),[54,55,66,67] Addison's disease,[68] and myasthenia gravis.[69]

Two studies have now shown that CTLA-4 confers susceptibility to the production of thyroid antibodies. Our group has shown strong evidence for linkage between the CTLA-4 gene region and the production of thyroid antibodies with a maximum LOD score (MLS) of 4.2.[70] Recently, another report has described an association between the G allele of the CTLA-4 A/G_{49} SNP and thyroid autoantibody diathesis.[71] Since the development of TAbs often represents the preclinical stage of AITD[72] it is possible that CTLA-4 predisposes, nonspecifically, to the development of thyroid autoimmunity. Additional genetic and/or environmental factors must be necessary for the development of the specific GD/HT phenotypes.[65]

Several studies have also examined whether CTLA-4 polymorphisms influence disease severity. Heward et al[61] reported that the CTLA-4 A/G_{49} SNP G allele was associated with more severe thyrotoxicosis at diagnosis (as reflected by higher free T4 levels). Similar findings were reported by Park et al[73] but not by Zaletel et al.[71] In addition, CTLA-4 has been shown to be associated with GD in children.[74] Taken together, these studies suggest that CTLA-4 may influence both the initiation of AITD, and the severity of the phenotype. CTLA-4 polymorphisms have also been tested for association with GO with conflicting results.[8,71,73,75,76] Vaidya et al[48] reported linkage to the CTLA-4 gene region on chromosome 2q33 in families with GD using nonparametric linkage analysis. The linkage became stronger when families with AITD, rather than just GD, were included in the study, again demonstrating that CTLA-4 most likely confers general susceptibility to thyroid autoimmunity and not to a specific AITD phenotype. As discussed earlier, and in keeping with the view that the CTLA-4 gene predisposes to thyroid autoimmunity rather than to one specific disease, we found strong linkage between the CTLA-4 gene region and Tabs.[70]

As mentioned, the region on chromosome 2q33 containing the CTLA-4 gene harbors in addition the CD28 and ICOS genes and it is unclear whether the CTLA-4 gene itself or another immune regulatory gene in the region was involved in the genetic susceptibility to AITD. Recently, we tested additional genes and markers in the 2q33 region, and the strongest association was with the CTLA-4 markers.[70] These results were in keeping with results obtained in T1DM.[77,78] However, in order to exclude other immune regulatory genes on 2q33 and to confirm that CTLA-4 is the susceptibility gene in this region studies using densely maps of markers in this region are needed.

The CD40 Gene

Two linkage studies, one by our group[79] and one by Pearce et al[80] have shown evidence that a locus on 20q11 was linked with GD. This GD locus was not linked to HT, since analysis of the data for the HT families gave strongly negative LOD scores. Moreover, in families with GD- and HT-affected individuals, the locus was linked only with GD, demonstrating its high specificity for GD.[78,79] The CD40 gene, an important regulator of B cell function, is located within the linked region on chromosome 20q11 and, therefore, it was a likely positional candidate gene for GD. CD40 is a transmembrane glycoprotein that is expressed predominantly on B cells, but also on monocytes, dendritic cells, epithelial cells and other cells (reviewed in ref. 81). It is a member of the tumor necrosis factor receptor superfamily and it binds to a ligand (CD40L or CD154) which is expressed mainly on activated T cells. Binding of CD40L to CD40 induces B cells to proliferate and to undergo immunoglobulin isotype switching.[82] CD40 has been shown to play an important role in the regulation of humoral immunity, central and peripheral T-cell tolerance, and APC function (reviewed in ref. 83). Moreover, in vivo blockade of CD40 has been shown to suppress the induction of experimental autoimmune thyroiditis.[84] Therefore, we tested whether CD40 was the GD susceptibility gene on chromosome 20q11. Sequencing of the CD40 gene revealed a C/T SNP in the promoter region of the gene. Analysis of the CD40 promoter region SNP in 154 Caucasian GD patients and 118 Caucasian controls showed an association between the CC genotype and GD but with a low relative risk of 1.6.[85] TDT analysis also showed preferential transmission of the C allele of the CD40 promoter SNP to affected individuals.[85] Other investigators which found evidence for linkage in this region have not found an association between this SNP and GD in their dataset (Pearce, personal communication) and it is possible that other polymorphisms in the CD40 gene, or another gene in linkage disequilibrium with CD40, is the GD susceptibility gene.

Table 3. Transmission disequilibrium test for markers D8S284, Tgms1, and Tgms2 in 102 AITD families

Marker	Allele/Haplotype	Transmitted	Untransmitted	p-Value
D8S284	3	54	34	**0.03**
	9	6	16	**0.03**
	all others	111	121	NS*
Tgms2	3	48	34	NS
	4	14	4	**0.02**
	7	32	52	**0.02**
	all others	62	66	NS
D8S284/Tgms1	3/3	32	12	**0.002**
	all others	101	121	NS

*NS: not significant; Tgms1: microsatellite marker located in intron 10 of the Tg gene; Tgms2: microsatellite marker located in intron 27 of the Tg gene

Other Immune Related Genes

Other immune related genes tested for association with GD include the T cell receptor β chain,[21,86,87] the IgG heavy chain (IgH) gene,[88,89] the IL-1 receptor antagonist gene,[90-93] tumor necrosis factor α (TNFα) gene,[47] interferon γ gene,[94] the transporters associated with antigen presentation (TAP) genes,[95] and the IL-4 gene.[96] However, none of these have produced replicable associations with GD. The vitamin D binding protein, which may have some immune modulatory functions, has also been reported to be associated with GD.[97] This result needs to be confirmed and it cannot be excluded that other genes in linkage disequilibrium with these genes are the susceptibility genes at these loci.

Thyroid Associated Genes

The Thyroglobulin (Tg) Gene

Two studies have found evidence for linkage between a locus on chromosome 8q24 and AITD. Our group has shown strong evidence for linkage at the Tg gene locus with an MLS of 3.5 between D8S514 and D8S284.[98] Recently, another study in Japanese sib-pairs identified a major AITD locus on 8q24 very close to the locus which we identified.[99] Since the Tg gene was located within this linked region we proceeded to analyze the Tg gene directly. We identified two new Tg microsatellites in intron 10 (designated Tgms1) and intron 27 (designated Tgms2). Linkage analysis using Tgms2 gave a 2-point LOD score of 2.1 and a multipoint LOD score of 2.9, confirming that it was the Tg gene linked with AITD.[98]

We then used the same two Tg microsatellites to test whether the Tg gene was associated as well as linked with AITD. Using an unselected group of 190 Caucasian GD patients and 134 age- and sex-matched Caucasian controls we found only a weak association between Tgms2 and AITD ($p=0.05$, RR=1.4).[98] However, the association was more impressive when the probands from the linked families (n=32) were used ($p=0.004$, RR=2.3). TDT analysis also showed an association of Tgms2 with AITD ($p=0.02$, Table 3), but with a different allele, suggesting that Tgms2 was in linkage disequilibrium with another polymorphism of the Tg gene. These results have been replicated recently in a U.K. dataset.[100] As in our study, the U.K. study also showed a significant association between Tgms2 and AITD ($p< 0.001$). Moreover, the same Tgms2 allele that we found to be associated with AITD was found to be associated by Collins et al.[100] Thus, the Tg gene was both linked and associated with AITD and, therefore, is an important AITD susceptibility gene. However, it remains possible that another gene on

8q24 in linkage disequilibrium with Tg was the AITD susceptibility gene responsible for the observed linkage and association at this locus.

The TSH Receptor (TSHR) Gene

The hallmark of GD is the production of the TSHR antibodies. Therefore, the TSHR gene was long thought to be a likely candidate gene for GD. Three common germline SNPs of the TSHR have been described.[101] Two of them are located in the extracellular domain of the TSHR: an aspartic acid to histidine substitution at position 36 (D36H), and a proline to threonine substitution at position 52 (P52T). The third SNP is a substitution of glutamic acid for aspartic acid (D727E) within the intracellular domain of the receptor. Most studies on the contribution of the TSHR gene to the genetic susceptibility to GD have focused on the two SNPs in the extracellular domain of the TSHR[102-107] because this domain is the major site for TSH and TSHR antibody binding. Amino acid changes in the extracellular domain of the TSHR could theoretically change the amino acid sequence of TSHR T-cell epitopes.[108] Initial studies suggested that the P52T SNP was associated with GD in females.[102] However, other authors were unable to confirm the association between the P52T SNP and GD in Caucasians.[103-107] The D36H SNP has also been reported not to be associated with GD.[105] Linkage studies in GD families using three microsatellite markers within introns 2 and 7 of the TSHR gene were also negative in Caucasians.[109,110] Recently, the D727E SNP was reported to be associated with GD in a Caucasian Russian population,[111] but these results were not replicated in a subsequent study.[112] We also recently tested whether the D727E SNP was associated with GD, but did not show an association between the D727E SNP and GD, and did not show an effect of the D727E SNP on the GD phenotype or disease severity.[113] In addition, the frequency of the G allele was not increased in patients with more severe forms of GD (i.e., ophthalmopathy and goiter) and in patients with early disease onset. Our own study and other negative TSHR studies have not excluded a weak association between GD and the TSHR gene since very large datasets may be needed to detect associations with low RRs. We, therefore, performed a meta-analysis combining our data with the data reported in the previous 2 negative TSHR studies. The results showed a weak association between the D727E SNP E allele and GD ($p = 0.03$, $RR = 1.6$).[113] Therefore, at this time it remains possible that the TSHR is indeed a minor susceptibility gene for GD.

The Thyroid Peroxidase (TPO) Gene

The TPO gene was tested for linkage and association with AITD in two studies using a microsatellite inside the TPO gene. However, these studies showed no evidence of linkage and/or association of the TPO gene with AITD.[114,115] Therefore, the TPO gene is not a major susceptibility gene for AITD.

The Effect of Ethnicity on the Development of AITD

The HLA Gene (Table 4)

As previously mentioned, HLA-DR3 is associated with GD in Caucasians. The HLA genes were also shown to be associated with GD in non-Caucasians, albeit the associated alleles were different (Table 4). Studies in the Japanese population have shown associations of GD with HLA-B35.[116,117] However, other both class I and II HLA alleles have also been reported to be increased in Japanese GD patients.[118-120] In Chinese an increased frequency of HLA-Bw46 has been reported.[121-125] It is interesting that in Asians the HLA associations are with class I genes while in Caucasians they are with class II genes. This may imply that other nonHLA genes in the region in linkage disequilibrium with class II genes are the susceptibility genes in Asians. In contrast, DR3 is believed to be the causative gene in Caucasians (see below). In African-Americans an increased frequency of HLA DRB3*0202 has been reported (Table 4).[126] Interestingly, one study of a mixed population in Brazil showed association with HLA-DR3 implying that this

Table 4. Some HLA association studies in AITD performed in non-Caucasian populations

Country	Ethnic Group	Dis.	No. of Patients	HLA Allele(s)	RR/p-Value	Reference
Hong Kong	Chinese	GD	132	Bw46	4.8	176
Hong Kong	Chinese	GD	97	B46	2.3	122
				DR9	2.2	
				DQB1*0303	3.2	
Singapore	Chinese	GD	35	B46	8.2	123
Singapore	Chinese	GD	159	Bw46	4.2	125
Japan	Japanese	GD	33	Bw35	p< 0.02	116
Japan	Japanese	GD	106	B46	p< 0.0004	118
Japan	Japanese	GD	76	A2	2.86	177
				DPB1*0501	5.32	
Korea	Korean	GD	128	B13	3.8	178
				DR5	4.4	
				DRw8	2.3	
India	Asian	GD	57	B8	4.1	179
	Indian			DQw2	5.4	
USA	African-American	GD	73	No association		180
USA	African-American	GD	49	DRB3*0202	3.6	181
South Africa	African	GD	103	DR1	3.5	182
				DR3	2.4	
China	Chinese	HT	53	DRw9	p< 0.05	129
Japan	Japanese	HT	99	DRw53	3.33	128

*RR: relative risk

allele may confer susceptibility in other ethnic groups and not just Caucasians.[127] Alternatively, this Brazilian population may have been mostly of European ancestry.

HLA association studies in HT also have not been consistent in non-Caucasian ethnic groups, e.g., HLA-DRw53 in Japanese,[128] and HLA-DR9 in Chinese[129](Table 4). In addition, Linkage studies of HLA in AITD have been consistently negative in non Caucasians, including Chinese[130] and Japanese.[99] The negative linkage studies imply that HLA are also minor AITD genes in non-Caucasians.

The CTLA-4 Gene

The association between GD and the CTLA-4 3' UTR microsatellite and A/G_{49} SNP has been consistent across populations of different ethnic backgrounds such as Japanese,[60,131] and Koreans.[73] As was reported in Caucasians,[62] the C/T_{-318} SNP of CTLA-4 has not been associated with GD in Chinese.[62] It has also been reported that the frequency of the G allele and the GG genotype of the CTLA-4 A/G_{49} SNP was significantly higher in GD patients who did not go into remission after five years on anti-thyroid medications in Japanese.[132] Similarly, CTLA-4 has been reported to be associated with HT in non-Caucasians including Japanese.[131,133] Although no linkage study has been reported in non-Caucasians, the association of CTLA-4 across populations of different ethnic backgrounds shows that it is an important susceptibility gene for thyroid autoimmunity.

Other Immune Related Genes

The IgH gene was found to be associated with GD in the Japanese.[134,135] However, these results have not been reproduced in Caucasians.[88,89] This might imply that the IgH gene may contribute to the susceptibility to GD only in the Japanese if a founder effect exists. Alternatively, these could result from random event due to sampling small populations. Recently, the TNF α gene[136] and the vitamin D receptor, which may have some immune modulatory functions, has been reported to be associated with GD in Japanese.[137] A C/T SNP in the promoter region of the CD40 gene also has been reported to be associated with GD in Koreans.[138] These results need to be confirmed and it cannot be excluded that other genes in linkage disequilibrium with these genes are the susceptibility genes at these loci. Other immune related genes such as the interferon γ gene have not been tested yet in non-Caucasians, and warrant further studies.

The Tg Gene

A Japanese whole genome screen in 123 Japanese sib-pair families identified two loci giving strong evidence for linkage [i.e., MLS >2.0]. One of these loci is located on chromosome 8q24 and showed evidence for linkage with both AITD (MLS=2.31) and HT (MLS=3.77).[99] This locus is identical to the one found to be linked in Caucasians[98] and contains the Tg gene. Since the Tg locus was linked with AITD both in Caucasians and in Japanese, this supports that it is a major gene.

The TSHR Gene

An association between AITD and TSHR microsatellite markers has been reported in the Japanese.[131,133] However, these results have not been reproduced in Caucasians.[8,103-107] These results suggest that maybe TSHR gene contributes to the susceptibility to GD only in Japanese especially if there is a founder effect. For example, NOD2 mutations in Crohn's disease were shown only in Caucasians, and not in Japanese.[139]

Mechanisms by Which Genes Can Induce Thyroid Autoimmunity

The HLA Gene

The mechanisms by which HLA molecules confer susceptibility to autoimmune diseases are now beginning to be understood. T cells recognize and respond to an antigen by interacting with a complex between an antigenic peptide and an HLA molecule (reviewed in ref. 140). It is thought that different HLA alleles have different affinities for peptides from autoantigens (e.g., thyroid antigens) which are recognized by T cell receptors on cells which have escaped tolerance.[141] Thus, certain alleles may permit the autoantigenic peptide to fit into the antigen binding groove inside the HLA molecule and to be recognized by the T-cell receptor while others may not.[142] This would determine, if an autoimmune response to that antigen will develop.

Studies on the structure of HLA polymorphisms associated with T1DM provided strong evidence in support of this hypothesis. Sequencing of the HLA DQ genes showed that an aspartic residue at position 57 of the DQβ chain played a key role in the genetic susceptibility to T1DM.[143] Individuals who did not have Asp^{57} on both of their DR alleles were at high risk for T1DM (RR >50).[144] Moreover, it has been shown that an aspartic acid at position 57 on the DQβ chain influences the antigen binding properties of the HLA-DQαβ heterodimer.[143,145] Lack of aspartic acid at position 57 on the DQβ chain permitted immunogenic insulin peptides to fit into the antigen binding groove inside the HLA molecule and to be recognized by the T-cell receptor.[146,147] In contrast, the presence of aspartic acid at position 57 of the DQ β chain prevented insulin peptides from fitting, and hence prevented autoantigen presentation to the T-cell receptor.[142] It is possible that similar mechanisms may be involved in the association of DR3 with GD. Indeed, we have preliminary data showing that specific amino acids in the

DR3 binding pocket predispose to GD,[29] supporting this notion are HLA-DR binding studies that have shown a higher affinity of HLA-DR3 to TSHR immunodominant peptides than to TSHR nonimmunodominant peptides.[148]

For thyroid autoantigens to be presented by HLA molecules to T-cells, a mechanism of autoantigen presentation must exist within the thyroid gland or the draining lymph nodes of the gland. One potential intrathyroidal mechanism not utilizing professional APCs may be through expression of HLA class II molecules on thyrocytes.[149-151] Unlike in normal thyroids, the thyroid epithelial cells from patients with GD and HT have been shown to express HLA class II antigen molecules similar to those normally expressed on APCs such as macrophages and dendritic cells.[151,152] This aberrant expression of HLA class II molecules on thyroid cells may initiate thyroid autoimmunity via direct thyroid autoantigen presentation[153] or a secondary event following cytokine secretion by invading T cells. Consistent with the former possibility was the fact that thyroid cell MHC class II antigen expression could be induced by certain viral infections in vitro,[154,155] and that mice constitutively expressing thyroid cell MHC class II antigens developed thyroiditis after immunization with human Tg.[42] Furthermore, a murine model of GD has been shown to depend on TSHR antigen presentation on cells expressing MHC class II molecules.[156,157] Coculture of PBMC from GD patients with homologous thyrocytes induced T cell activation,[158] as well as interferon-γ production and thyroid cell HLA class II antigen expression.[159] Such cytokine secretion may be the common cause of HLA class II antigen expression by thyroid cells in AITD.[150,160,161]

The CTLA-4 Gene

The CTLA-4 gene polymorphisms have also been studied for their effects on CTLA-4 function. CTLA-4 is an important costimulatory molecule that participates in the presentation of peptides to T-cells. APCs activate T cells by presenting to the T cell receptor an antigenic peptide bound to an HLA class II protein on the cell surface. However, a second signal is also required for T cell activation and these costimulatory signals may be provided by the APCs themselves or other local cells.[50] The co stimulatory signals are provided by a variety of proteins (e.g., B7-1, B7-2, CD40) which are expressed on APCs and interact with receptors (CD28, CTLA-4, and CD40L) on the surface of CD4+ T-lymphocytes during antigen presentation.[50] Whereas, the binding of B7 to CD28 on T cells costimulates T cell activation, the higher affinity binding of B7 to CTLA-4 down regulates T-cell activation and induces tolerance. The suppressive effects of CTLA-4 on T cell activation have raised the possibility that the CTLA-4 polymorphisms associated with AITD decreased its expression and/or function thereby promoting the development of autoimmunity.[67]

As discussed earlier, two CTLA-4 polymorphisms have been shown to be associated with AITD, a 3' UTR microsatellite and an A/G polymorphism in the leader sequence of the gene. One recent study examined the effects of the A and G alleles of the CTLA-4 A/G_{49} SNP on the inhibitory function of CTLA-4. The authors showed that blocking of CTLA-4 on T cells isolated from individuals with the G allele had less effect on reducing the inhibitory function of CTLA-4 than blocking CTLA-4 on T cells isolated from individuals with the A allele.[162] This could imply that the A and G alleles of the CTLA-4 leader sequence influenced its function and/or expression. Xu et al have examined the effects of the CTLA-4 A/G_{49} SNP using an in vitro assay by transfecting T-cell lines lacking CTLA-4 with CTLA-4 cDNA having the A or the G allele. When T cells were transfected with CTLA-4 cDNA carrying the G or A allele there was no difference in the expression and inhibitory function of CTLA-4.[163] This means that the A and G alleles of the CTLA-4 A/G_{49} SNP did not directly influence its function. Other polymorphisms in linkage disequilibrium with the A/G SNP must be responsible for the association of CTLA-4 with AITD. Indeed, preliminary data in myathenia gravis showed that the AT microsatellite at the 3' UTR of the CTLA-4 gene influenced the half life of the CTLA-4 mRNA.[164,165] This could provide an attractive explanation for the association between the short alleles of the AT microsatellite and AITD, as well as other autoimmune diseases.

Hypothetical Mechanisms by Which Tg Could Induce Susceptibility to AITD

As mentioned above the Tg gene is linked and associated with AITD.[98,99] Therefore, Tg may be a susceptibility gene for AITD. In order to demonstrate that Tg is indeed the AITD susceptibility gene on chromosome 8q24 we have sequenced the gene in patients and controls and identified sequence variants which are associated with AITD.[166] The Tg gene may predispose to AITD in a number of ways, for example: (1) Sequence changes in Tg may change its antigenicity making it more immunogenic; (2) Sequence changes in Tg may change its interaction with HLA class II molecules; (3) Sequence changes in Tg may influence its degradation by cathepsin S in endosomes, a process which has been recently shown to play an important role in development of autoimmunity.[167] In addition, alterations in Tg could possibly explain interactions between genetic and environmental factors in the etiology of AITD, since Tg is iodinated to form thyroid hormones, and dietary iodine may influence the development of AITD.[168-170] Indeed, as noted above, the Tg hormonogenic sites were shown to contain the autoepitopes in experimental autoimmune thyroiditis, albeit the role of iodine is still controversial in experimental thyroiditis.[171,172]

Conclusion

The AITD are complex diseases believed to be caused by the combined effects of multiple susceptibility genes and environmental triggers. There are sufficient epidemiologic data to support an important genetic contribution to the development of AITD, and in the past few years several loci and genes have shown evidence for linkage and/or association with AITD. The genetic susceptibility to AITD seems to involve several genes with varying effects. With the completion of the human genome project and the establishment of large SNP databases the identification of additional AITD susceptibility genes will become more feasible.

The AITD loci identified so far show that some putative AITD susceptibility genes may be immune related genes which increase the susceptibility to autoimmunity in general (e.g., HLA, CTLA-4) while others may be specific to AITD (e.g., TSHR, Tg). The next step in investigating the role of these genes in the development of AITD is by functional studies and genotype-phenotype correlations. Preliminary functional studies have been performed for HLA[148] and CTLA-4.[162,163] More functional studies are needed for these and other genes which have shown association with AITD.

It is most likely that the susceptibility genes for AITD interact and that their interactions may influence disease phenotype and severity.[109] The molecular basis for the interactions between susceptibility genes in complex diseases is unknown. These interactions could represent the cumulative effect of increased statistical risk, or alternatively, there may be molecular interactions between the susceptibility genes or their products which ultimately determine disease phenotype. Another unresolved question is how do environmental factors interact with susceptibility genes to modify the risk for disease, as well as the disease phenotype. We are slowly progressing towards identification of the AITD susceptibility genes and once they are identified we will begin to understand the underlying molecular mechanisms by which they induce thyroid autoimmunity.

Acknowledgements

We thank Drs. Terry F. Davies and David A. Greenberg for their teaching, support and ever ready help in our joint studies. This work was supported in part by grants DK61659 & DK58072 from NIDDKD (to YT).

References

1. Davies TF. Graves' Diseases: Pathogenesis. In: Braverman LE, Utiger RD, eds. Werner and Ingbar's The Thyroid: A Fundamental and Clinical Text. Philadelphia: Lippincott Williams and Wilkens, 2000:518-530.
2. Weetman AP. Chronic autoimmune thyroiditis. In: Braverman LE, Utiger RD, eds. Werner and Ingbar's the thyroid. Philadelphia: Lippincott-Raven, 1996:738-748.
3. Brix TH, Kyvik KO, Hegedus L. What is the evidence of genetic factors in the etiology of Graves' disease? A brief review. Thyroid 1998; 8:727-734.
4. Tomer Y, Barbesino G, Greenberg DA et al. The immunogenetics of autoimmune diabetes and autoimmune thyroid disease. Trends Endocrinol Metab 1997; 8:63-70.
5. Bartels ED. Twin examinations: Heredity in Graves' disease. Copenhagen: Munksgaad, 1941:32-36.
6. Martin L. The heredity and familial aspects of exophathalmic goitre and nodular goitre. Q J Med 1945; 14:207-219.
7. Hall R, Stanbury JB. Familial studies of autoimmune thyroiditis. Clin Exp Immunol 1967; 2:719-725.
8. Villanueva RB, Inzerillo AM, Tomer Y et al. Limited genetic susceptibility to severe graves' ophthalmopathy: No role for ctla-4 and evidence for an environmental etiology. Thyroid 2000; 10:791-798.
9. Risch N. Linkage strategies for genetically complex traits. II. The power of affected relative pairs. Am J Hum Genet 1990; 46:229-241.
10. Vyse TJ, Todd JA. Genetic analysis of autoimmune disease. Cell 1996; 85:311-318.
11. Brix TH, Christensen K, Holm NV et al. A population-based study of Graves' diseases in Danish twins. Clin Endocrinol 1998; 48:397-400.
12. Brix TH, Kyvik KO, Christensen K et al. Evidence for a major role of heredity in Graves' disease: A population- based study of two Danish twin cohorts. J Clin Endocrinol Metab 2001; 86:930-934.
13. Ringold DA, Nicoloff JT, Kesler M et al. Further evidence for a strong genetic influence on the development of autoimmune thyroid disease: The California twin study. Thyroid 2002; 12:647-653.
14. Brix TH, Kyvik KO, Hegedus L. A population-based study of chronic autoimmune hypothyroidism in Danish twins. J Clin Endocrinol Metab 2000; 85:536-539.
15. Phillips DI, Osmond C, Baird J et al. Is birthweight associated with thyroid autoimmunity? A study in twins. Thyroid 2002; 12:377-380.
16. Todd JA, Acha-Orbea H, Bell JI et al. A molecular basis for MHC class II— associated autoimmunity. Science 1988; 240:1003-1009.
17. Bech K, Lumholtz B, Nerup J et al. HLA antigens in Graves' disease. Acta Endocrinol 1977; 86:510-516.
18. Farid NR, Stone E, Johnson G. Graves' disease and HLA: Clinical and epidemiologic associations. Clin Endocrinol (Oxf) 1980; 13:535-544.
19. Farid NR. Graves' disease. In: Farid NR, ed. HLA in Endocrine and Metabolic Disorders. Academic Press, 1981:85-143.
20. Farid NR, Sampson L, Noel EP et al. A study of human D locus related antigens in Graves' disease. J Clin Invest 1979; 63:108-113.
21. Mangklabruks A, Cox N, DeGroot LJ. Genetic factors in autoimmune thyroid disease analyzed by restriction fragment length polymorphisms of candidate genes. J Clin Endocrinol Metab 1991; 73:236-244.
22. Volpe R. Immunology of human thyroid disease. In: Volpe R, ed. Autoimmunity in endocrine disease. Boca Raton: CRC Press, 1990:73.
23. Heward JM, Allahabadia A, Daykin J et al. Linkage disequilibrium between the human leukocyte antigen class II region of the major histocompatibility complex and Graves' disease: Replication using a population case control and family-based study. J Clin Endocrinol Metab 1998; 83:3394-3397.
24. Barlow ABT, Wheatcroft N, Watson P et al. Association of HLA- DQA1*0501 with Graves' disease in English caucasian men and women. Clin Endocrinol 1996; 44:73-77.
25. Yanagawa T, Mangklabruks A, Chang YB et al. Human histocompatibility leukocyte antigen-DQA1*0501 allele associated with genetic susceptibility to Graves' disease in a caucasian population. J Clin Endocrinol Metab 1993; 76:1569-1574.
26. Marga M, Denisova A, Sochnev A et al. Two HLA DRB 1 alleles confer independent genetic susceptibility to Graves disease: Relevance of cross- population studies. Am J Med Genet 2001; 102:188-191.
27. Zamani M, Spaepen M, Bex M et al. Primary role of the HLA class II DRB1*0301 allele in Graves disease. Am J Med Genet 2000; 95:432- 437.

28. Villanueva R, Greenberg DA, Davies TF et al. Sibling recurrence risk in autoimmune thyroid disease. Thyroid 2003; 13:761-764.
29. Ban Y, Davies TF, Greenberg DA et al. Potential role of HLA-DR-74 arginine in the genetic susceptibility to Graves' disease. San Francisco, CA: The 84th Annual Meeting of the Endocrine Society, 2002.
30. Segni M, Pani MA, Pasquino AM et al. Familial clustering of juvenile thyroid autoimmunity: Higher risk is conferred by human leukocyte antigen DR3- DQ2 and thyroid peroxidase antibody status in fathers. J Clin Endocrinol Metab 2002; 87:3779-3782.
31. Schleusener H, Schwander J, Fischer C et al. Prospective multicentre study on the prediction of relapse after antithyroid drug treatment in patients with Graves' disease. Acta Endocrinol (Copenh) 1989; 120:689-701.
32. Dahlberg PA, Holmlund G, Karlsson FA et al. HLA-A, -B, -C and -DR antigens in patients with Graves' disease and their correlation with signs and clinical course. Acta Endocrinol (Copenh) 1981; 97:42-47.
33. McKenna R, Kearns M, Sugrue D et al. HLA and hyperthyroidism in Ireland. Tissue Antigens 1982; 19:97-99.
34. Allannic H, Fauchet R, Lorcy Y et al. A prospective study of the relationship between relapse of hyperthyroid Graves' disease after antithyroid drugs and HLA haplotype. J Clin Endocrinol Metab 1983; 57:719-722.
35. Kendall-Taylor P, Stephenson A, Stratton A et al. Differentiation of autoimmune ophthalmopathy from Graves' hyperthyroidism by analysis of genetic markers. Clin Endocrinol (Oxf) 1988; 28:601-610.
36. Rapoport B, Alsabeh R, Aftergood D et al. Elephantiasic pretibial myxedema: Insight into and a hypothesis regarding the pathogenesis of the extrathyroidal manifestations of Graves' disease. Thyroid 2000; 10:685-692.
37. Irvine WJ, Gray RS, Morris PJ et al. HLA in primary atrophic hypothyroidism and Hashimoto goitre. J Clin Lab Immunol 1978; 3:193-195.
38. Farid NR, Sampson L, Moens H et al. The association of goitrous autoimmune thyroiditis with HLA-DR5. Tissue Antigens 1981; 17:265-268.
39. Moens H, Farid NR, Sampson L et al. Hashimoto's thyroiditis is associated with HLA-DRw3. N Engl J Med 1978; 299:133-134.
40. Tandon N, Zhang L, Weetman AP. HLA associations with Hashimoto's thyroiditis. Clin Endocrinol (Oxf) 1991; 34:383-386.
41. Ban Y, Davies TF, Greenberg DA et al. The influence of human leucocyte antigen (HLA) genes on autoimmune thyroid disease (AITD): Results of studies in HLA-DR3 positive AITD families. Clin Endocrinol (Oxf) 2002; 57:81-88.
42. Kong YC, Lomo LC, Motte RW et al. HLA-DRB1 polymorphism determines susceptibility to autoimmune thyroiditis in transgenic mice: Definitive association with HLA- DRB1*0301 (DR3) gene. J Exp Med 1996; 184:1167-1172.
43. Wu Z, Stephens HAF, Sachs JA et al. Molecular analysis of HLA-DQ and -DP genes in caucasoid patients with Hashimoto's thyroiditis. Tissue Antigens 1994; 43:116- 119.
44. Badenhoop K, Schwartz G, Walfish PG et al. Susceptibility to thyroid autoimmune disease: Molecular analysis of HLA-D region genes identifies new markers for goitrous Hashimoto's thyroiditis. J Clin Endocrinol Metab 1990; 71:1131-1137.
45. Bode HH, Dorf ME, Forbes AP. Familial lymphocytic thyroiditis: Analysis of linkage with histocompatibility and blood group. J Clin Endocrinol Metab 1973; 37:692-697.
46. Roman SH, Greenberg DA, Rubinstein P et al. Genetics of autoimmune thyroid disease: Lack of evidence for linkage to HLA within families. J Clin Endocrinol Metab 1992; 74:496-503.
47. Barbesino G, Tomer Y, Concepcion ES et al. Linkage analysis of candidate genes in autoimmune thyroid disease. I. Selected immunoregulatory genes. J Clin Endocrinol Metab 1998; 83:1580-1584.
48. Vaidya B, Imrie H, Perros P et al. The cytotoxic T lymphocyte antigen- 4 is a major Graves' disease locus. Hum Mol Genet 1999; 8:1195-1199.
49. Shields DC, Ratanachaiyavong S, McGregor AM et al. Combined segregation and linkage analysis of Graves' disease with a thyroid autoantibody diathesis. Am J Hum Genet 1994; 55:540-554.
50. Reiser H, Stadecker MJ. Costimulatory B7 molecules in the pathogenesis of infectious and autoimmune diseases. N Engl J Med 1996; 335:1369-1377.
51. Hutloff A, Dittrich AM, Beier KC et al. ICOS is an inducible T-cell costimulator structurally and functionally related to CD28. Nature 1999; 397:263-266.
52. Coyle AJ, Lehar S, Lloyd C et al. The CD28-related molecule ICOS is required for effective T cell-dependent immune responses. Immunity 2000; 13:95-105.
53. Yanagawa T, Hidaka Y, Guimaraes V et al. CTLA-4 gene polymorphism associated with Graves' disease in a caucasian population. J Clin Endocrinol Metab 1995; 80:41-45.

54. Nistico L, Buzzetti R, Pritchard LE et al. The CTLA-4 gene region of chromosome 2q33 is linked to, and associated with, type 1 diabetes. The Belgian Diabetes Registry. Hum Mol Genet 1996; 5:1075-1080.
55. Donner H, Rau H, Walfish PG et al. CTLA4 alanine-17 confers genetic susceptibility to Graves' disease and to type 1 diabetes mellitus. J Clin Endocrinol Metab 1997; 82:143- 146.
56. Kotsa K, Watson PF, Weetman AP. A CTLA-4 gene polymorphism is associated with both Graves' disease and autoimmune hypothyroidism. Clin Endocrinol 1997; 46:551-554.
57. Kouki T, Gardine CA, Yanagawa T et al. Relation of three polymorphisms of the CTLA-4 gene in patients with Graves' disease. J Endocrinol Invest 2002; 25:208-213.
58. Nithiyananthan R, Heward JM, Allahabadia A et al. Polymorphism of the CTLA-4 gene is associated with autoimmune hypothyroidism in the United Kingdom. Thyroid 2002; 12:3-6.
59. Braun J, Donner H, Siegmund T et al. CTLA-4 promoter variants in patients with Graves' disease and Hashimoto's thyroiditis. Tissue Antigens 1998; 51:563-566.
60. Yanagawa T, Taniyama M, Enomoto S et al. CTLA4 gene polymorphism confers susceptibility to Graves' disease in Japanese. Thyroid 1997; 7:843-846.
61. Heward JM, Allahabadia A, Armitage M et al. The development of Graves' disease and the CTLA-4 gene on chromosome 2q33. J Clin Endocrinol Metab 1999; 84:2398-2401.
62. Heward JM, Allahabadia A, Carr-Smith J et al. No evidence for allelic association of human CTLA-4 promoter polymorphism with autoimmune thyroid disease in either population- based case-control or family-based studies. Clin Endocrinol 1998; 49:331-334.
63. Donner H, Braun J, Seidl C et al. Codon 17 polymorphism of the cytotoxic T lymphocyte antigen 4 gene in Hashimoto's thyroiditis and Addison's disease. J Clin Endocrinol Metab 1997; 82:4130-4132.
64. Petrone A, Giorgi G, Mesturino CA et al. Association of DRB1*04-DQB1*0301 haplotype and lack of association of two polymorphic sites at CTLA-4 gene with Hashimoto's thyroiditis in an Italian population. Thyroid 2001; 11:171-175.
65. Tomer Y. Unraveling the genetic susceptibility to autoimmune thyroid diseases: CTLA-4 takes the stage. Thyroid 2001; 11:167-169.
66. Marron MP, Raffel LJ, Garchon HJ et al. Insulin-dependent diabetes mellitus (IDDM) is assocaited with CTLA4 polymorphisms in multiple ethnic groups. Hum Mol Genet 1997; 6:1275-1282.
67. Ueda H, Howson JM, Esposito L et al. Association of the T-cell regulatory gene CTLA4 with susceptibility to autoimmune disease. Nature 2003; 423:506-511.
68. Vaidya B, Imrie H, Geatch DR et al. Association analysis of the cytotoxic T lymphocyte antigen-4 (CTLA- 4) and autoimmune regulator-1 (AIRE1) genes in sporadic autoimmune Addison's disease. J Clin Endocrinol Metab 2000; 85:688-691.
69. Huang D, Liu L, Noren K et al. Genetic association of Ctla-4 to myasthenia gravis with thymoma. J Neuroimmunol 1998; 88:192-198.
70. Tomer Y, Greenberg DA, Barbesino G et al. CTLA-4 and not CD28 is a susceptibility gene for thyroid autoantibody production. J Clin Endocrinol Metab 2001; 86:1687-1693.
71. Zaletel K, Krhin B, Gaberscek S et al. The influence of the exon 1 polymorphism of the cytotoxic T lymphocyte antigen 4 gene on thyroid antibody production in patients with newly diagnosed graves' disease. Thyroid 2002; 12:373-376.
72. Vanderpump MPJ, Tunbridge WMG, French JM et al. The incidence of thyroid disorders in the community: A twenty-year follow-up of the Whickham survey. Clin Endocrinol (Oxf) 1995; 43:55-68.
73. Park YJ, Chung HK, Park DJ et al. Polymorphism in the promoter and exon 1 of the cytotoxic T lymphocyte antigen-4 gene associated with autoimmune thyroid disease in Koreans. Thyroid 2000; 10:453-459.
74. Yung E, Cheng PS, Fok TF et al. CTLA-4 gene A-G polymorphism and childhood Graves' disease. Clin Endocrinol (Oxf) 2002; 56:649-653.
75. Allahabadia A, Heward JM, Nithiyananthan R et al. MHC class II region, CTLA4 gene, and ophthalmopathy in patients with Graves' disease. Lancet 2001; 358:984-985.
76. Vaidya B, Imrie H, Perros P et al. Cytotoxic T lymphocyte antigen-4 (CTLA-4) gene polymorphism confers susceptibility to thyroid associated orbitopathy [letter]. Lancet 1999; 354:743- 744.
77. Marron MP, Zeidler A, Raffel LJ et al. Genetic and physical mapping of a type 1 diabetes susceptibility gene (IDDM12) to a 100-kb phagemid artificial chromosome clone containing D2S72-CTLA4-D2S105 on chromosome 2q33. Diabetes 2000; 49:492-499.
78. Wood JP, Pani MA, Bieda K et al. A recently described polymorphism in the CD28 gene on chromosome 2q33 is not associated with susceptibility to type 1 diabetes. Eur J Immunogenet 2002; 29:347-349.
79. Tomer Y, Barbesino G, Greenberg DA et al. A new Graves disease-susceptibility locus maps to chromosome 20q11.2. Am J Hum Genet 1998; 63:1749-1756.

80. Pearce SH, Vaidya B, Imrie H et al. Further evidence for a susceptibility locus on chromosome 20q13.11 in families with dominant transmission of Graves disease [letter]. Am J Hum Genet 1999; 65:1462-1465.
81. Durie FH, Foy TM, Masters SR et al. The role of CD40 in the regulation of humoral and cell-mediated immunity. Immunol Today 1994; 15:406- 411.
82. Banchereau J, Bazan F, Blanchard D et al. The CD40 antigen and its ligand. Annu Rev Immunol 1994; 12:881-922.
83. Foy TM, Aruffo A, Bajorath J et al. Immune regulation by CD40 and its ligand GP39. Annu Rev Immunol 1996; 14:591-617.
84. Carayanniotis G, Masters SR, Noelle RJ. Suppression of murine thyroiditis via blockade of the CD40-CD40L interaction. Immunology 1997; 90:421-426.
85. Tomer Y, Concepcion E, Greenberg DA. A C/T single nucleotide polymorphism in the region of the CD40 gene is associated with Graves' disease. Thyroid 2002; 12:1129-1135.
86. Demaine A, Welsh KI, Hawe BS et al. Polymorphism of the T cell receptor beta-chain in Graves' disease. J Clin Endocrinol Metab 1987; 65:643-646.
87. Weetman AP, So AK, Roe C et al. T-cell receptor alpha chain V region polymorphism linked to primary autoimmune hypothyroidism but not Graves' disease. Human Immunology 1987; 20:167-173.
88. Roman SH, Hubbard M, Rubinstein P. Failure to confirm standard HLA and Gm immunogenetic typing as a predictor of familial autoimmune thyroid disease. Seattle, WA: The 74th Annual Meeting of the Endocrine Society, 1989.
89. Fakhfakh F, Maalej A, Makni H et al. Analysis of immunoglobulin VH and TCR cbeta polymorphisms in a large family with thyroid autoimmune disorder. Exp Clin Immunogenet 1999; 16:185-191.
90. Blakemore AIF, Watson PF, Weetman AP et al. Association of Graves' disease with an allele of the interleukin-1 receptor antagonist gene. Journal of Clinical Endocrinology and Metabolism 1995; 80:111-115.
91. Cuddihy RM, Bahn RS. Lack of an association between alleles of interleukin-1 alpha and interleukin-1 receptor antagonsit genes and Graves' disease in a north American Caucasian population. J Clin Endocrinol Metab 1996; 81:4476-4478.
92. Muhlberg T, Kirchberger M, Spitzweg C et al. Lack of association of Graves' disease with the A2 allele of the interleukin-1 receptor antagonist gene in a white European population. Eur J Endocrinol 1998; 138:686-690.
93. Heward J, Allahabadia A, Gordon C et al. The interleukin-1 receptor antagonist gene shows no allelic association with three autoimmune diseases. Thyroid 1999; 9:627-628.
94. Siegmund T, Usadel KH, Donner H et al. Interferon-gamma gene microsatellite pollymorphisms in patients with Graves' disease. Thyroid 1998; 8:1013-1017.
95. Rau H, Nicolay A, Usadel KH et al. Polymorphisms of TAP1 and TAP2 genes in Graves' disease. Tissue Antigens 1997; 49:16-22.
96. Heward JM, Nithiyananthan R, Allahabadia A et al. No association of an interleukin 4 gene promoter polymorphism with Graves' disease in the United Kingdom. J Clin Endocrinol Metab 2001; 86:3861-3863.
97. Pani MA, Regulla K, Segni M et al. A polymorphism within the vitamin D-binding protein gene is associated with Graves' disease but not with Hashimoto's thyroiditis. J Clin Endocrinol Metab 2002; 87:2564-2567.
98. Tomer Y, Greenberg DA, Concepcion E et al. Thyroglobulin is a thyroid specific gene for the familial autoimmune thyroid diseases. J Clin Endocrinol Metab 2002; 87:404-407.
99. Sakai K, Shirasawa S, Ishikawa N et al. Identification of susceptibility loci for autoimmune thyroid disease to 5q31-q33 and Hashimoto's thyroiditis to 8q23-q24 by multipoint affected sib-pair linkage analysis in Japanese. Hum Mol Genet 2001; 10:1379-1386.
100. Collins JE, Heward JM, Carr-Smith J et al. Association of a rare thyroglobulin gene microsatellite variant with autoimmune thyroid disease. J Clin Endocrinol Metab. 2003; 88:5039-5042.
101. Tonacchera M, Pinchera A. Thyrotropin receptor polymorphisms and thyroid diseases. J Clin Endocrinol Metab 2000; 85:2637-2639.
102. Cuddihy RM, Dutton CM, Bahn RS. A polymorphism in the extracellular domain of the thyrotropin receptor is highly associated with autoimmune thyroid disease in females. Thyroid 1995; 5:89-95.
103. Kotsa KD, Watson PF, Weetman AP. No association between a thyrotropin receptor gene polymorphism and Graves' disease in the female population. Thyroid 1997; 7:31-33.
104. Allahabadia A, Heward JM, Mijovic C et al. Lack of association between polymorphism of the thyrotropin receptor gene and Graves' disease in United Kingdom and Hong Kong Chinese patients: case control and family-based studies. Thyroid 1998; 8:777-780.

105. Simanainen J, Kinch A, Westermark K et al. Analysis of mutations in exon 1 of the human thyrotropin receptor gene: High frequency of the D36H and P52T polymorphic variants. Thyroid 1999; 9:7-11.
106. Kaczur V, Takacs M, Szalai C et al. Analysis of the genetic variability of the 1st (CCC/ACC, P52T) and the 10th exons (bp 1012-1704) of the TSH receptor gene in Graves' disease. Eur J Immunogenet 2000; 27:17-23.
107. Chistyakov DA, Savost'anov KV, Turakulov RI et al. Complex association analysis of graves disease using a set of polymorphic markers. Mol Genet Metab 2000; 70:214-218.
108. Rapoport B, Chazenbalk GD, Jaume JC et al. The thyrotropin (TSH) receptor: Interaction with TSH and autoantibodies. Endocr Rev 1998; 19:673-716.
109. Tomer Y, Barbesino G, Greenberg DA et al. Mapping the major susceptibility loci for familial Graves' and Hashimoto's diseases: Evidence for genetic heterogeneity and gene interactions. J Clin Endocrinol Metab 1999; 84:4656-4664.
110. De Roux N, Shields DC, Misrahi M et al. Analysis of the thyrotropin receptor as a candidate gene in familial Graves' disease. J Clin Endocrinol Metab 1996; 81:3483-3486.
111. Chistiakov DA, Savost'anov KV, Turakulov RI et al. Further studies of genetic susceptibility to Graves' disease in a Russian population. Med Sci Monit 2002; 8:CR180-CR184.
112. Muhlberg T, Herrmann K, Joba W et al. Lack of association of nonautoimmune hyperfunctioning thyroid disorders and a germline polymorphism of codon 727 of the human thyrotropin receptor in a European Caucasian population. J Clin Endocrinol Metab 2000; 85:2640-2643.
113. Ban Y, Greenberg DA, Concepcion ES et al. A germline single nucleotide polymorphism at the intracellular domain of the human thyrotropin receptor does not have a major effect on the development of Graves' disease. Thyroid 2002; 12:1079-1083.
114. Pirro MT, De Filippis V, Di Cerbo A et al. Thyroperoxidase microsatellite polymorphism in thyroid disease. Thyroid 1995; 5:461-464.
115. Tomer Y, Barbesino G, Keddache M et al. Mapping of a major susceptibility locus for Graves' disease (GD-1) to chromosome 14q31. J Clin Endocrinol Metab 1997; 82:1645-1648.
116. Kawa A, Nakamura S, Nakazawa M et al. HLA-BW35 and B5 in Japanese patients with Graves' disease. Acta Endocrinol (Copenh) 1977; 86:754-757.
117. Inoue D, Sato K, Enomoto T et al. Correlation of HLA types and clinical findings in Japanese patients with hyperthyroid Graves' disease: Evidence indicating the existence of four subpopulations. Clin Endocrinol (Oxf) 1992; 36:75-82.
118. Onuma H, Ota M, Sugenoya A et al. Association of HLA-DPB1*0501 with early-onset Graves' disease in Japanese. Hum Immunol 1994; 39:195-201.
119. Katsuren E, Awata T, Matsumoto C et al. HLA class II alleles in Japanese patients with Graves' disease: Weak associations of HLA-DR and -DQ. Endocr J 1994; 41:599-603.
120. Ohtsuka K, Nakamura Y. Human leukocyte antigens associated with hyperthyroid Graves ophthalmology in Japanese patients. Am J Ophthalmol 1998; 126:805-810.
121. Chan SH, Yeo PP, Lui KF et al. HLA and thyrotoxicosis (Graves' disease) in Chinese. Tissue Antigens 1978; 12:109-114.
122. Cavan DA, Penny MA, Jacobs KH et al. The HLA association with Graves' disease is sex-specific in Hong Kong Chinese subjects. Clin Endocrinol (Oxf) 1994; 40:63-66.
123. Chan SH, Lin YN, Wee GB et al. Human leucocyte antigen DNA typing in Singaporean Chinese patients with Graves' disease. Ann Acad Med Singapore 1993; 22:576-579.
124. Tan S, Chan S, Lee B et al. HLA association in Singapore children with Grave's disease. Metabolism 1988; 37:518-519.
125. Yeo PP, Chan SH, Thai AC et al. HLA Bw46 and DR9 associations in Graves' disease of Chinese patients are age- and sex-related. Tissue Antigens 1989; 34:179-184.
126. Chen QY, Nadell D, Zhang XY et al. The human leukocyte antigen HLA DRB3*020/DQA1*0501 haplotype is associated with Graves' disease in African Americans. J Clin Endocrinol Metab 2000; 85:1545-1549.
127. Maciel LM, Rodrigues SS, Dibbern RS et al. Association of the HLA-DRB1*0301 and HLA-DQA1*0501 alleles with Graves' disease in a population representing the gene contribution from several ethnic backgrounds. Thyroid 2001; 11:31-35.
128. Honda K, Tamai H, Morita T et al. Hashimoto's thyroiditis and HLA in Japanese. J Clin Endocrinol Metab 1989; 69:1268-1273.
129. Hawkins BR, Lam KSL, Ma JTC et al. Strong association between HLA-DRw9 and Hashimoto's thyroiditis in Southern Chinese. Acta Endocrinol 1987; 114:543-546.
130. Hawkins BR, Ma JT, Lam KS et al. Analysis of linkage between HLA haplotype and susceptibility to Graves' disease in multiple-case Chinese families in Hong Kong. Acta Endocrinol (Copenh) 1985; 110:66-69.

131. Akamizu T, Sale MM, Rich SS et al. Association of autoimmune thyroid disease with microsatellite markers for the thyrotropin receptor gene and CTLA-4 in Japanese patients. Thyroid 2000; 10:851-858.
132. Kinjo Y, Takasu N, Komiya I et al. Remission of Graves' hyperthyroidism and A/G polymorphism at position 49 in exon 1 of cytotoxic T lymphocyte-associated molecule-4 gene. J Clin Endocrinol Metab 2002; 87:2593-2596.
133. Sale MM, Akamizu T, Howard TD et al. Association of autoimmune thyroid disease with a microsatellite marker for the thyrotropin receptor gene and CTLA-4 in a Japanese population. Proc Assoc Am Physicians 1997; 109:453-461.
134. Nagataki S. The interaction of MHC and Gm in liability to autoimmune thyroid disease. Mol Biol Med 1986; 3:73-84.
135. Nakao Y, Matsumoto H, Miyazaki T et al. IgG heavy chain allotypes (Gm) in atrophic and goitrous thyroiditis. Clin Exp Immunol 1980; 42:20-26.
136. Kamizono S, Hiromatsu Y, Seki N et al. A polymorphism of the 5' flanking region of tumour necrosis factor alpha gene is associated with thyroid-associated ophthalmopathy in japanese. Clin Endocrinol (Oxf) 2000; 52:759-764.
137. Ban Y, Taniyama M, Ban Y. Vitamin D receptor gene polymorphism is associated with Graves' disease in the Japanese population. J Clin Endocrinol Metab 2000; 85:4639-4643.
138. Kim TY, Park YJ, Hwang JK et al. A C/T Polymorphism in the 5'-untranslated region of the CD40 gene is associated with Graves' Disease in Koreans. Thyroid. 2003; 13:919-925.
139. Yamazaki K, Takazoe M, Tanaka T et al. Absence of mutation in the NOD2/CARD15 gene among 483 Japanese patients with Crohn's disease. J Hum Genet 2002; 47:469-472.
140. Buus S, Sette A, Grey HM. The interaction between protein-derived immunogenic peptides and Ia. Immunol Rev 1987; 98:115-141.
141. Nelson JL, Hansen JA. Autoimmune disease and HLA. CRC Crit Rev Immunol 1990; 10:307-328.
142. Faas S, Trucco M. The genes influencing the susceptibility to IDDM in humans. J Endocrinol Invest 1994; 17:477-495.
143. Aitman TJ, Todd JA. Molecular genetics of diabetes mellitus. Baillière's Clin Endocrinol Metab 1995; 9:631-656.
144. Morel PA, Dorman JS, Todd JA et al. Aspartic acid at position 57 of the HLA-DQ beta-chain protects against type I diabetes: A family study. Proc Natl Acad Sci USA 1988; 85:8111-8115.
145. Brown JH, Jardetzky T, Gorga JC et al. Three-dimensional structure of the human class II histocompatibility antigen HLA-DR1. Nature 1993; 364:33-39.
146. Lee KH, Wucherpfennig KW, Wiley DC. Structure of a human insulin peptide- HLA-DQ8 complex and susceptibility to type 1 diabetes. Nat Immunol 2001; 2:501-507.
147. Wucherpfennig KW. Insights into autoimmunity gained from structural analysis of MHC- peptide complexes. Curr Opin Immunol 2001; 13:650-656.
148. Sawai Y, DeGroot LJ. Binding of human thyrotropin receptor peptides to a Graves' disease- predisposing human leukocyte antigen class II molecule. J Clin Endocrinol Metab 2000; 85:1176-1179.
149. Hanafusa T, Pujol Borrell R, Chiovato L et al. Aberrant expression of HLA-DR antigen on thyrocytes in Graves' disease: Relevance for autoimmunity. Lancet 1983; 2:1111-1115.
150. Bottazzo GF, Pujol Borrell R, Hanafusa T et al. Role of aberrant HLA- DR expression and antigen presentation in induction of endocrine autoimmunity. Lancet 1983; 2:1115-1119.
151. Davies TF. Cocultures of human thyroid monolayer cells and autologous T cells: Impact of HLA class II antigen expression. J Clin Endocrinol Metab 1985; 61:418-422.
152. Londei M, Lamb JR, Bottazzo GF et al. Epithelial cells expressing aberrant MHC class II determinants can present antigen to cloned human T cells. Nature 1984; 312:639-641.
153. Davies TF, Piccinini LA. Intrathyroidal MHC class II antigen expression and thyroid autoimmunity. Endocrinol Metab Clin North Am 1987; 16:247-268.
154. Neufeld DS, Platzer M, Davies TF. Reovirus induction of MHC class II antigen in rat thyroid cells. Endocrinology 1989; 124:543-545.
155. Belfiore A, Mauerhoff T, Pujol Borrell R et al. De novo HLA class II and enhanced HLA class I molecule expression in SV40 transfected human thyroid epithelial cells. J Autoimmun 1991; 4:397-414.
156. Shimojo N, Kohno Y, Yamaguchi K et al. Induction of Graves-like disease in mice by immunization with fibroblasts transfected with the thyrotropin receptor and a class II molecule. Proc Natl Acad Sci USA 1996; 93:11074-11079.
157. Kita M, Ahmad L, Marians RC et al. Regulation and transfer of a murine model of thyrotropin receptor antibody mediated Graves' disease. Endocrinology 1999; 140:1392-1398.
158. Davies TF, Bermas B, Platzer M et al. T-cell sensitization to autologous thyroid cells and normal non specific suppressor T-cell function in Graves' disease. Clin-Endocrinol (Oxf) 1985; 22:155-167.

159. Eguchi K, Otsubo T, Kawabe K et al. The remarkable proliferation of helper T cell subset in response to autologous thyrocytes and intrathyroidal T cells from patients with Graves' disease. Isr J Med Sci 1987; 70:403-410.
160. Migita K, Eguchi K, Otsubo T et al. Cytokine regulation of HLA on thyroid epithelial cells. Clin Exp Immunol 1990; 82:548-552.
161. Weetman AP, McGregor AM. Autoimmune thyroid disease: Further developments in our understanding. Endocr Rev 1994; 15:788-830.
162. Kouki T, Sawai Y, Gardine CA et al. CTLA-4 Gene polymorphism at position 49 in exon 1 reduces the inhibitory function of CTLA-4 and contributes to the pathogenesis of Graves' Disease. J Immunol 2000; 165:6606-6611.
163. Xu Y, Graves P, Tomer Y et al. CTLA-4 and autoimmune thyroid disease: Lack of influence of the A49G signal peptide polymorphism on functional recombinant human CTLA-4. Cell Immunol 2002; 215:133.
164. Huang D, Giscombe R, Zhou Y et al. Dinucleotide repeat expansion in the CTLA-4 gene leads to T cell hyper- reactivity via the CD28 pathway in myasthenia gravis. J Neuroimmunol 2000; 105:69-77.
165. Holopainen PM, Partanen J. Technical note: Linkage disequilibrium and disease-associated CTLA-4 gene polymorphisms. J Immunol 2001; 167:2457-2458.
166. Ban Y, Greenberg DA, Concepcion ES et al. Amino acid substitutions in the thyroglobulin gene confer susceptibility to autoimmune thyroid disease. Philadelphia, PA: The 85th Annual Meeting of the Endocrine Society, 2003.
167. Saegusa K, Ishimaru N, Yanagi K et al. Cathepsin S inhibitor prevents autoantigen presentation and autoimmunity. J Clin Invest 2002; 110:361-369.
168. Bagchi N, Brown TR, Urdanivia E et al. Induction of autoimmune thyroiditis in chickens by dietary iodine. Science 1985; 230:325-327.
169. Kahaly GJ, Dienes HP, Beyer J et al. Iodide induces thyroid autoimmunity in patients with endemic goitre: A randomised, double-blind, placebo-controlled trial. Eur J Endocrinol 1998; 139:290-297.
170. Papanastasiou L, Alevizaki M, Piperingos G et al. The effect of iodine administration on the development of thyroid autoimmunity in patients with nontoxic goiter. Thyroid 2000; 10:493-497.
171. Kong YC, McCormick DJ, Wan Q et al. Primary hormonogenic sites as conserved autoepitopes on thyroglobulin in murine autoimmune thyroiditis. Secondary role of iodination. J Immunol 1995; 155:5847-5854.
172. Hutchings PR, Cooke A, Dawe K et al. A thyroxine-containing peptide can induce murine experimental autoimmune thyroiditis. J Exp Med 1992; 175:869-872.
173. Stenszky V, Kozma L, Balazs C et al. The genetics of Graves' disease: HLA and disease susceptibility. J Clin Endocrinol Metab 1985; 61:735-740.
174. Weetman AP, So AK, Warner CA et al. Immunogenetics of Graves' ophthalmopathy. Clinical Endocrinology 1988; 28:619-628.
175. Chen QY, Huang W, She JX et al. HLA-DRB1*08, DRB1*03/DRB3*0101, and DRB3*0202 are susceptibility genes for Graves' disease in North American Caucasians, whereas DRB1*07 is protective. J Clin Endocrinol Metab 1999; 84:3182-3186.
176. Hawkins BR, Ma JT, Lam KS et al. Association of HLA antigens with thyrotoxic Graves' disease and periodic paralysis in Hong Kong Chinese. Clin Endocrinol (Oxf) 1985; 23:245-252.
177. Dong RP, Kimura A, Okubo R et al. HLA-A and DPB1 loci confer susceptibility to Graves' disease. Hum Immunol 1992; 35:165-172.
178. Cho BY, Rhee BD, Lee DS et al. HLA and Graves' disease in Koreans. Tissue Antigens 1987; 30:119-121.
179. Tandon N, Mehra NK, Taneja V et al. HLA antigens in Asian Indian patients with Graves' disease. Clin Endocrinol (Oxf) 1990; 33:21-26.
180. Sridama V, Hara Y, Fauchet R et al. HLA immunogentic heterogenity in Black American pateitns with Graves' disease. Arch Intern Med 1987; 147:229-231.
181. Chen QY, Nadell D, Zhang XY et al. The human leukocyte antigen HLA DRB3*020/DQA1*0501 haplotype is associated with Graves' disease in African Americans. J Clin Endocrinol Metab 2000; 85:1545-1549.
182. Omar MA, Hammond MG, Desai RK et al. HLA class I and II antigens in South African blacks with Graves' disease. Clin Immunol Immunopathol 1990; 54:98-102.

Chapter 5

Central and Peripheral Nervous System Diseases

Dorothée Chabas, Isabelle Cournu-Rebeix and Bertrand Fontaine

Abstract

Immune diseases of the central and peripheral nervous system constitute an heterogeneous group of disorders which share a significative implication of the immune system in pathophysiology. Multiple sclerosis (MS), Guillain Barré syndrome (GBS) and chronic inflammatory demyelinating polyneuropathy (CIDP) are considered of autoimmune origin, with an unidentified candidate auto-antigen. Many investigations have been performed to find genetic associations or linkage with genes encoding proteins involved in immune regulation. The only significant positive result is the HLA, especially class II molecules, whereas other genes like cytokines or chemokines did not give reproductive results. Myasthenia gravis (MG) is an antigen specific autoimmune disease (antibodies against acetyl choline receptors (AchR)), mainly mediated by the humoral immunity, but also associated with thymus changes, allowing a rough classification into different subsets of patients. In MG, it was possible to identify a genetic association to HLA and AchR genes, suggesting a direct participation of these molecules to disease initiation and development. Finally, narcolepsy is a disease of possible autoimmune origin, as suggested by its tight association with HLA alleles, although the primary antigenic target remains unknown.

Multiple Sclerosis

Multiple Sclerosis, an Autoimmune Disease of Central Nervous System

Multiple sclerosis [MS] is an autoimmune and inflammatory demyelinating disease of the central nervous system, affecting 0.25-6 ‰ of the general population.[1-3] It was first described over a century ago, and is the main disabling disease in young adults, although its origin is still unknown. MS is characterized by relapsing episodes of neurologic impairment followed by remissions (relapsing remitting MS). In approximately half of the patients the disease evolves into a progressive phase (secondary progressive MS). In a minority of patients progressive neurologic deterioration without remission occurs from the disease onset (primary progressive MS). MS diagnosis is based on clinical and radiological criteria (magnetic resonance imaging). In some cases a lumbar puncture might also be needed. Disabling relapses—severe optic neuritis, acute myelitis, oculomotor troubles, facial weakness, ataxia or sphincter disturbances—retreated by intravenous injections of high doses of corticosteroids. In relapsing remitting MS, immunomodulatory treatments like interferon beta and copolymer reduce the risk of relapses by 30%. Immunosuppressors might also be used in aggressive forms of the disease.

Immunogenetics of Autoimmune Disease, edited by Jorge Oksenberg and David Brassat.

Table 1. Genome-wide linkage studies in multiple sclerosis

Author	Population	Number and Type of Families	Markers	Regions of Interest
Sawcer et al, 1996	U.K.	128 sibs	311	6p21, 1cen, 5cen, 7p, 12p, 17q22, 22q
Haines et al, 1996	U.S.A.	52 sibs	443	6p21, 2p23, 3q22-24, 4q31-qter, 5q13- q23, 6q27, 7q11-q22, 9p22, 9q34.3, 10q21-22, 11p15, 12q23-q24, 13q33-34, 16p13, 18p11, 19q13
Ebers et al, 1996	Canada	61 sibs	257	6p21, 2p21, 3, 5p, 11q, X
Kuokkanen et al, 1997	Finland	16 extended pedigrees	328	6p21, 17q21-q24
Coraddu et al, 2001	Sardinia	49 sibs	327	1q31, 10q23, 11p15
Broadley et al, 2001	Italy	40 sibs	322	1q42, 1q44, 2q36, 5q33, 6pter, 6q22, 10cen, 15q21
Ban et al, 2002	Australia	54 sibs	397	2p13, 4q26, 6q26, Xp21-11

Influence of Genetic Factors on Multiple Sclerosis

The pathological mechanism underlying MS is considered to be autoimmune attack of the myelin sheat, mediated by both cellular and humoral immunity.[4] Recent data have also suggested that MS is a degenerative disease affecting axons[5] and oligodendrocytes.[6]

Genetic and environmental factors influence susceptibility to MS, but MS is not a genetically inherited disease. The role of environmental factors has been suggested by the results of migrant studies. Migrants tend to have a MS risk of the region where they lived their first 15 years of life. Genetic contribution has been suggested by the observation that the risk of MS in a family with a MS patient is higher than in the general population or in families of adoptees. For example, the relative-risk of MS is increased by 20-40 folds in sibs of MS patients. Finally, the higher MS concordance rate in monozygote twins (6-40%) vs dizygote twins (2.7-4.7%) also supports the influence of MS susceptibility genetic factors .

Genome Wide Analysis in Multiple Sclerosis

In 1996, the first three genome-wide linkage studies in MS were published. Since then, four additional scans have been performed. These data identified numerous regions with "nominal" or "suggestive" linkage (Table 1). The conclusion of these studies was that MS genetic susceptibility was under the control of multiple genes, each of them with a modest contribution to the increase of the relative risk to develop the disease (increased relative-risk between 1 and 2). The number of genes, their relative contribution and their mode of inheritance remain unknown.

Candidate Genes in Multiple Sclerosis

Given the strong and reproducible linkage findings on chromosome 6p region containing HLA, and the known participation of HLA molecules to antigen presentation in dysimmune diseases, many HLA association studies were performed in MS. More specifically, a genetic association was found between MS and a chromosomal region containing HLA class II molecules.[7-9] In most Caucasian populations, this region was defined by the serological marker DR2 and the molecular haplotype HLA-DRB1*1501-DQA1*0102-DQB1*0602 (HLA DR15). This haplotype confers an increased risk of developing MS (4 fold) and accounts for

20% of MS predisposing genes. However, because of a strong linkage disequilibrium in this region, it has not been possible to further narrow the chromosomal region conferring predisposition.

In MS, the strategy for choosing candidate genes has privileged pathophysiology rather than linkage peak location. The list of candidate genes studied in MS is long. None of them has been reproducibly found in all studied populations,[10-15] (http://www.ucsf.edu/msdb/r_ms_candidate_genes.htlm). As MS is an autoimmune disease involving T and B cell mediated inflammation and targeting myelin proteins, many immune genes like cytokine, chemokine, T-cell receptor, immunoglobulin and myelin genes have been investigated. However these studies have been disappointing, as no functional candidates have consistently demonstrated any association with MS. Some data support the hypothesis that some genes may confer susceptibility in a single population, as the myelin basic protein (MBP) gene in Finland.[16] Some of these genes have been repeatedly studied with contradictory results. Among them, the CTLA-4 gene encodes a costimulatory molecule involved in the immune response down-regulation. Genetic association with CTLA-4 had been observed for several other dysimmune disorders, like type 1 diabetes and auto-immune thyroiditis. For both disorders, a peak association was found with a noncoding region of the gene correlating with a decreased gene transcription.[17] The several studies on MS have conflicting results.[18] The gene encoding ICAM-1 has also been extensively studied since its protein product plays a key-role in the blood-brain-barrier breakdown observed in active MS. If a gene association with MS was initially reported in Poland,[19] it was not confirmed in other populations, although a rare haplotype was observed using larger samples of families of French origin, suggesting a protection to MS[20] in that particular population.

In addition to genetic susceptibility, some data support the hypothesis that genetic factors might play a role in specific MS features like age at onset, clinical form, severity or response to treatment. This field has been less extensively explored and studies are scarce and far from being conclusive, although there are evidence supporting the hypothesis that severity in MS might be, at least partly, influenced by genes encoding TNF, interleukins or ApoE

Myasthenia Gravis

Myasthenia Gravis, an Autoimmune Disease Targeting the Neuromuscular Junction

Acquired autoimmune generalized myasthenia gravis (MG) is the most common disorder of neuromuscular transmission with an annual incidence rate ranging from 0,25 to 2,00 per 100 000.[24] MG is characterized by a post-synaptic blockage of nervous transmission, causing painless weakness and fatigability of striated muscle. It can be life-threatening when bulbar or respiratory muscles are involved.[25] In typical MG, both the target autoantigen, the muscle acetylcholine receptor (AChR), and the pathogenic effectors, autoantibodies directed against AchR (AchR Ab), are clearly identified.[26] These autoantibodies are highly specific and their presence in the serum of most MG patients (80 to 90%) is a key element of diagnosis.[27]

Despite this well known common effector (AChR Ab) and although most patients with myasthenia gravis share common features, MG is an heterogeneous disorder (Table 2). Remarkably, the thymus of MG patients is often abnormal with benign or malignant alteration, hyperplasia or thymoma respectively. According to these thymic changes, characteristic subsets of patients can be delineated.[29] Thymus hyperplasia is preferentially observed in females (sex ratio F:M=4:1) with an age of onset before 40 years and with high titers of anti-AChR Ab. Thymoma occurs equally in males and females, and is often associated with severe clinical symptoms. A subset of patients with thymoma also presents a detectable titer of autoantibodies directed against titin and ryanodine receptor (RyR). Titin plays an important role in muscle fiber elasticity and is the major molecular target of anti-striated muscle antibodies.[30] RyR is an ion channel pivotal in striated muscle excitation-contraction coupling by releasing Ca^{2+} from intracellular stores such as sarcoplasmic reticulum. Anti-RyR antibodies target an epitope

Table 2. Heterogeneity of myasthenia gravis

	Thymus Hyperplasia	Normal Thymus	Thymoma
Seropositives Patients (S+) 90%	45% of S+ patients	30% of S+ patients	25% of S+ patients
	Sex ratio: F:M=4:1 Onset <40 years High Anti-AChR Ab **HLA-DR3B8A1** haplotype **HLA DR3**+ 60% of MG patients	**Anti-titin Ab+** Onset >60 years Moderate Anti-AChR Ab HLA-DR7 **Anti-titin Ab-** Clinical and biological heterogeneity **HLA-DR3**	Sex ratio: F:M=1:1 Moderate Anti-AChR Ab Severe clinical symptoms **Anti-titin Ab+** **Anti-Ryanodine Ab +** **HLA-DR15** (DR2-Dw2-DQ1)
Seropositives Patients (S-) 10%	Anti-AChR Ab- Young patients **Anti-MusK Ab+** (70% of S-patients)		

involved in channel regulation, and inhibit Ca2+ release from sarcoplasmic reticulum.[31] Finally, among seronegative patients (no detectable serum AChR Ab), 70% produce antibodies directed against MuSK, which is a tyrosine kinase receptor involved in the neuromuscular junction development.

Genetic Contribution of HLA and the Antigen to Myasthenia Gravis

On a genetic point of view, despite the paucity of families with multiple affected siblings, a complex mode of inheritance has been proposed. Reproducible association studies have suggested an involvement of the HLA complex in the pathogenesis of the disease (Table 2). Initially, class I alleles, B8 and A1, and subsequently class II alleles, DR3 and Dw3, were implicated. Other HLA-linked genes, including complement (C4) and TNF alpha were also associated with the disease.[36] This has led to the conclusion that an extended ancestral haplotype, HLA-A1B8DRB1*0301DRB3*0101DQA1*0501 was associated with myasthenia gravis, and more specifically with thymus hyperplasia. This haplotype is also known to be involved in other human autoimmune disease, like systemic lupus erythematosus, celiac disease, type I diabetes and autoimmune thyroiditis, suggesting it could also predispose to non antigen-specific immune dysregulation.[37]

MG patients with normal thymus and expressing anti-titin antibodies, displayed a different association to those with thymus hyperplasia or without anti-titin antibodies:[38] a positive association with HLA-DR7 and a negative association with HLA-DR3 respectively. Dr3 and DR7 or associated alleles of closely linked genes could therefore have opposing effects on the phenotype of MG patients.[28]

Conflicting data have been obtained in MG patients with thymoma. Associations with both HLA class II and class I loci have been reported, like HLA-DR 15 alleles (DR2-Dw2-DQ1) in females.

In MG, the knowledge of the autoantigenic target provides a rare opportunity to investigate a genetic contribution of genes encoding for the self-antigen. The muscle AchR is made of five subunits, two α, one β, one δ and one γ or ε. The α subunit is of particular immunological interest, as it contains the main immunogenic region on its N-terminal extra-cellular domain, and is directly involved in acetylcholine binding.[39] Genetic studies of the CHRNA1 gene encoding the α-subunit concluded to an association between this gene and myasthenia gravis.

Therefore, a three-gene model was suggested: a particular epitope of the AChR α -subunit would be presented to immune cells by a class II HLA heterodimer containing the α-chain encoded by DQA1*0101, whereas a locus associated with DR3 haplotype would determine a nonantigen specific immune dysregulation.[28]

Other Candidate Genes

Others immune genes have been associated with MG : IL1β,[40] CTLA-4,[41] the kappa chain Km allotype and only in patients with high titers of anti-AChR antibodies IL10.[44] Studies of the antigen T cell receptor α and β loci,[45] the IL1 receptor antagonist,[40] IL6,[46] IL4,[47] beta-2 adrenergic receptor have shown no association with myasthenia gravis.

Guillain Barré Syndrome

Guillain Barré Syndrome, an Acute Autoimmune Disease of Peripheral Nervous System

Guillain Barré syndrome (GBS) is an acute inflammatory polyneuropathy with an annual incidence rate worldwide of 0.4-1.7/100,000 population. It is characterized by a limb symmetrical ascending weakness evolving over a period of several days to weeks, associated with paresthesias and numbness, cranial nerve palsies, and reduced or absent tendon reflexes. Symptoms can progress to total motor paralysis and disturbances of autonomic functions, and patients may die from respiratory failure. Laboratory findings usually show an elevated protein content in the cerebrospinal fluid, with no pleiocytosis. Electromyographic studies show demyelination features, like slowed conduction velocity, or conduction block in motor nerves, and prolonged distal latencies and F responses. Axonal damage may also be present, sometimes early in the disease. Pathological studies show perivascular inflammatory infiltrates with periveinous demyelination and a variable degree of wallerian degeneration. GBS is classified into several subtypes based on clinical and pathologic criteria, with acute inflammatory demyelinating polyneuropathy (AIDP) and acute motor axonal neuropathy (AMAN) being the most common forms observed. Plasma exchange and intravenous immunoglobulins are the gold standard therapies for GBS.[52,53]

GBS is considered an autoimmune disease mediated by T and B cells directed against the peripheral myelin sheats.[52-54] T cell reaction is specifically directed against the specific peripheral myelin protein P2, while diverse anti-myelin antibodies mediate demyelination in vitro or can be detected in the serum of GBS patients (like anti-GQ1b and anti-GM1 antibodies).

A mild respiratory or gastrointestinal infection preceded the symptoms by 1 to 3 weeks in about 60% of the patients. *Campylobacter jejuni* is the most frequent identifiable preceding infection. All attempts to isolate a virus or microbial agent from nerves have yet failed, suggesting a possible mechanism of molecular mimicry, rather than a direct nerve infection.

Genetic Susceptibility of Guillain Barré Syndrome

GBS is a sporadic disease, although rare cases of familial GBS have been reported.[55-59] Regarding the immunological aspects, a few studies attempted to find immunogenetic factors influencing susceptibility to GBS, susceptibility to *Campylobacter jejuni* associated GBS, or susceptibility to various clinical forms of the disease.

HLA Influence on Guillain Barré Syndrome

To better understand the pathogenesis of GBS and host susceptibility to developing the disease, the distribution of HLA antigens has been investigated in population of GBS patients using either DNA-based methods, or serotyping. In a few studies from the 80's using serotyping methods,[58,60,61] the distribution of HLA molecules appeared different in GBS patients compared with controls, although none of these studies could ever be repeated, especially using DNA-based methods, later in the 90's (Table 3).[62-66] Interestingly, if HLA distribution does not appear to influence directly susceptibility to GBS, class II molecules like HLA-DQ or HLA-DR, influence the specific susceptibility to AIDP[67-69] or AMAN,[67,68] suggesting different

Table 3. HLA association studies in Guillain Barré syndrome

	Reference	HLA Allele or Serotype
Significant Association		
GBS	Hafez 1985	A3, B8
	Kaslow 1984	A11 less common
	Gorodezky 1983	DR3
AIDP	Magira 2003	DQ beta RLD(55-57)/ ED(70-71) and DR betaE(9)V(11)H(13)
	Magira 2003	protection : DO beta RPD(55-57)
	Guo 2002	A33, DR15 and DO5
	Monos 1997	DRB1*1301
AMAN	Guo 2002	B15, B35
	Monos 1997	DRB1*1301-03 and DRB1*1312
Association with preceding	Koga 1998	B54 and Cw1
CJ infection	Rees 1995	DQB1*03
Profound weakness	Winer 1988	DR2
No or Non Significant Association		
GBS	Ma 1998	DRB1, DQB1
	Koga 1998	HLA-class I (A, B and Cw), HLA-class II (DRB1 and DQB1)
	Hillert 1991	DR, -DO or -DP alleles, or HLA-DR-DQ haplotypes
	Winer 1988	HLA cII and cIII type HLA antigen
	Latovitzki 1979	HLA-A, B and C
Association with preceding CJ infection	Li 2000	DQA1*0302
Association with GM1 IgG	Li 2000	DQA1*0301

immunological pathways supporting the distinct clinical presentations. Only two studies demonstrated that HLA molecules (HLA B15, B35, and HLA-DQB1) may influence the association with a preceding *Campylobacter jejuni* infection, suggesting that immunogenetics factors may influence the host response to *Campylobacter jejuni* in GBS.[65,70] Although these data were never confirmed.[71] Finally, there are not enough data allowing us to conclude regarding the influence of HLA genes on the clinical severity or the association with anti-GM1 antibodies.[63,71]

Other Candidate Genes in Guillain Barré Syndrome

A few studies aimed to identify genes involved in the immune response, or in neurodegeneration, and associated with GBS (Table 4). An association was found with the IL10 promotor, TNF alpha or the constant region of kappa chains of immunoglobulins. Interestingly, certain alleles located in IgG receptor gene (FcgammaR) were either associated with less severe disease, or favorizing a higher risk for severe disease, suggesting a direct influence of IgG in the development of the disease. Although roughly, none of these data were ever repeated in other papers, suggesting that we should interpret them carefully.

Finally, it is of interest to notice that GBS might sometimes be mistaken for other peripheral neurological disorders of genetic origin (Table 4), like Charcot-Marie-Tooth, hereditary neuropathy with liability to pressure palsies, or hypokalaemic periodic paralysis, even though inflammation is not typical in those particular cases.

Table 4. Genes implicated in Guillain Barré syndrome (besides HLA, see Table 3)

Genes Associated with CGS			
Myhr 2003	IL10 promotor	-592 CC and -819CC genotypes	Associated with IL10 up-regulation
Pandey 2003	Constant region of Kappa chains	Increased frequency of KM3 homozygosity Decrease frequency of KM1/KM3 heterozygosity	
Van der Pol 2000	Leukocyte receptors for IgG	Fcγ RIIa-H131 homozygosity	
Ma 1998	TCR α-chain constant and β-chain variable		
Association with Preceding CJ Infection			
Ma 1998	Tumor necrosis factor	(TNFa2) allele	Associated with TNFα up-regulation
McCombe 1985	Alpha-1 antitrypsin	M3 allele	
Association with Less Severe Disease			
Vedeler 2000	Leukocyte receptors for IgG	FcγRIIIB NA1/NA1 homozygosity	High affinity for IgG3 and IgG1
Higher Risk for Severe Disease			
Van der Pol 2000	Leukocyte receptors for IgG	Fcγ RIIa-H131 homozygosity	
No Association with GBS			
Pritchard 2003	Cholesterol transport protein apolipoprotein E	Apolipoprotein E	
Differential Diagnosis with Genetic Disorders			
Vital 2003	Charcot-Marie-Tooth	PMP22 gene duplication (CMT type 1A)	
Korn-Lubetzki 2002	Hereditary neuropathy with liability to pressure palsies	Deletion at chromosomal locus 17p12	
Warren 1998	Hypokalaemic periodic paralysis	Mutation in the skeletal muscle voltage-gated calcium channel alpha-1 subunit (CACNL1A3)	

Chronic Inflammatory Demyelinating Polyneuropathy (CIDP)

CIDP, a Chronic Autoimmune Disease of Peripheral Nervous System

CIDP is an acquired, immune mediated peripheral neuropathy.[72] It is considered an autoimmune attack targeting the myelin sheaths of peripheral nerves, even though the supportive evidence remains incomplete.[73] Demyelination is partly mediated by the humoral immunity, as 29% of patients produce antibodies directed against the myelin protein P0, 15% against the ganglioside GM1 located in the nodes of Ranvier, 5% against the ganglioside LM1 located in the myelin sheath, and some against acidic glycolipids. 32% of patients have a history of preceding nonspecific upper respiratory or gastrointestinal tract infection or vaccination within 6 weeks of their first neurological symptoms, suggesting a possible mechanism of molecular mimicry at the origin of CIDP. This hypothesis is independently supported by the fact that human nerve fibers share epitopes with infectious agents like *Campylobacter jejuni*, *Haemophilus influenzae* and CMV.

The distinction between CIDP and GBS (see above) was primarily based on the notable chronic evolution and the corticosteroid responsiveness of CIDP. The prevalence of CIDP is probably underestimated, and recent surveys report a prevalence of 1 to 7.7 per 100 000 population. It is a clinically heterogeneous disease and there are no generally agreed-on clinical diagnostic criteria:[72] the clinical presentation may consist of a symmetric or multifocal, motor and/or sensory neuropathy, affecting either the proximal or distal portions of the nerve. CSF analysis shows an isolated elevated protein level. Electrophysiology confirms demyelination with slowed conduction velocities, sometimes limited to proximal regions, and sometimes associated with axonal loss. Pathological studies, when they are done, show hallmarks of demyelination, sometimes associated with distal axon degeneration. Finally, a favorable response to therapy –polyvalent immunoglobulins or plasmapheresis- consisting of stabilization or improvement of the neuropathy, would confirm the diagnosis.

Immunogenetic Factors Influencing CIDP

Disease heterogeneity and various associations with preceding infections and antibody responses may be secondary to immunogenetic factors influencing the host immune response. However, immunogenetic susceptibility studies have not been conclusive so far.

In 1979, 16 patients with "chronic relapsing polyneuritis" showed a definite association with HLA-AW30 and AW31 serotypes, and probable association with HLA-B8 and HLA-DW3, although the sampling size was small.[62] Later, in 1990, thirty-one CIDP patients were typed for HLA-A, -B and -C antigens serologically and for HLA-DR, -DQ and -DP class II genes by RFLP analysis.[74] The study showed only a slight association with HLA-B8 and identified a stronger association with HLA-Cw7. One year later, the expression of class II antigen was studied in sural nerve biopsies from patients with chronic demyelinating polyradiculoneuropathy (CIDP) and other neuropathies. In CIDP there was a marked increase in class II expression on Schwann cells, whereas class II expression was mainly restricted to endothelial and perineurial cells in the control nerves. Increased endoneurial expression of class II antigen was found to correlate with elevated cerebrospinal fluid (CSF) protein levels but not with other clinical variables or demyelination as defined by electrophysiologic criteria or teased fiber analysis. The increased expression of class II antigen on Schwann cells may be indicative of a local activation of antigen presentation in the autoimmune process of demyelination, but does not define MHC genes as CIDP susceptibility genes.

Narcolepsy

Narcolepsy, a Sleep Disorder of Potential Autoimmune Origin

Narcolepsy is a neurological disease affecting specifically the generation of sleep.[75-78] It affects 0.03-0.1% of the general population in Western Europe and North America. It usually begins in young adulthood and affects men and women equally. Clinically, it is typically characterized by a tetrad of symptoms, fully present in only 10-15% of patients. Excessive daytime sleepiness is a constant symptom, due to an inability to maintain wakefulness in daytime. Cataplexy (70%), a specific symptom, is a sudden loss of muscle tone in response to emotional arousal, in particular laughter. Sleep paralysis (25%), and hypnagogic hallucinations (30%) (dream-like episodes at the time of going to sleep), like cataplexy, are considered intrusions of rapid eye movement (REM) sleep into wakefulness.

The diagnosis of narcolepsy is mainly clinical combined with sleep recording, where electroencephalography (EEG) is recorded with electromyography (EMG) and eye movements. During the multiple sleep latency test (MSLT), latencies to falling asleep are measured during 4 to 5 short naps taken during daytime, and the presence or absence of a REM sleep transition is recorded. Narcoleptic patients typically have short mean sleep latencies (MSL) (=8 minutes) and 2 or more sleep onset REM periods (SOREMPs) during naps.

Hypocretin Deficiency Linked to HLA in Narcolepsy

Recently, genetic studies of a dog model of inherited narcolepsy, in combination with mouse and human studies, have shown that deficiency in hypocretin (also called orexin[79,80]) peptide neurotransmission is key to the pathophysiology.[81-83] Hypocretin neurons in small number are normally located in the lateral and perifornical hypothalamus, and send projections throughout the brain, particularly to regions involved in sleep regulation.[84] In human narcoleptic brain, there is a global loss of hypocretin,[85,86] and narcoleptic patients have low cerebrospinal fluid hypocretin concentration.[87-89] A hypocretin-1 concentration lower than 110 pg/ml has a positive predictive value of 94%. It is almost specific for patients suffering narcolepsy-cataplexy and carrying the Human Leukocyte Antigen allele HLA-DQB1*0602. Although rare narcoleptic patients without cataplexy or without HLA-DQB1*0602 may also have low hypocretin levels. Human narcolepsy is a sporadic disease, with no significant association with single-nucleotide polymorphisms in the preprohypocretin gene, nor in the hcrtr1 and hcrtr2 genes. Only one case of narcolepsy was related to a mutation in the hcrt gene, and this patient had a particularly severe disease.[85] Moreover, no genetic mutation was found in multiplex families.

The Autoimmune Hypothesis of Narcolepsy

The hypothesis that narcolepsy might be of autoimmune origin is based on its tight association with human leukocyte antigen (HLA) markers DR2 and DQB1*0602, greater than HLA association with known autoimmune disorders such as multiple sclerosis (see above).[90,91] The peripubertal onset of narcolepsy, together with the reported low concordance rate in monozygotic twins and the complex genetic susceptibility in family studies also argued in favor of this hypothesis. But stronger biological studies are needed to support the hypothesis of a cellular or humoral activation of autoimmunity in narcolepsy.

Association of HLA with Narcolepsy

The influence of genetic factors on narcolepsy were reviewed in reference 90.

Serological Typing Studies

Early studies reported a significant association of narcolepsy-cataplexy with HLA class I Bw35 in Japanese patients while in Caucasians, an increased frequency of HLA-Bw7 but not Bw35 was observed.[92,93] The study of class II antigens discovered stronger associations:[94] all Japanese narcoleptic patients share two serologically defined HLA class II antigens, DR2 and DQ1[92,94-96] like 90-95% of Caucasians.[97] A lower (60%) DR2 association was observed in African Americans, while all were DQ1, suggesting interethnic differences.[98]

High Resolution Typing Studies

Common HLA haplotype combinations found in narcoleptic subject in three ethnic groups are displayed in Table 5.[90]

HLA-DQB1*0602

In African-Americans patients, narcolepsy is more tightly associated with DQB1*0602 (a subtype of DQ1/DQ6) than with HLA-DRB1*15 (a subtype of DR15/DR2). In African Americans, DQB1*0602 can be found in association with DR2, DR5, and DR6. A third of African-American narcoleptic patients carry DQB1*0602 independently of DR2. In Caucasians and Japanese, DQB1*0602 is almost always associated with DR-B1*15 because of a linkage disequilibrium between these two alleles. In African Americans, fewer patients are DQB1*0602 positive independently of DR2, because of the absence of linkage disequilibrium in that group.[99]

Table 5. Common HLA haplotype combinations found in narcoleptic subjects in three ethnic groups (according to ref. 90)

		Japanese		Caucasians		African Americans	
Haplotype 1	Haplotype 2	% narcoleptic (n=105)	% control-HW (n=698)	% narcoleptic (n=238)	% control-HW (n=146)	% narcoleptic (n=77)	% control-HW (n=243)
DRB1-DQA1-DQB1	**DRB1-DQA1-DQB1**						
15-0102-0602	15-0102-0602	15.2	0.4	18.1	1.6	14.3	1.8
15-0102-0602	11-05-0301	6.7	0.2	10.9	2.5	6.5	1.9
15-0102-0602	04-03-0302	7.6	0.8	9.2	1.4	2.6	1.2
15-0102-0602	13-0102-0604	6.7	0.8	6.3	1.7	2.6	0.7
15-0102-0602	04-03-0301	1.9	0.0	7.6	0.9		
15-0102-0602	04-03-0401	19.0	1.7				
15-0102-0602	12-0601-0301	6.7	0.2				
15-0102-0602	08-0401-0402	2.9	0.1				
15-0102-0602	12-05-0301	3.8	0.3				
15-0102-0602	08-03-0302	2.9	0.2				
15-0102-0602	11-0102-0602					6.5	0.0
DQA1-DQB1	**DRB1**						
0102-0602	15	20.0	2.0	19.4	1.9	15.6	2.5
0102-0602	04	30.5	3.0	17.6	2.4	2.6	2.1
0102-0602	11	6.7	0.3	11.3	2.6	19.5	3.9
0102-0602	12	11.4	0.6	0.8	0.3	7.8	1.8
0102-0602	08	8.6	1.7	3.4	0.5	5.4	1.6

Table continued on next page

Table 5. Continued

		Japanese		Caucasians		African Americans	
Haplotype 1	**Haplotype 2**	**% narcoleptic (n=105)**	**% control-HW (n=698)**	**% narcoleptic (n=238)**	**% control-HW (n=146)**	**% narcoleptic (n=77)**	**% control-HW (n=243)**
DQA1-DQB1	**DQB1**						
/0102-0602	0602	15.2	0.4	18.1	1.6	24.7	3.0
0102-0602	0301	20.0	1.3	23.1	4.2	22.1	6.0
0102-0602	0302	10.5	1.2	9.2	1.4	26.0	1.6
0102-0602	0402	4.8	0.4	3.4	0.4	3.9	2.0
0102-0602	0604	6.7	0.8	6.3	1.7	3.9	1.1
0102-0602	0303	9.5	2.0	3.4	1.0	0.0	0.6
0102-0602	0401	19.0	1.7				
DQA1-DQB1	**DQA1**						
0102-0602	0102	23.8	1.4	26.9	3.0	32.5	6.2
0102-0602	03	42.9	5.3	18.5	2.4	5.2	4.7
0102-0602	05	11.4	1.1	22.3	6.9	28.6	6.3
0102-0602	06	6.7	0.3				

The highest susceptibility for narcolepsiy is found in homozygous allelic combination 15-0102-0602/15-0102-0602 among different ethnic groups. Relative risks for DQB1*0602/0301 combination were approximately half of those with the homozygous allelic combination HLA-DQB1*0602. DR11, DR12, DR4 alleles also have increased disease susceptibility.

HLA-DQB1*0602 is therefore the major HLA susceptibility allele for narcolepsy: the majority of patients (88-98%) with clear cataplexy are HLA-DQB1*0602 positive across ethnic groups, with corresponding values in control population (12% in Japanese, 25% in Caucasian and 38% in African Americans) (Table 5).[97] More precisely DQB1*0602 increases directly the susceptibility for cataplexy, as only 41% of narcoleptic patients without cataplexy are DQB1*0602 positive, and normal people sharing this allele have a slightly shorter REM sleep latency. Moreover DQB1*0602 homozygotes have a 2-4 higher risk of developing the disease than heterozygotes.[100]

Complementation of HLA-DQA1 and DQB1

Unusual DRB1*X, DQA1*0102, DQB1*0602 haplotypes have been identified in Caucasian narcoleptic patients with cataplexy. In contrast, no unusual DRB1*1501, DQA1*X, DQB1*X haplotypes have ever been observed in these patients. In all narcolepsy susceptibility DR-DQ haplotypes identified, both DQA1*0102 and DQB1*0602 are present, suggesting complementation of HLA-DQA1 and DQB1 in mediating susceptibility. Although DQB1*0602 is almost in complete linkage disequilibrium with DQA1*0102, a number of DR-DQ haplotypes with DQA1*0102 but without DQB1*0602, as rare haplotypes with DQB1*0602 but without DQA1*0102, exist in the general population, but these are not seen in narcolepsy. Therefore, DQA1*0102 and DQB1*0602 may be important for disease predisposition.[97,101]

Sequencing of HLA Alleles

Although HLA-DQ alleles influence narcolepsy, they do not have mutations in narcoleptic patients. Sequencing analysis of the HLA-DRB1, DQA1 and DQB1 genes has shown no difference between narcoleptic patients and controls.[97,102-104] And numerous microsatellite polymorphisms have been identified in the HLA-DQ region, around DQB1*0602 and DQA1*0102, with no difference between DQB1*0602 narcoleptic patients and controls.[105-107]

Other HLA Protecting or Favorizing Genes

A recent interethnic study has shown that other HLA genes than DQB1*0602 are associated with narcolepsy, either positively or negatively.[102] A higher risk is observed in heterozygotes coexpressing DQB1*0602 with either DQB1*0301, DQA1*06, DRB104, DRB1*08, DRB1*11 or DRB1*12 than other DQB1*0602 heterozygotes. On the contrary, heterozygotes carrying either DQB1*0601, DQB1*0501 or DQA1*01 have a relative lower risk. There is no clear explanation why some alleles are favorizing narcolepsy and some are protective. For example DQB1*0602 and DQB1*0601 are very similar but the first is favorizing, and the second protecting. These alleles may participate to the HLA susceptibility in the DQB1*0602 negative narcoleptic population (10% of the patients). For example a particularly high proportion of these patients carry the susceptibility allele DQB1*0301.

An alignment study of the susceptibility and protective DRB1, DQA1 and DQB1 alleles[108] showed that in HLA-DQB1, residues Y30, D57 and maybe A38 appear to be essential susceptibility amino acid. Although regarding DRB1 and DQA1, no particular susceptibility amino acid was identified.

TNF Alpha and Narcolepsy

One recent study suggests a significant association between the TNF-α(-857T) homozygote haplotype and narcolepsy and an increased rate of the rare haplotype DRB1*1501/TNF-α(-857T), suggesting that TNF-α is implicated in the disease.[109,110] In parallel, an association of narcolepsy with the TNF-α receptor gene TNFR2 (TNFR2-196R) has been demonstrated in Japanese narcoleptic patient.[111] This suggests that an inflammatory mechanism implicating the TNF-α pathway may directly contribute to narcolepsy.

References

1. Steinman L. Multiple sclerosis: A coordinated immunological attack against myelin in the central nervous system. Cell 1996; 85(3):299-302.
2. Compston A, Ebers G, Lassmann H et al. Mc Alpine's Multiple Sclerosis. 3rd ed. 1998.
3. McDonald WI, Compston A, Edan G et al. Recommended diagnostic criteria for multiple sclerosis: Guidelines from the International Panel on the diagnosis of multiple sclerosis. Ann Neurol 2001; 50(1):121-127.
4. Steinman L. Multiple sclerosis: A two-stage disease. Nature Immunology 2001; 2(9):762-764.
5. Trapp BD, Peterson J, Ransohoff RM et al. Axonal transection in the lesions of multiple sclerosis [see comments]. N Engl J Med 1998; 338(5):278-285.
6. Lucchinetti CF, Brueck W, Rodriguez M et al. Multiple sclerosis: Lessons from neuropathology. Semin Neurol 1998; 18(3):337-349.
7. Jersild C, Fog T. Histocompatibility (HL-A) antigens associated with multiple sclerosis. Acta Neurol Scand Suppl 1972; 51:377.
8. Clerget-Darpoux F, Govaerts A, Feingold N. HLA and susceptibility to multiple sclerosis. Tissue Antigens 1984; 24(3):160-169.
9. Yaouanq J, Semana G, Eichenbaum S et al. Evidence for linkage disequilibrium between HLA-DRB1 gene and multiple sclerosis. The French Research Group on Genetic Susceptibility to MS. Science 1997; 276(5313):664-665.
10. Wansen K, Pastinen T, Kuokkanen S et al. Immune system genes in multiple sclerosis: Genetic association and linkage analyses on TCR beta, IGH, IFN-gamma and IL-1ra/IL-1 beta loci. J Neuroimmunol 1997; 79(1):29-36.
11. Feakes R, Chataway J, Sawcer S et al. Susceptibility to multiple sclerosis and the immunoglobulin heavy chain gene cluster. Ann Neurol 1998; 44(6):984.
12. Mertens C, Brassat D, Reboul J et al. A systematic study of oligodendrocyte growth factors as candidates for genetic susceptibility to MS. French Multiple Sclerosis Genetics Group. Neurology 1998; 51(3):748-753.
13. Reboul J, Mertens C, Levillayer F et al. Cytokines in genetic susceptibility to multiple sclerosis:A candidate gene approach. French Multiple Sclerosis Genetics Group. J Neuroimmunol 2000; 102(1):107-112.
14. Oksenberg JR, Baranzini SE, Barcellos LF et al. Multiple sclerosis: Genomic rewards. J Neuroimmunol 2001; 113(2):171-184.
15. Kantarci OH, de Andrade M, Weinshenker BG. Identifying disease modifying genes in multiple sclerosis. J Neuroimmunol 2002; 123(1-2):144-159.
16. Pihlaja H, Rantamaki T, Wikstrom J et al. Linkage disequilibrium between the MBP tetranucleotide repeat and multiple sclerosis is restricted to a geographically defined subpopulation in Finland. Genes Immun 2003; 4(2):138-146.
17. Ueda H, Howson JM, Esposito L et al. Association of the T-cell regulatory gene CTLA4 with susceptibility to autoimmune disease. Nature 2003; 423(6939):506-511.
18. Alizadeh M, Babron MC, Birebent B et al. Genetic interaction of CTLA-4 with HLA-DR15 in multiple sclerosis patients. Ann Neurol 2003; 54(1):119-122.
19. Mycko MP, Kwinkowski M, Tronczynska E et al. Multiple sclerosis: The increased frequency of the ICAM-1 exon 6 gene point mutation genetic type K469. Ann Neurol 1998; 44(1):70-75.
20. Cournu-Rebeix I, Genin E, Lesca G et al. Intercellular adhesion molecule-1: A protective haplotype against multiple sclerosis. Genes Immun 2003; 4(7):518-523.
21. Weinshenker BG, Wingerchuk DM, Liu Q et al. Genetic variation in the tumor necrosis factor alpha gene and the outcome of multiple sclerosis. Neurology 1997; 49(2):378-385.
22. Schrijver HM, Crusius JB, Uitdehaag BM et al. Association of interleukin-1beta and interleukin-1 receptor antagonist genes with disease severity in MS. Neurology 1999; 52(3):595-599.
23. Schmidt S, Barcellos LF, DeSombre K et al. Association of polymorphisms in the apolipoprotein E region with susceptibility to and progression of multiple sclerosis. Am J Hum Genet 2002; 70(3):708-717.
24. Vincent A, Palace J, Hilton-Jones D. Myasthenia gravis. Lancet 2001; 357(9274):2122-2128.
25. Engel AG. Myasthenia gravis and myasthenic syndromes. Ann Neurol 1984; 16(5):519-534.
26. Patrick J, Lindstrom J. Autoimmune response to acetylcholine receptor. Science 1973; 180(88):871-872.
27. Lindstrom JM, Seybold ME, Lennon VA et al. Antibody to acetylcholine receptor in myasthenia gravis. Prevalence, clinical correlates, and diagnostic value. Neurology 1976; 26(11):1054-1059.
28. Garchon HJ. Genetics of autoimmune myasthenia gravis, a model for antibody-mediated autoimmunity in man. J Autoimmun 2003; 21(2):105-110.

29. Compston DA, Vincent A, Newsom-Davis J et al. Clinical, pathological, HLA antigen and immunological evidence for disease heterogeneity in myasthenia gravis. Brain 1980; 103(3):579-601.
30. Gautel M, Lakey A, Barlow DP et al. Titin antibodies in myasthenia gravis: Identification of a major immunogenic region of titin. Neurology 1993; 43(8):1581-1585.
31. Ogawa Y, Kurebayashi N, Murayama T. Ryanodine receptor isoforms in excitation-contraction coupling. Adv Biophys 1999; 36:27-64.
32. Mossman S, Vincent A, Newsom-Davis J. Myasthenia gravis without acetylcholine-receptor antibody: A distinct disease entity. Lancet 1986; 1(8473):116-119.
33. Hoch W, McConville J, Helms S et al. Auto-antibodies to the receptor tyrosine kinase MuSK in patients with myasthenia gravis without acetylcholine receptor antibodies. Nat Med 2001; 7(3):365-368.
34. Fritze D, Herrman Jr C, Naeim F et al. HL-A antigens in myasthenia gravis. Lancet 1974; 1(7851):240-242.
35. Carlsson B, Wallin J, Pirskanen R et al. Different HLA DR-DQ associations in subgroups of idiopathic myasthenia gravis. Immunogenetics 1990; 31(5-6):285-290.
36. Hjelmstrom P, Peacock CS, Giscombe R et al. Polymorphism in tumor necrosis factor genes associated with myasthenia gravis. J Neuroimmunol 1998; 88(1-2):137-143.
37. Price P, Witt C, Allcock R et al. The genetic basis for the association of the 8.1 ancestral haplotype (A1, B8, DR3) with multiple immunopathological diseases. Immunol Rev 1999; 167:257-274.
38. Giraud M, Beaurain G, Yamamoto AM et al. Linkage of HLA to myasthenia gravis and genetic heterogeneity depending on anti-titin antibodies. Neurology 2001; 57(9):1555-1560.
39. Tzartos SJ, Barkas T, Cung MT et al. Anatomy of the antigenic structure of a large membrane autoantigen, the muscle-type nicotinic acetylcholine receptor. Immunol Rev 1998; 163:89-120.
40. Huang D, Pirskanen R, Hjelmstrom P et al. Polymorphisms in IL-1beta and IL-1 receptor antagonist genes are associated with myasthenia gravis. J Neuroimmunol 1998; 81(1-2):76-81.
41. Huang D, Liu L, Noren K et al. Genetic association of Ctla-4 to myasthenia gravis with thymoma. J Neuroimmunol 1998; 88(1-2):192-198.
42. Gilhus NE, Pandey JP, Gaarder PI et al. Immunoglobulin allotypes in myasthenia gravis patients with a thymoma. J Autoimmun 1990; 3(3):299-305.
43. Demaine A, Willcox N, Janer M et al. Immunoglobulin heavy chain gene associations in myasthenia gravis: New evidence for disease heterogeneity. J Neurol 1992; 239(1):53-56.
44. Huang DR, Zhou YH, Xia SQ et al. Markers in the promoter region of interleukin-10 (IL-10) gene in myasthenia gravis: Implications of diverse effects of IL-10 in the pathogenesis of the disease. J Neuroimmunol 1999; 94(1-2):82-87.
45. Mantegazza R, Oksenberg JR, Baggi F et al. Increased incidence of certain TCR and HLA genes associated with myasthenia gravis in Italians. J Autoimmun 1990; 3(4):431-440.
46. Huang D, Zheng C, Giscombe R et al. Polymorphisms at - 174 and in the 3' flanking region of interleukin-6 (IL-6) gene in patients with myasthenia gravis. J Neuroimmunol 1999; 101(2):197-200.
47. Huang D, Xia S, Zhou Y et al. No evidence for interleukin-4 gene conferring susceptibility to myasthenia gravis Genetic association of Ctla-4 to myasthenia gravis with thymoma Polymorphisms in IL-1beta and IL-1 receptor antagonist genes are associated with myasthenia gravis. J Neuroimmunol 1998; 92(1-2):208-211.
48. Xu BY, Huang D, Pirskanen R et al. beta2-adrenergic receptor gene polymorphisms in myasthenia gravis (MG). Clin Exp Immunol 2000; 119(1):156-160.
49. Asbury AK, Cornblath DR. Assessment of current diagnostic criteria for Guillain-Barre syndrome. Ann Neurol 1990; 27(Suppl):S21-24.
50. Asbury AK. Guillain-Barre syndrome:Historical aspects. Ann Neurol 1990; 27 (Suppl):S2-6.
51. Feasby TE, Gilbert JJ, Brown WF et al. An acute axonal form of Guillain-Barre polyneuropathy. Brain 1986; 109 (Pt 6):1115-1126.
52. Hartung HP, Pollard JD, Harvey GK et al. Immunopathogenesis and treatment of the Guillain-Barre syndrome—Part II. Muscle Nerve 1995; 18(2):154-164.
53. Hartung HP, Pollard JD, Harvey GK et al. Immunopathogenesis and treatment of the Guillain-Barre syndrome—Part I. Muscle Nerve 1995; 18(2):137-153.
54. Saida K. The immunopathology of Guillain-Barre syndrome. Curr Opin Neurol 1996; 9(5):329-333.
55. Yuki N, Tsujino Y. Familial Guillain-Barre syndrome subsequent to Campylobacter jejuni enteritis. J Pediatr 1995; 126(1):162.
56. Korn-Lubetzki I, Steiner I, Brenner T et al. Familial inflammatory demyelinating polyneuropathy:A Guillain-Barre syndrome variant without autoimmune predilection. J Neurol Neurosurg Psychiatry 1994; 57(8):1008-1009.
57. Davidson DL, O'Sullivan AF, Morley KD. HLA antigens in familial Guillain-Barre syndrome. J1992; 55(6):508-509.

58. MacGregor GA. Familial Guillain-Barre syndrome. Lancet 1965; 2(7425):1296.
59. Wilmshurst JM, Pohl KR, Vaughan RW et al. Familial Guillain-Barre syndrome. Eur J Neurol 1999; 6(4):499-503.
60. Kaslow RA, Sullivan-Bolyai JZ, Hafkin B et al. HLA antigens in Guillain-Barre syndrome. Neurology 1984; 34(2):240-242.
61. Hafez M, Nagaty M, Al-Tonbary Y et al. HLA-antigens in Guillain-Barre syndrome. J Neurogenet 1985; 2(4):285-290.
62. Latovitzki N, Suciu-Foca N, Penn AS et al. HLA typing and Guillain-Barre syndrome. Neurology 1979; 29(5):743-745.
63. Winer JB, Briggs D, Welsh K et al. HLA antigens in the Guillain-Barre syndrome. J Neuroimmunol 1988; 18(1):13-16.
64. Hillert J, Osterman PO, Olerup O. No association with HLA-DR, -DQ or -DP alleles in Guillain-Barre syndrome. J Neuroimmunol 1991; 31(1):67-72.
65. Koga M, Yuki N, Kashiwase K et al. Guillain-Barre and Fisher's syndromes subsequent to Campylobacter jejuni enteritis are associated with HLA-B54 and Cw1 independent of anti-ganglioside antibodies. J Neuroimmunol 1998; 88(1-2):62-66.
66. Ma JJ, Nishimura M, Mine H et al. HLA and T-cell receptor gene polymorphisms in Guillain-Barre syndrome. Neurology 1998; 51(2):379-384.
67. Monos DS, Papaioakim M, Ho TW et al. Differential distribution of HLA alleles in two forms of Guillain-Barre syndrome. J Infect Dis 1997; 176 (Suppl 2):S180-182.
68. Guo L, Wang W, Li C et al. The association between HLA typing and different subtypes of Guillain Barre syndrome. Zhonghua Nei Ke Za Zhi 2002; 41(6):381-383.
69. Magira EE, Papaioakim M, Nachamkin I et al. Differential distribution of HLA-DQ beta/DR beta epitopes in the two forms of Guillain-Barre syndrome, acute motor axonal neuropathy and acute inflammatory demyelinating polyneuropathy (AIDP): Identification of DQ beta epitopes associated with susceptibility to and protection from AIDP. J Immunol 2003; 170(6):3074-3080.
70. Rees JH, Vaughan RW, Kondeatis E et al. HLA-class II alleles in Guillain-Barre syndrome and Miller Fisher syndrome and their association with preceding Campylobacter jejuni infection. J Neuroimmunol 1995; 62(1):53-57.
71. Li H, Yuan J, Hao H et al. HLA alleles in patients with Guillain-Barre syndrome. Chin Med J (Engl) 2000; 113(5):429-432.
72. Latov N. Diagnosis of CIDP. Neurology 2002; 59(12 Suppl 6):S2-6.
73. Kieseier BC, Dalakas MC, Hartung HP. Immune mechanisms in chronic inflammatory demyelinating neuropathy. Neurology 2002; 59(12 Suppl 6):S7-12.
74. Vaughan RW, Adam AM, Gray IA et al. Major histocompatibility complex class I and class II polymorphism in chronic idiopathic demyelinating polyradiculoneuropathy. J Neuroimmunol 1990; 27(2-3):149-153.
75. Aldrich MS. Diagnostic aspects of narcolepsy. Neurology 1998; 50(2 Suppl 1):S2-7.
76. Bassetti C. Narcolepsy. Curr Treat Options Neurol 1999; 1(4):291-298.
77. Bassetti C, Aldrich MS. Narcolepsy. Neurol Clin 1996; 14(3):545-571.
78. Overeem S, Mignot E, Gert van Dijk J et al. Narcolepsy: Clinical features, new pathophysiologic insights, and future perspectives. J Clin Neurophysiol 2001; 18(2):78-105.
79. Sakurai T, Amemiya A, Ishii M et al. Orexins and orexin receptors: A family of hypothalamic neuropeptides and G protein-coupled receptors that regulate feeding behavior. Cell 1998; 92(5):1 page following 696.
80. Sakurai T, Moriguchi T, Furuya K et al. Structure and function of human prepro-orexin gene. J Biol Chem 1999; 274(25):17771-17776.
81. Lin L, Faraco J, Li R et al. The sleep disorder canine narcolepsy is caused by a mutation in the hypocretin (orexin) receptor 2 gene. Cell 1999; 98(3):365-376.
82. Chemelli RM, Willie JT, Sinton CM et al. Narcolepsy in orexin knockout mice: Molecular genetics of sleep regulation. Cell 1999; 98(4):437-451.
83. Hara J, Beuckmann CT, Nambu T et al. Genetic ablation of orexin neurons in mice results in narcolepsy, hypophagia, and obesity. Neuron 2001; 30(2):345-354.
84. Peyron C, Tighe DK, van den Pol AN et al. Neurons containing hypocretin (orexin) project to multiple neuronal systems. J Neurosci 1998; 18(23):9996-10015.
85. Peyron C, Faraco J, Rogers W et al. A mutation in a case of early onset narcolepsy and a generalized absence of hypocretin peptides in human narcoleptic brains. Nat Med 2000; 6(9):991-997. taf/dynapage.taf?file=/ncb/medicine/v996/n999/full/nm0900_0991.html taf/dynapage.taf?file=/ncb/medicine/v0906/n0909/abs/nm0900_0991.html.
86. Thannickal TC, Moore RY, Nienhuis R et al. Reduced number of hypocretin neurons in human narcolepsy. Neuron 2000; 27(3):469-474.

87. Nishino S, Ripley B, Overeem S et al. Hypocretin (orexin) deficiency in human narcolepsy. Lancet 2000; 355(9197):39-40.
88. Ripley B, Overeem S, Fujiki N et al. CSF hypocretin/orexin levels in narcolepsy and other neurological conditions. Neurology 2001; 57(12):2253-2258.
89. Mignot E, Lammers GJ, Ripley B et al. The role of cerebrospinal fluid hypocretin measurement in the diagnosis of narcolepsy and other hypersomnias. Arch Neurol 2002; 59(10):1553-1562.
90. Chabas D, Taheri S, Renier C et al. The genetics of narcolepsy. Annu Rev Genomics Hum Genet 2003; 4:459-483.
91. Mignot E, Tafti M, Dement WC et al. Narcolepsy and immunity. Adv Neuroimmunol 1995; 5(1):23-37.
92. Juji T, Satake M, Honda Y et al. HLA antigens in Japanese patients with narcolepsy. All the patients were DR2 positive. Tissue Antigens 1984; 24(5):316-319.
93. Seignalet J, Billiard M. Possible association between HLA-B7 and narcolepsy. Tissue Antigens 1984; 23(3):188-189.
94. Lin L, Hungs M, Mignot E. Narcolepsy and the HLA region. J Neuroimmunol 2001; 117(1-2):9-20.
95. Honda Y, Juji T, Matsuki K et al. HLA-DR2 and Dw2 in narcolepsy and in other disorders of excessive somnolence without cataplexy. Sleep 1986; 9(1):133-142.
96. Matsuki K, Juji T, Tokunaga K et al. Human histocompatibility leukocyte antigen (HLA) haplotype frequencies estimated from the data on HLA class I, II, and III antigens in 111 Japanese narcoleptics. J Clin Invest 1985; 76(6):2078-2083.
97. Mignot E, Hayduk R, Black J et al. HLA DQB1*0602 is associated with cataplexy in 509 narcoleptic patients. Sleep 1997; 20(11):1012-1020.
98. Neely S, Rosenberg R, Spire JP et al. HLA antigens in narcolepsy. Neurology 1987; 37(12):1858-1860.
99. Matsuki K, Grumet FC, Lin X et al. DQ (rather than DR) gene marks susceptibility to narcolepsy. Lancet 1992; 339(8800):1052.
100. Pelin Z, Guilleminault C, Risch N et al. HLA-DQB1*0602 homozygosity increases relative risk for narcolepsy but not disease severity in two ethnic groups. US Modafinil in Narcolepsy Multicenter Study Group. Tissue Antigens 1998; 51(1):96-100.
101. Mignot E, Lin L, Rogers W et al. Complex HLA-DR and -DQ interactions confer risk of narcolepsy-cataplexy in three ethnic groups. Am J Hum Genet 2001; 68(3):686-699.
102. Lock CB, So AK, Welsh KI et al. MHC class II sequences of an HLA-DR2 narcoleptic. Immunogenetics 1988; 27(6):449-455.
103. Mignot E, Lin X, Arrigoni J et al. DQB1*0602 and DQA1*0102 (DQ1) are better markers than DR2 for narcolepsy in Caucasian and black Americans. Sleep 1994; 17(8 Suppl):S60-67.
104. Uryu N, Maeda M, Nagata Y et al. No difference in the nucleotide sequence of the DQ beta beta 1 domain between narcoleptic and healthy individuals with DR2,Dw2. Hum Immunol 1989; 24(3):175-181.
105. Ellis MC, Hetisimer AH, Ruddy DA et al. HLA class II haplotype and sequence analysis support a role for DQ in narcolepsy. Immunogenetics 1997; 46(5):410-417.
106. Kadotani H, Faraco J, Mignot E. Genetic studies in the sleep disorder narcolepsy. Genome Res 1998; 8(5):427-434.
107. Singh SM, George CF, Ott RN et al. IgH (mu-switch and gamma-1) region restriction fragment length polymorphism in human narcolepsy. J Clin Immunol 1996; 16(4):208-215.
108. Hungs M, Lin L, Okun M et al. Polymorphisms in the vicinity of the hypocretin/orexin are not associated with human narcolepsy. Neurology 2001; 57(10):1893-1895.
109. Hohjoh H, Nakayama T, Ohashi J et al. Significant association of a single nucleotide polymorphism in the tumor necrosis factor-alpha (TNF-alpha) gene promoter with human narcolepsy. Tissue Antigens 1999; 54(2):138-145.
110. Hohjoh H, Terada N, Miki T et al. Haplotype analyses with the human leucocyte antigen and tumour necrosis factor-alpha genes in narcolepsy families. Psychiatry Clin Neurosci 2001; 55(1):37-39.
111. Hohjoh H, Terada N, Kawashima M et al. Significant association of the tumor necrosis factor receptor 2 (TNFR2) gene with human narcolepsy. Tissue Antigens 2000; 56(5):446-448.

Chapter 6

Immunogenetics of Rheumatoid Arthritis, Systemic Sclerosis and Systemic Lupus Erythematosus

Allison Porter and J. Lee Nelson

Abstract

The autoimmune rheumatologic diseases discussed in this chapter include rheumatoid arthritis (RA), systemic sclerosis (SSc), also called scleroderma, and systemic lupus erythematosus (SLE). Historically the terms connective-tissue diseases or collagen-vascular diseases have sometimes been used in considering diseases such as RA, SSc and SLE, because fibrinoid degeneration especially in collagen and vascular tissues is often found and was thought to contribute to clinical manifestations of these disorders. The predominant current view is that autoimmunity underlies the pathogenesis of these disorders, with normal tissues, cells and proteins the target of self-directed immune reactivity. Genetic susceptibility to autoimmune rheumatologic diseases is clearly multifactorial involving combinations of many different genes. More than three decades of research, however, indicates HLA genes most often make the strongest genetic contribution. Although the mechanism(s) by which particular HLA genes increase or decrease risk of a disease are not known it is not difficult to appreciate a central role since the products of HLA genes, HLA molecules, are intimately involved in the process of presenting both foreign and self antigens to T cells. For some diseases very specific HLA sequences have been identified and for others extended stretches of genes within the greater major histocompatibility complex (MHC) are implicated. More recently candidate genes other than those in the MHC have been identified for RA, SSc and SLE. Some implicated genes are known to be involved in other aspects of immune regulation while for other candidate genes the functions are as yet unknown.

Rheumatoid Arthritis (RA)

RA is a relatively common disorder, with a prevalence of about 1 percent in the U.S. and an estimated incidence of 500 per million.[1] The hallmark feature of RA is chronic symmetrical inflammatory arthritis. RA is found in virtually all populations worldwide, but is further increased in some populations, for example among certain Native American populations, and decreased in others, for example some African populations. RA can begin at any age including in children, but is increasingly frequent with advancing age both in women and in men at least into the '60s or early '70s.[1] RA affects women two to three times more often than men. The autoantibody rheumatoid factor (RF) is found in the peripheral blood of 80 to 90% of patients with RA. RFs are autoantibodies that react with the Fc fragment of immunoglobulin G (IgG). RFs are generally considered a marker of RA rather than directly pathogenic since they do not correlate with disease activity and are sometimes found in other diseases and in

Immunogenetics of Autoimmune Disease, edited by Jorge Oksenberg and David Brassat.

Table 1. American College of Rheumatology revised criteria for classification of RA

1. Morning stiffness	Stiffness in and around the joints lasting 1 hour before maximal improvement.
2. Soft-tissue swelling or fluid	At least 3 joint areas with simultaneous soft-tissue swelling or fluid (not bony overgrowth alone). The 14 possible joint areas are right or left PIP, MCP, wrist, elbow, knee, ankle, and MTP joints.
3. Swollen joint	At least one joint area swollen above is in a wrist, MCP, or PIP.
4. Symmetric involvement	Simultaneous involvement of the same joint areas (as in 2) on both sides of the body (bilateral involvement of PIP, MCP, or MTP is acceptable without absolute symmetry).
5. Subcutaneous nodules	Subcutaneous nodules over bony prominences or extensor surfaces.
6. Rheumatoid factor	Demonstration of abnormal amounts of rheumatoid factor by any method that has been positive in fewer than 5% of normal control subjects.
7. Radiographic changes	Radiographic changes typical of RA on posteroanterior wrist radiographs, including erosions or unequivocal bony decalcification localized to or most marked adjacent to the involved joints (osteoarthritic changes alone do not qualify).

The diagnosis of RA is based on the combination of 4 or more of the above criteria. Disease must be continuous for at least 6 weeks. A physician must observe the signs and symptoms of criteria 2, 3, 4, and 5. The table is adapted from the 1987 American Rheumatism Association revised classification of rheumatoid arthritis.[2] PIP: proximal interphalangeal joint, MCP: metacarpalphalangeal joint, MTP: metatarsalphalangeal joint

normal individuals. A positive RF test is just one of the criteria for RA for which 4 of 7 criteria are required according to the American College of Rheumatology criteria[2] (Table 1).

Concordance of RA in monozygotic twins is 15% and 4% in dizygotic twins.[1] Heritable factors are estimated to account for approximately 60% of RA cases.[3] The HLA region clearly provides the single most important contribution to genetic risk of RA. However, less than 50% of the genetic risk of RA is estimated as attributable to HLA genes. Recent studies have identified additional candidate genes both within the greater MHC and on other chromosomes.

HLA Associations with RA

An HLA association with RA was first identified in 1977.[4] The initial description was of the cellularly defined HLA specificity "Dw4", although subsequent studies were done using serological techniques i.e., with antibodies to HLA molecules used as reagents. Numerous reports followed that described the serologic specificity DR4 as increased in RA patients in a wide diversity of populations worldwide. The magnitude of RA risk associated with DR4 varies depending upon the population studied, for example among Native American Chippewas the relative risk is 14.6 but among southern Spaniards 1.8.[5,6]

In earlier studies it became apparent using cellular techniques with homozygous typing cells in addition to serological reagents that DR4 was actually a family of molecules. In the late 1980s DNA-based typing began to replace both serological and cellular techniques, resulting in the appreciation of an even greater number of different variants within the HLA-DR4 family. As information evolved it became clear that only some alleles (variant forms) of DR4 are associated with risk of RA. At the same time alleles of different HLA DR families were also identified in association with RA including DRB1*0101, DRB1*1402 and DRB1*1001. As of the present, the alleles that have been reported as significantly associated with RA include DRB1*0401, *0404, *0405, *0101, *1001 and *1402 (the latter only in meta analysis). These

```
        60        70        80        90
        YWNSQKDLLEQRRAAVDTYCRHNYGVVESFT
*0401   -----------K--------------G----
*0402   -------I--DE-------------------
*0403   --------------E----------------
*0404   -------------------------------
*0405   --------------------------G----
*0408^  --------------------------G----
*0101   --------------------------G----
*1402   --------------------------G----
*1001   ----------R---------------G----
```

^0408 is uncommon; statistical significance not reported.

Figure 1. The RA-associated DRβ1 "shared epitope" sequence.

alleles encode similar amino acid sequences from positions 70 through 74 of the DRβ1 chain of the DR molecule. The similar sequence is referred to as the "shared epitope" and is thought to be the underlying "unit" of HLA defined susceptibility to RA.[7,8] The sequences include QKRAA (DRB1*0401 previously called "Dw4") and QRRAA (DRB1*0404, *0405, *0101, previously called Dw14, Dw15 and Dw1 respectively), with a conservative substitution of an arginine (latter group) for a lysine (former), both of which carry a positive charge (Fig. 1). An extension of the shared epitope hypothesis added the sequence RRRAA which is encoded by DRB1*1001 (previously called "DwSHY"), found in a variety of populations including Spanish, Greeks, Asian Indians and Zimbabweans, in which a positively charged arginine replaces the uncharged polar amino acid glutamine at position 70.

Limitations of the RA Shared Epitope Hypothesis

Although there is ample support for the shared epitope hypothesis it is important to recognize a number of limitations of the shared epitope hypothesis in RA. First, the associations with DRB1*0101 are not uniformly observed and even differ within the same racial/ethnic population and DRB1*1402, reported among Native Americans, was highly prevalent among healthy individuals (up to 80% of healthy controls) without a statistically significant difference among RA patients compared to controls in any single study. Second, according to the shared epitope hypothesis DRB1*0102 would be expected to be associated with RA, but to date no study has shown a significant increase of DRB1*0102 in RA patients compared to controls. Third, the shared epitope hypothesis does not explain the association with DRB1*09 now described in several populations.[9] Finally, and most importantly, the shared epitope hypothesis fails to explain the synergistic effect of particular combinations of alleles reported in numerous HLA studies of RA.

Combinations of HLA-DR Molecules and Protective Effects

An unexpectedly high frequency of patients with a particular combination of DR4 variants was first reported in juvenile onset RA.[10] The combination described was "Dw4" and "Dw14", now known to correspond to DRB1*0401 for the former and to DRB1*0404 and DRB1*0408 for the latter. Subsequent studies noted the interesting role of DRB1*0404 as a synergistic risk factor when present along with other DRB1 alleles containing the shared epitope.[11-13] The ability of DRB1*0404 to confer risk independent of any other shared epitope containing allele has been more controversial.[11-14] The unsuitability of an oversimplified view in which shared epitope copies are counted ranging from 0 to 2 is more than evident in studies from multiple groups demonstrating increasing hierarchies of risk associated with particular combinations of DRB1 alleles. Thus assessment of HLA associated risk must also consider at a minimum the HLA DR molecule on which the shared epitope resides and the DRB1 allele of the second haplotype. Directing analysis to particular combinations of HLA DR molecules the spectrum of RA risk was as high as 49 or as low as 3 in one study.[12]

Other studies have identified particular HLA molecules that are associated with resistance to RA. Among Caucasian populations a protective effect has often been found for genes encoding HLA-DR15 molecules (e.g., DRB1*1501). Among Japanese, a protective effect has been identified in association with DRB1*0803.[15] In the Japanese population DRB1*0405 is the allele that confers risk of RA and interestingly, in this population among more than 200 patients no RA patient was identified who had DRB1*0405 and *0803, suggesting that the protective effect of DRB1*0803 was actually dominant over the DRB1*0405 susceptibility allele in this population. These observations again emphasize that both haplotypes need to be considered in evaluating HLA-associated risk of RA.

Differences in HLA Associations According to Gender and to Age of Onset

Although gender is an established variable in RA with more women affected than men, most studies have not conducted analyses stratified according to gender. When separate analyses have been examined differences in HLA-associations have been reported in men and women. Several studies have found an especially marked increase of the DRB1*0401,*0404 genotype among male RA patients,[16] with one report describing a difference in relative risk of 90 compared to 16.7 in men and women with this genotype respectively.[13] Other reports have described decreasing HLA association strength with increasing age at disease onset.[17]

Susceptibility or Severity?

RA manifests in a wide spectrum with self-limited spontaneously resolving disease on one end and severe progressive disease on the other. A question that arises is whether HLA genes are associated with RA because they increase susceptibility to disease or whether their contribution is in selecting for individuals who will have continuous and/or more severe disease. A number of earlier studies suggested RA patients who had DR4, and especially those with two copies of DR4, were likely to have more severe RA. However, results of other studies were variable. Differences in study populations and differences in measures of disease "severity" offer some explanation for variability in results. In fact the term "severity" has been equated to a multitude of different outcome measures. For example, "severity" has been measured by extraarticular disease manifestations such as leukocytoclastic vasculitis or Felty's syndrome (both of which are uncommon), joint replacement surgery (which can be influenced by other factors such as socioeconomic status), need for second line mediations, decreased functional capacity and radiographic changes. The rapidity with which an individual develops joint damage may also be considered a measure of severity. Other measures that have been equated to "severity" are not actually manifestations of severity but rather suggest severity by inference, e.g., presence of rheumatoid nodules or rheumatoid factor-positivity. Differences in the population examined may also introduce variability. As noted above gender impacts disease risk and may also impact disease manifestations. Consistent with this possibility, a study of radiographic erosions when stratified by gender found that DR4 correlated with severity of erosions only in females with onset under the age of 50.[18]

More recently the suggestion was put forward that two copies of the shared epitope are associated with more severe RA. However, the data in the reports[19,20] showed that for two of three severity measures a worse outcome was associated not with two copies of the shared epitope but rather with two copies of HLA-DR4 (measures of severity included extra-articular disease, history of joint surgery, presence of nodules). Not surprisingly, when a multitude of studies followed, asking whether severity correlated with 0, 1, or 2 copies of the shared epitope sequence, the results were conflicting. Moreover, as described above, earlier studies had clearly identified that shared epitope sequences are not equal since effects clearly differ depending both on the particular HLA molecule on which the shared epitope sequence resides and by the particular combination of HLA alleles in an individual's genotype.

HLA-DQ and RA

It has been difficult to determine the role of DQ in susceptibility to RA owing primarily to linkage disequilibrium patterns of class II genes. Some have argued that DQ is not relevant to RA susceptibility since the same DQ molecules are observed in linkage disequilibrium with RA-associated and non RA-associated DRB1 alleles (for example DRB1*0401 and DRB1*0402 are both in linkage disequilibrium with DQB1*03). However, this is not necessarily a valid argument since particular DQ molecules could be contributory when accompanied by a primary DRB1 susceptibility allele but have no independent effect. Extensive studies in collagen induced arthritis, an experimental model of RA where the contribution of DR and DQ molecules to some extent can be separated has lent support to a potential role for DQ in RA.[21] However, the role of DQ in RA susceptibility and/or severity remains controversial.

Mechanisms by Which Particular HLA Molecules Might Contribute to Disease

How HLA molecules associated with RA might contribute to disease pathogenesis remains unknown. A number of possibilities have been proposed. One possibility is that HLA molecules encoding the shared epitope preferentially bind particular arthritogenic peptides. This explanation appears unlikely given the wide array of peptides that can be bound by various HLA molecules. A second possibility is that predisposition to RA occurs because of the way in which particular HLA molecules have shaped the TCR receptor repertoire. A third possibility is that specific DRB1 alleles affect antigen processing.[22] Another possibility suggests the shared epitope becomes a target due to molecular mimicry by infectious agents.[23] In one multi-step model of molecular mimicry it has been proposed that T cells with low affinity for self DR peptides (i.e., RA-associated QKRAA sequence) are positively selected, that the QKRAA amino acid sequence is shared by the bacterial heat shock protein dnaJ, and GP110 protein of Epstein Barr virus, and that exposure to such bacterial proteins results in expansion of the T cells. Thereafter immune response could continue in the joints due to expression of heat shock proteins resembling dnaJ, mechanical stress, and epitope spreading. In this model human dnaJ homologues become the eventual target of T lymphocytes that have been positively selected by the self peptide (QKRAA), later triggered by exogenous antigens.[23] Another model incorporates the observation that in addition to presenting peptides from foreign antigens, HLA molecules have been found to present peptides derived from other (self) HLA molecules.[24] In this model,[21] DQ presents a peptide derived from a self DRβ1 molecule. A model in which DQ presents peptides derived from DRβ1 offers one possible explanation for the observation that remission of RA frequently occurs during pregnancy in association with fetal disparity from the mother for HLA class II antigens, especially DQ.[25]

Non HLA Genes in Risk of RA

In addition to genes encoding classical HLA molecules the HLA complex includes more than 100 expressed genes, many of which are known to have immunologic functions. While some reports describing genes in the HLA complex other than those encoding the classical HLA molecules were subsequently attributed to linkage disequilibrium with classical HLA genes, for example TAP2 genes and DMA, evidence has strengthened for a potential role for others. The largest number of studies have investigated the cluster of tumor necrosis factor (TNF) genes in the HLA class III region. Polymorphisms in genes encoding TNF or TNF receptors are particularly attractive candidates in RA because TNF plays a central role in the pro-inflammatory cascade of cytokines. Moreover, recent years have seen a major advance in treatment of RA with agents directed at TNF. Although there has been considerable variability in reports, support for a role for TNF genes has accrued. A particularly large study in Japanese RA cases and controls used single nucleotide polymorphism (SNP) typing and found an association that localized to a region containing the TNF receptor II gene.[26] Other studies from the U.S. used microsatellite markers across the entire HLA complex, conducted haplotypic rather than single marker analyses, and identified a stretch of genes associated with RA that spans the TNF cluster on haplotypes encoding A1-B8-DR3—an ancestral haplotype that is not known to be associated with RA.[27] The 13th International HLA Working Group used an approach by which cases and controls were matched for their DRB1-DQB1 haplotypes, thereby essentially "controlling for" any effect of DRB1 and DQB1 and in a preliminary report also described an association in the TNF region on DR3 containing haplotypes.[28] Other MHC genes that have been implicated include MICA and DQB2.[9] MICA encodes the ligand for the NKG2D receptor which is present on some subsets of natural killer cells, CD8 T cells and γδ T cells. DQB2 is an interesting gene that is not a pseudogene, but for which the protein expression has not been well studied. Complement genes are also located in the MHC class III region and an earlier report described an increased frequency of C4B null alleles in patients with Felty's syndrome with or without DRB1*0401.[29]

Beginning in 1998 the results of whole genome scans, including genes on chromosome 6 but outside of the MHC complex, as well as other chromosomes have been reported. Most of the larger genome scans have been conducted using European, U.S. or Japanese populations. Some studies have been conducted with families, often with identification of affected sibling pairs or trios, while others have been conducted as association studies investigating unrelated RA cases and controls. Similar to studies of other complex diseases, results have been difficult to replicate across studies, and interpretation is often hampered by insufficient power to detect weaker gene associations as well as heterogeneity in the disease phenotype. A recent metaanalysis[30] examined four of the major RA genome-wide linkage studies deriving from France,[31] the U.K.,[32] the U.S.[33] and Japan.[34] Although 4 regions of particular interest were identified at 6p, 16cen, 6q and 12p, results did not replicate across studies. After weighting results according to study size, the metaanalysis found the strongest association was with16p, which although ranked in the top 25% among all 4 studies, was not highlighted in any single study. One candidate gene in this region is metalloproteinase gene MMP2. More recently a large case control study from Japan using SNP markers identified a highly significant association at 1p.[35] The study was especially noteworthy because the PADI type 4 gene identified as increased in RA is associated with antibodies to citrullinated peptide in RA sera implying the RA-associated PADI4 haplotype increases production of citrullinated peptides that act as autoantigens in RA.

Scleroderma and Systemic Sclerosis (SSc) (Table 2)

Scleroderma is characterized by thickening and tethering of the skin ("scleros" meaning hardening and derma skin). Scleroderma is first classified according to whether it is localized or systemic. Localized scleroderma includes morphea and linear scleroderma and is not considered further here. The classification systemic sclerosis (SSc) indicates there is a combination of scleroderma skin changes and some form of internal organ involvement. SSc is subcategorized into two distinct subtypes: limited or diffuse. Diffuse SSc includes skin thickening that extends proximal to the elbows or knees whereas with limited SSc skin thickening is confined to the distal extremities below the elbows and knees. In addition to skin changes in the fingers and hands, skin involvement is generally evident on the face even in limited SSc. SSc often involves the gastrointestinal tract. Diffuse SSc often affects the lungs, heart and kidneys. Most all patients with SSc also have Raynauds phenomenon, a three-phase color change usually in the fingers but sometimes in the toes from white to blue to red associated with vasospasm followed by reperfusion.

Table 2. The classification and subsets of scleroderma and systemic sclerosis

Systemic Sclerosis
- Diffuse cutaneous involvement
  - Symmetrical and widespread skin changes
  - Affects both distal and proximal extremities and often trunk and face
  - Often rapid progression of skin thickening and early visceral disease
- Limited cutaneous involvement:
  - Symmetrical restricted skin thickening
  - Affects distal extremities (often confined to fingers) and face
  - Prolonged delay in internal manifestations (i.e., pulmonary arterial hypertension, biliary cirrhosis)
  - Also referred to as CREST syndrome (calcinosis, Raynaud's phenomenon, esophageal hypomotility, sclerodactyly, and telangectasias)
- With "overlap": typical features of another autoimmune disease (e.g., Sjögren's syndrome, polymyositis/dermatomyositis, or SLE)

Localized Scleroderma
- Morphea: single or multiple (generalized plaques)
- Linear scleroderma: with or without cortical thickening of long bones; includes scleroderma *en coup de sabre,* with or without facial hemiatrophy

Scleroderma-Like
- Eosinophilic fasciitis
- Eosinophilia-myalgia syndrome
- Toxic oil syndrome

Pathogenic changes of SSc are evident in three major areas that include vascular abnormalities, immunological abnormalities, and disordered collagen synthesis (Table 3). The primary event is thought to be vascular affecting small arteries and arterioles with endothelial cell proliferation and thickening in the intimal layer. Early in the disease skin biopsies usually show mononuclear cell infiltrates in the dermis. Another hallmark feature of SSc is increased fibroblast activity with resultant overproduction of collagen evident mostly in the dermis leading to hyalinization, obliteration of small blood vessels, and loss of dermal appendages and thinning of the epidermis. Increased fibrinogen and fibrin are found in vessels, and the lumina of the vessels are often occluded by fibrosis. Vessels that remain may dilate and become visible in the skin as telangiectases.

SSc is an uncommon disease with incidence estimates ranging from 2 to 30 per million new cases per year. The peak incidence of SSc in women occurs between 45 to 65 years and the female-to-male ratio is about 3-4:1.[1] The prevalence of disease is variable with higher rates described in the U.S. and Australia, for example, than in Europe or Japan. A significant difference in concordance between monozygotic and dizgotic twins has not been shown, but the number of twins identified has been small. However, studies from Australia[36] and also from the U.S.[37] have found an increase of SSc among first-degree relatives (e.g., 1.4% vs expected of 0.009% in Australian study).

HLA Associations with SSc and SSc Related Autoantibodies

Many studies of HLA associations with SSc have been conducted with categorization of patients according to whether they have diffuse or limited SSc since these subsets are very clinically distinct and limited SSc rarely evolves into diffuse SSc. The two subsets also have different autoantibodies, with antibodies to topoisomerase I (ATA) found in the former and to centromere (ACA) in the latter. Other HLA studies have investigated HLA associations according to whether a patient has ATA or ACA autoantibodies. Since there are few exceptions to ATA occurring with diffuse and ACA with limited SSc these studies also reflect the clinical

Table 3. Clinical characteristics of SSc clinical subsets

Signs and Symptoms	Diffuse SSc	Limited SSc
Skin involvement	Proximal and distal extremities/ trunk, neck/face	Distal extremities, face/neck
Disease progression	Often fast	Slow
Fatigue, anorexia, weight loss	Common	Uncommon
Arthralgias	Associated with contractures	Sometimes
Tendon friction rubs	Possible	Absent
Organ involvement	Interstitial fibrosis Pulmonary hypertension Cardiac hypertrophy/dilatation Renal crisis Severe GE reflux Intestinal dysmotility Sicca syndrome	Interstitial fibrosis not common Pulmonary hypertension Biliary cirrhosis Severe GE reflux Intestinal dysmotility CREST syndrome Sicca syndrome
Associated autoantibodies	Scl-70 (anti-topoisomerase I), RNA polymerase III	Anti-centromere
Other	Raynaud's	Raynaud's

Abbreviations: GE (gastroesophageal) and CREST (Calcinosis, Raynaud's syndrome, Esophageal dysmotility, Scleroderma, Telangiectasias)

disease subset. However, although ATA and ACA are very specific neither is very sensitive, found in a minority of SSc patients, hence results from studies utilizing clinical and autoantibody categorizations can be considered only in part as overlapping.

Diffuse SSc and Antibodies to Topoisomerase I

The most consistently described HLA associations have been with diffuse SSc and ATA with an increase of HLA-DR11 in Caucasian populations and of DR15 in Japanese. In earlier studies an increase of "DR5" was described but is expected to represent DR11 which typed as "DR5" with earlier serological reagents. An increase of DR11 has been found in numerous Caucasian populations including from the U.K., U.S., Canada, Greece, Australia and Mexicans whereas in Asians (Japanese and Thai) the predominant association is with DR15.[37] There is some debate as to whether the particular allelic variant encoding DR11 is important or not with some studies finding a particular increase of DRB1*1104 while others reporting no disproportionate representation of any DRB1*11 allele. Among Japanese the association has been attributed to a DRB1*1502 haplotype, that also includes DRB5*0102, DQA1*0103 and DQB1*0601. An increase of DRB1*0802 has also been reported among Japanese.[38] Although DR8 is relatively common in the Japanese population (in contrast to Caucasians) the DR8 allelic variant DRB1*0803 is about twice as common as DRB1*0802; thus it is of interest that DRB1*0802 differs from DRB1*0803 in having a charged amino acid, aspartic acid, at position 57 (versus a serine), and at position 67, phenylalanine (versus an isoleucine). An increase of DRB1*08 has also been reported in American Blacks.[37] Finally, a recent study of a Native North American population with an especially high prevalence of diffuse SSc reported an increase of DRB1*1602, on a haplotype that also contains DQA1*0501 and DQB1*0301.[39] When stratified according to gender, another report described a significant increase of DQA1*0501, only in men with diffuse SSc.[40]

DRB1 allele	Amino acid number 67	68	69	70	71	72	73	74
0101, 0102, 0404, 0405, 0408, 1402, 1406	L	L	E	Q	R	R	A	A
1101, 1104	*F*	-	-	*D*	-	-	-	-
1103,1111	*F*	-	-	*D*	*E*			
1601	*F*	-	-	*D*	-	-	-	-
0801 0802 0804 0805	*F*	-	-	*D*	-	-	-	*L*
1202	*F*	-	-	*D*	-	-	-	-
0103, 0402, 0414, 1102, 1301-2, 1304, 1308, 1317	I	-	-	D	E	-	-	-
1501 1502, 1209	I	-	-	-	A	-	-	-
1303,1310	I	-	-	D	K			
0401 0413	-	-	-	-	K	-	-	-
0403,0406,0407	-	-	-	-	-	-	-	E
0803,0810	I	-	-	D	-	-	-	L
1201,1203	I	-	-	D	-	-	-	-
1401,4,5,7,8,10,11,14				R	-	-	-	E
1403,12				D				L
0301	-	-	-	-	K	-	G	R
0701	I	-	-	D	-	-	G	Q
0901	F	-	-	R	-	-	-	E
1001	-	-	-	R	-	-	-	-
1602								
DRB5 allele								
****0101, 0102 ^***	*F*	-	-	*D*	-	-	-	-
*0202,0203 ^^	I	-	-	-	A			
DRB3~	-	-	-	-	K	-	G	R or Q
DRB4 #	-	-	-	R	-	-	-	E

^ DRB5 encodes DR51 molecules with this sequence when the DRB1*02 allele is either DRB1*1501 or *1502
^^ DRB5 encodes DR51 molecules with this sequence when the DRB1*02 allele is either DRB1*1601 or *1602
# DRB4 encodes DR53 molecules, which are co-expressed with haplotypes that have DRB1*04, *07 or *09
~ DRB3 encodes DR52 molecules, which are co-expressed with haplotypes that have DRB1*03, *11, *12, *13 and *14

Figure 2. Amino acid sequence shared by some DRβ1 and DRβ5 alleles in diffuse SSc.

Consistent with reports for diffuse SSc when patients with ATA have been studied an increase of DR11 has been described in Caucasians (U.S., U.K., Finland, Germany) and DR15 in Japanese. Again some studies have reported a preferential increase in the DRB1*1104 allele while others have not. Two studies from the U.K., in addition to concurring with an association of DRB1*11 with ATA, described a significant association of ATA with DPB1*0301,[41] and of antibodies to RNA polymerases with DQB1*0201.[42] Among Japanese, ATA is associated with DRB1*1502, a haplotype that also includes the DRB5*0102 allele.[38] With respect to genes conferring protection from SSc, it is striking that no study in any population has described diffuse SSc or ATA with any haplotype in the DRB4* family (DRB1*04, *07, *09).

Although there is no shared amino acid sequence in the DRB1 genes described above, an often overlooked observation is that DRB3, DRB4 and DRB5 genes also encode for molecules expressed on the cell surface that sometimes share amino acid sequences with DRB1 encoded molecules. DRB3, DRB4 and DRB5 encode DR52, DR53 and DR51 molecules respectively. All haplotypes with DRB1*15 or *16 include a DRB5 gene, DRB5*01 or *02 respectively. Since DRB1*15 is always accompanied by DRB5*02, the amino acid sequence "FLED" is also expressed on these haplotypes from positions 67-70. Interestingly the "FLED" sequence is expressed by the DRβ1 chain also from positions 67-70 on DRB1*11 haplotypes and also by DRB1*0802, another allele described as increased in Japanese. The DRβ1 chain of the Amerindian DRB1*1602 haplotype shares the latter three amino acids with L instead of the F at the initial position 67, and would be expected to also have a DRB5 allele although the DRB5 allele was not reported. Thus, a similar sequence encoded by DRβ1 or alternatively by DRβ5 could potentially contribute to diffuse SSc (Fig. 2).

There is considerable support for a role for DQB1 especially among SSc patients with ATA. DQB1 associations have been described in patients with ATA, in Caucasians with DQB1*0301[43] and in Japanese with DQB1*0301 and DQB1*0601.[44] The findings are

DQB1 alleles	Amino acid number 71	72	73	74	75	76	77
0501, 0502, 0503	A	R	A	S	V	D	R
0601 - 0604	***T***	-	-	***E***	***L***	-	***T***
0301 - 0303	***T***	-	-	***E***	***L***	-	***T***
0201	K	-	-	A	-	-	-
0401, 0402	D	-	-	-	-	-	T

Figure 3. Shared amino acid sequences "TRAELDT" of some DQβ1 alleles associated with antibodies to Topoisomerase I.

consistent with the above description of DRB1 since in Caucasian populations DQB1*0301 is in linkage disequilibrium with DRB1*11 and in Japanese, DQB1*0601 is in linkage disequilibrium with DRB1*1502. Reveille et al have proposed that the primary association of ATA antibodies is with the DQB1 encoded amino acid sequence "TRAELDT" encoded by DQB1*0301 and DQB1*0601 from positions 71 through 77 (Fig. 3). Support for this hypothesis has been generated by studies in U.S. populations[45] and in Japanese[44] This sequence is found on DQβ1 chains encoded by DQB1*0301, *0302, *0303, *0601, *0602, *0603 and *0604. Studies have been conflicting as to whether tyrosine at position 26 or at position 30 of DQβ1 are also contributory.[42,44]

Limited SSc and Antibodies to Centromere

HLA associations with limited SSc have been less consistent than those with diffuse SSc. Some reports describe an increase of DR1 (U.S., U.K., Germany), others DR11 (Australia), DR3 (U.S.), and still others no significant association.[37] Although studies using DNA typing techniques to examine patients with limited SSc are few, more than 10 different studies have examined patients who are positive for ACA. The overall consensus is that ACA associations are strongest with DQB1 alleles. The primary alleles identified in association with ACA are DQB1*0501[46,47] and DQB1*0301.[48] A protective effect of DQB1*0201 has also been reported.[47] The DQB1*0501 and DQB1*0301 alleles have no similarity of the third hypervariable region. However, both lack a leucine at position 26 leading to the hypothesis that the ACA response is associated with DQB1 alleles lacking leucine at position 26,[48] however, studies in Japanese as well as another U.S. population did not find an association with the absence of leucine at position 26.[46] Two studies found no significant association with any DPB1 allele.

Considered together studies to date have not generated a model in which a common sequence of DQβ1 can be attributed to the ACA response. Of potential interest, in a study from Japan,[46] higher titers of ACA correlated with some allelic variants at DRB1 raising the possibility that both DQB1 and DRB1 genes may be contributory and interactive in contributing to ACA production.

Finally it should be noted that despite significant HLA associations with SSc disease subsets and with SSc associated antibodies, unlike RA where most studies show that the majority of patients have the RA-associated shared epitope sequence, in SSc both when categorized by clinical disease type and by autoantibody, despite significant HLA associations the majority of patients are negative for the identified disease-associated HLA allele.

Non HLA Genes in Risk of SSc

Genome wide studies of SSc are challenging because large numbers are needed whereas the disease has a low prevalence and familial aggregation is uncommon in SSc. Some earlier studies implicated complement genes (HLA class III region) in SSc. Significant advances have been made in identifying nonMHC (and MHC) genes by genome wide studies of a Native American Indian group (Choctaws) with a particularly high prevalence of SSc.[39] Initial studies identified a SNP that was strongly associated with SSc near the fibrillin 1 gene on chromosome 15q.[49] This is of interest in SSc because fibrillin 1 abnormalities could lead to enhanced release of bound latent TGFβ and other cytokines. In a recent report from the same group 17 microsatellite markers were identified with significant associations with SSc in this population.[50] Interestingly, the microsatellite markers on chromosome 1 (1p21.2 and lq32-42) and 14 (14q21) have also been reported in association with SLE and the microsatellite markers 7p12-11, 19q13, 1p21.2 and Xp11.4 have been reported in association with autoimmune diseases other than SSc such as RA. Studies of other autoimmune diseases have shown a similar phenomenon i.e., association of a single microsatellite maker with more than one autoimmune disease, suggesting some genes may predispose generally to autoimmunity. The 17 microsatellite markers significantly associated with SSc included 11 different chromosomes with 2 or more on 1, 6, 7, 19 and X and 1 on 5, 8, 14, 15, 20 and 22.

An overview of candidate genes that have been described in association with SSc include a number that are attractive candidates in the pathogenesis of SSc.[37] As discussed above endothelial injury and increased collagen are hallmark features of SSc. Polymorphisms have been implicated in SSc in the osteonectin gene, a protein secreted by endothelial cells in response to injury, and in the COL1A1 and 2 and genes, which function in increased output of type 1 collagen. Similarly differences in SSc patients have been described in genes in the TGFβ family, genes that are involved in fibrotic disorders with increased extracellular matrix and in the TNF family, that invoke proinflammaotry cytokine responses. Polymorphisms in IL4-R and CXCR2 have also been described, with IL-4 known to activate and induce B cell differentiation promoting Th2 cytokines and CXCR2, a member of the IL-8 receptor family, with IL-8 known to be a potent chemotractant for neutrophils which are implicated in the pathogenesis of pulmonary fibrosis in SSc.

Systemic Lupus Erythematosus (SLE)

SLE is an autoimmune disease that frequently involves multiple organs as well as the hematopoietic system including the skin, joints, kidneys, lungs, serous membranes, central nervous system and other organs. SLE is a protean disease expressing a wide variability in clinical signs, symptoms and course with waxing and waning over time. SLE effects approximately 1 in 1500 individuals in the general population with an incidence of approximately 2.5 per 100,000 per year.[1] These estimates, however, somewhat underestimate the clinical magnitude of SLE in that for every two patients with definite SLE, there is likely another with possible or probable SLE. SLE is primarily a disease of young women. The female to male ratio varies according to age of onset from a low of 2 to 1 for age 0-9 to a high of 8 to 1 for ages 30 to 39. Ethnicity impacts the risk of SLE with American Blacks at higher risk as well as Afro Caribbeans living in the U.K.

The American College of Rheumatology has established criteria for the diagnosis of SLE,[51] which are summarized in Table 4. The diagnosis of SLE requires 4 of 11 criteria. It is easy to appreciate that the spectrum of this disease is wide and variable since some patients have life-threatening involvement of internal organs whereas others have limited problems with skin rash, sun sensitivity, joint pains and a positive ANA. The extraordinary diversity in the clinical manifestations of SLE (Table 5) have made studies and clinical trials challenging and required the cooperation of international groups of investigators to establish consensus criteria, for example by which to judge ongoing disease activity in SLE patients.

Table 4. The American College of Rheumatology criteria for classification of SLE*

Criteria	Definition
1. Malar rash	Fixed erythema, flat or raised, over malar eminences, tending to spare nasolabial folds.
2. Discoid rash	Erythematous raised patches with keratotic scaling and follicular plugging
3. Photosensitivity	Skin rash resulting from unusual reaction to sunlight, by patient history or physician observation.
4. Oral ulcers	Oral or nasopharyngeal ulceration (observed by physician).
5. Arthritis	Nonerosive arthritis involving at least 2, peripheral joints, characterized by tenderness, swelling, or effusion.
6. Serositis	a. Pleuritis—history of pleuritic pain, rub heard by a physician, or pleural effusion, OR b. Pericarditis—documented by ECG, rub, or pericardial effusion.
7. Renal disorder	a. Persistent proteinuria greater than 0.5 g/day or 3+ if quantification not performed, OR b. Cellular casts—red cell, granular, tubular, or mixed.
8. Neurologic disorder	a. Seizures—in the absence of drugs or known metabolic derangement (i.e., uremia, ketoacidosis, electrolyte imbalance) OR b. Psychosis—in the absence of drugs or known metabolic derangement.
9. Hematologic disorder	a. Hemolytic anemia—with reticulocytosis, OR b. Leukopenia— < 4000/mm total on 2 or more occasions, OR c. Lymphopenia— < 1500/mm^3 on 2 or more occasions, OR d. Thrombocytopenia— < 100,000/mm^3 in the absence of offending drugs.
10. Immunologic disorder	a. Anti-DNA - antibody to native DNA in abnormal titer, OR b. Anti-Sm - presence of antibody to Sm nuclear antigen, OR c. Antiphospholipid antibodies based on (1) an abnormal serum level of IgG or IgM anticardiolipin antibodies, (2) a positive test for lupus anticoagulant, or (3) a false positive serologic test for syphilis for at least 6 months confirmed by *Treponema pallidum* immobilization or fluorescent treponemal antibody absorption test.**
11. Antinuclear antibody	An abnormal titer of ANA by immunofluorescence or equivalent assay in the absence of drugs associated with drug-induced lupus syndrome.

*The 1982 criteria were modified to reflect identification of primary antiphospholipid antibody syndrome as a distinct entity from SLE.[51] A patient must have at least 4 criteria serially or simultaneously. **Antibodies to cardiolipin are responsible for false-positive VDRL tests due to inclusion of cardiolipin as a test substrate.

SLE is a disease of complex pathogenesis, some aspects of which are beginning to be understood. The development of SLE is multifactorial and is thought to include exposure to one or a number of particular pathogens (infectious or noninfectious) in a genetically susceptible host at a susceptible time in life. No single contributory factor is likely to operate independently either in the initiation or persistence of SLE. SLE tissue damage results from products of T cells and B cells, including pathogenic autoantibodies and immune complexes. Although the normal immune response to exogenous antigens functions in SLE patients, there are increased numbers of antibody producing cells associated with hyperglobulinemia and a heightened response to a wide variety of autoantigens. Immune complexes that activate complement are thought to play an important role in SLE pathogenesis.

Table 5. The many manifestations of SLE

Dermatologic	Photosensitivity, mucous membrane ulcerations (mouth, nose, vagina, vulva), alopecia, livedo reticularis, malar (butterfly) rash, discoid and subacute cutaneous lesions
Musculoskeletal	Arthralgia, arthritis, myalgia, myositis, osteopenia, avascular necrosis of bone
Cardiac	Pericarditis, myocarditis, endocarditis, coronary artery disease
Eye	Sicca syndrome, episcleritis, retinal vasculitis
Gastrointestinal	Hepatomegaly
Hematologic	Anemia, leukopenia, lymphopenia, and thrombocytopenia
Lymphoid	Lymphadenopathy, splenomegaly
Neurologic	Headaches, seizures, cranial or peripheral neuropathies, psychosis, depression, chorea, transverse myelitis, strokes
Pulmonary	Pleuritis, pulmonary hypertension, pneumonitis, pulmonary emboli
Renal	Interstitial nephritis, glomerulonephritis
Vascular	Raynaud's phenomenon, periungual erythema, leg ulcers, vasculitis
Constitutional	Fatigue, fever, anorexia, and weight loss

A positive test for antinuclear antibodies (ANA) is one of the best-recognized immunologic features of SLE. A positive ANA test is not a sufficient criteria to define SLE since positive ANA tests occur in a variety of different diseases and are also present in a small percentage of the normal healthy population. Neither does the absence of a positive ANA test exclude the diagnosis of SLE since up to 10% of patients will have a negative test. Moreover, the ANA titer may be high while a patient is in remission or may decrease when there is continued disease activity. Why and how antinuclear antibodies arise remains unclear. Nuclear antigens are generally protected from antibody binding by virtue of their intracellular location. Thus other scenarios for ANA binding are invoked, such as entry of ANAs into damaged cells or expression of nuclear antigens on apoptotic blebs on the cell surface. ANAs might also bind to free nuclear antigens or cross-react with other tissue specific antigens. In either event, they may also form immune complexes that themselves act in producing some features of SLE.

In contrast to ANAs, a correlation with disease activity is often observed for antibodies to double-stranded DNA (anti-dsDNA) with SLE nephritis. Antibodies to dsDNA have been found to bind directly to renal structures. Other autoantibodies that have been linked more directly to disease pathogenesis are anti-SSA and -SSB antibodies (also known as anti-Ro and anti-La respectively). Considerable evidence suggests these antibodies can exert direct effects, binding to and damaging fetal cardiac tissue, resulting in congenital heart block in the offspring of women who carry antibodies to SSA and SSB.

The genetic contribution to SLE is well recognized. The λ_s (sibling risk divided by risk in the general population) is between 10 and 20.[52] Monozygotic twins have a concordance rate of 24-58%, whereas that of dizygotic twins is only 2-5%.[53] Overall studies indicate multiple susceptibility genes are contributory and disease modifying or protective genes likely also play a role.

HLA Associations with SLE

More than 25 years ago an association of SLE with HLA-DR2 and DR3 was first reported.[54] Since that time numerous reports in multiple populations confirmed this observation. In some Caucasian populations an increase of both DR2 and DR3 is found while in others only one or the other. Among Black patients in the U.S. an increase of DR3 and DR2 has also been found,[55] although not invariably.[56] Further studies conducted after DNA typing was instituted identified the two haplotypes associated with SLE as DRB1*03 along with DQA1*0501 and DQB1*0201,[57] particularly among Caucasians, and DRB1*1501 (encoding DR15 which is a "split" of DR2) along with DQA1*0102 and DQB1*0602.[58]

Determining the extent to which a specific HLA allele or a specific HLA locus confers susceptibility to SLE has been challenging due to strong linkage disequilibrium among HLA genes. The tendency for stretches of genes to be inherited "en bloc" also extends across the greater MHC region. Thus, for example, many Caucasians carry a haplotype encoding A1-Cw7-B8-TNFB*1-C2C-Bfs-C4AQ0-C4B1-DR3-DQ2.[52] Because of this it was initially thought that HLA-B8 was associated with SLE, although it later became apparent that the increase of B8 was due to linkage disequilibrium with DR3. Similarly, it has been difficult to determine whether the effect of other genes in the MHC, for example TNF, confer risk independent of the classical HLA genes.

It is worth noting that although significant associations have been reported in many different populations less than 50% of SLE patients have one or the other of these HLA molecules and the relative risk associated with DR3 and DR2 is modest, in the range of 2.0 to 3.0. Occasional modest protective effects have also been described, such as DRB1*04 in Japanese and B40 among Australians.[52] In contrast to other autoimmune diseases, there is no particular amino acid sequence that is encoded by both DRB1*15 and DRB1*03, nor by the DQA1 or DQB1 alleles in disequilibrium with either.

Complement

Substantial data implicates genes encoding complement components in SLE. Complement pathways mediate inflammatory responses contributing to both innate and adaptive immunity. The complement genes C2, C4A, C4B, and factor B are located on chromosome 6 within the MHC class III region. The complement deficiency with the strongest association to SLE is C1q, a complement component that participates in the clearance of apoptotic cells. In one study greater than 90% of individuals with complete C1q deficiency developed SLE.[59] The next strongest association to SLE is complete C4 deficiency. Complete C4 deficiency is comprised of four null alleles, two each of C4A and C4B, and, similar to homozygous C1q deficiency is rare. Approximately three-quarters of individuals with complete C4 deficiency develop SLE.[53] The C4A null allele is referred to as C4A*Q0 and is associated with SLE in virtually every population studied.[52] While C4A*Q0 is in linkage disequilibrium with the DRB1*03-B*08 haplotype, some studies have shown that this allele confers risk for SLE independent of its association with DRB1*03. The association between C4B*Q0 and SLE is not as great as that between C4A*Q0 and SLE. Finally, approximately 33% of individuals of European descent with complete C2 deficiency develop SLE. Complete C2 deficiency is more common than that of C1q or C4, but it confers a lower risk for SLE.

Non HLA Genes in Risk of SLE

The primary methods that have been used to search for genes involved in SLE have been linkage and asociation studies in families and case-control association studies. In murine studies, loci have been identified which contribute to murine lupus susceptibility and for which syntenic regions in the human genome might exist. Since the late 1990s at least six human whole genome and six targeted genome scans have been reported for SLE.[52,53] Studies have resulted in the identification of some genes predisposing to SLE that are found across different ethnic groups, while others appear to be limited to one population. According to the results of genome scans, the HLA region is significant but does not necessarily confer the greatest genetic risk of SLE.[53] Overall the studies indicate there may be additional nonMHC genes located on chromosomes 1q, 2q, 4p and 16q that contribute to SLE. Considered together, results of studies imply that SLE susceptibility is a result of the interactions of many genes.

A characteristic feature of SLE is tissue deposition of immune complexes consisting of antibodies complexed with antigens. Fcγ receptors bind the Fc region of IgG containing immune complexes (IC) and are found on the surfaces of mononuclear phagocytes. Inefficient or defective function of Fcγ receptors in clearing these complexes represents a pathway potentially contributing to SLE. There are three classes of Fcγ receptors encoded by chromosome 1q22-24: FcγR1, FcγRII, and FcγRIII.[52] The genes for FcγRIIA and FcγRIIIA have shown the greatest association with SLE, in addition to FcγRIIIB and FcγRIIB.

FcγRIIA has the allelic variations FcγRIIA-H131 with histidine and FcγRIIA-R131 with arginine at codon 131. R131 does not bind IgG2 as well as H131 and an initial report described an association with SLE for patients who were homozygous for the R131 genotype.[60] However, results were variable in other studies and in other ethnic groups.[52] FcγRIIIA (CD16) binds to IgG1 and IgG3, plays a role in cell death, and is expressed on mononuclear phagocytes, natural killer cells, and macrophages. SLE susceptibility has been associated with a T-G substitution at nucleotide 559 which results in a phenylalanine (F)-valine (V) substitution at amino acid 176. This particular amino acid is located in an important binding site, and F176/F176 homozygotes demonstrate a lower binding affinity for IgG than V176/V176 homozygotes. As a result, the clearance of IgG1 and IgG3 containing ICs is reduced in F176/F176 homozygotes and the risk of SLE is increased. An increase in F176/F176 has been observed in ethnically diverse populations.[61,52] The FcγRIIIB gene is expressed on neutrophils and the polymorphism NA1/NA2 has been implicated in SLE. In a study of Japanese the NA2 gene was over represented among patients with SLE, and the NA2/NA2 genotype was present in more than twice as many SLE patients as controls.[62] The NA2/NA2 genotype has a decreased efficiency of phagocytosis relative to the NA1/NA1 genotype. It has been hypothesized that FcγRIIb-NA1/2, FcγRIIB-I/T 232, and others may also play a role in SLE.[53] A recent report described an association of FcγRIIB-I/T 232 with SLE.[63] Further studies are needed to confirm this and other potential associations.

In a large study that included both Europeans and Mexicans another study of SLE described an association with PDCD1, a finding of special interest because PDCD1 is an inhibitory immunoreceptor that has a central role in peripheral tolerance.[64] Results from other studies point to a potential role for a number of other genes including angiotension converting enzyme FAS and FAS ligand, CTLA-4, and IL-10 but await confirmation and larger studies.[52,53]

References

1. In: Silman AJ, Hochberg MC, eds. Epidemiology of the Rheumatic Diseases. 2nd ed. Oxford: Oxford University Press, 2001.
2. Arnett FC, Edworthy SM, Bloch DA et al. The American Rheumatism Association 1987 revised criteria for the classification of rheumatoid arthritis. Arthritis Rheum 1988; 31(3):315-324.
3. MacGregor AJ, Snieder H, Rigby AS et al. Characterizing the quantitative genetic contribution to rheumatoid arthritis using data from twins. Arthritis Rheum 2000; 43:30-7.
4. Stastny P, Fink CW. HLA-Dw4 in adult and juvenile rheumatoid arthritis. Transplant Proc 1977; IX:1863-1866.
5. Harvey J, Lotze M, Arnett FC et al. Rheumatoid arthritis in a Chippewa band. II. Field study with clinical serologic and HLA-D correlations. J Rheumatol 1983; 10:28-32.
6. Sanchez B, Moreno I, Magarino R et al. HLA-DRw10 confers the highest susceptibility to rheumatoid arthritis in a Spanish population. Tissue Antigens 1990; 36:174-176.
7. Gregersen PK, Silver J, Winchester RJ. The shared epitope hypothesis. An approach to understanding the molecular genetics of susceptibility to rheumatoid arthritis. Arthritis Rheum 1987; 30:1205-1213.
8. Reveille JD. The genetic contribution to the pathogenesis of rheumatoid arthritis. Curr Opin Rheumatol 1998; 10:187-200.
9. Kochi Y, Yamada R, Kobayashi K et al. Analysis of single-nucelotide polymorphisms in Japanese rheumatoid arthritis patients shows additional susceptibility markers besides the classic shared epitope susceptibility sequences. Arthritis Rheum 2004; 50:63-71.
10. Nepom GT, Seyfried CE, Holbeck SL et al. Identification of HLA-Dw14 genes in DR4+ rheumatoid arthritis. Lancet 1986; 2:1002-1004.
11. Nelson JL, Mickelson EM, Masewicz SA et al. Dw14 (DRB1*0404) is a Dw4-dependent risk factor for rheumatoid arthritis. Tissue Antigens 1991; 38:145-151.

12. Wordsworth P, Pile KD, Buckely et al. HLA heterozygosity contributes to susceptibility to rheumatoid arthritis. Am J Hum Genet 1992; 51:585-91.
13. MacGregor A, Ollier W, Thomson W et al. HLA-DRB1*0401/0404 genotype and rheumatoid arthritis: Increased association in men, young age at onset, and disease severity. J Rheumatol 1995; 22:1032-6.
14. Gao X, Olsen NJ, Pincus T et al. HLA-DR alleles with naturally occurring amino acid substitutions and risk for development of rheumatoid arthritis. Arthritis Rheum 1990; 33:939-946.
15. Tsuchiya K, Kondo M, Kimura A et al. The DRB1 and/or the DQB1 locus controls susceptibility and DRB1 controls resistance to RA in the Japanese. HLA 1991. In: Tsuji K, Aizawa M, Sasazuki T, eds. New York: Oxford University Press, 1992; 2:509-512.
16. Meyer JM, Han J, Singh R et al. Sex influences on the penetrance of HLA shared-epitope genotypes for rheumatoid arthritis. Am J Hum Genet 1996; 58:371-83.
17. Jaraquemada D, Ollier W, Awad J et al. HLA and rheumatoid arthritis: A combined analysis of 440 British patients. Ann Rheum Dis 1986; 45:627-36.
18. Young A, Jaraquemada D, Awad J et al. Association of HLA-DR4/Dw4 and DR2/Dw2 with radiologic changes in a prospective study of patients with rheumatoid arthritis. Arthritis Rheum 1984; 27:20-5.
19. Weyand C, Hicok K, Conn D et al. The influence of HLA-DRB1 genes on disease severity in rheumatoid arthritis. Ann Int Med 1992; 117:801-6.
20. Weyand C, Xie C, Goronzy J. Homozygosity for the HLA-DRB1 allele selects for extraarticular manifestations in rheumatoid arthritis. J Clin Invest 1992; 89:2033-2039.
21. Zanelli E, Gonzalez-Gay MA, David CS. Could HLA-DRB1 be the protective locus in rheumatoid arthritis? Immunology Today 1995; 16:274-8.
22. Auger I, Escola J, Gorval et al. HLA-DR4 and HLA-DR10 motifs that carry susceptibility to rheumatoid arthritis bind 70-kD heat shock proteins. Nature Med 1996; 2:306-10.
23. Albani S, Keystone EC, Nelson JL et al. Positive selection in autoimmunity: Abnormal immune responses to a bacterial dnaJ antigenic determinant in patients with early rheumatoid arthritis. Nature Medicine 1995; 1:448-452.
24. Engelhard V. Structure of peptides associated with class I and class II MHC molecules. Annu Rev Immunol 1994; 12:181-207.
25. Nelson J, Hughes K, Smith A et al. Fetal HLA class II alloantigen disparity and the pregnancy induced amelioration of rheumatoid arthritis. N Engl J Med 1993; 329:466-71.
26. Shibue T, Tsuchiya N, Komata T et al. Tumor necrosis factor alpha 5'-flanking region, tumor necrosis factor receptor II, and HLA-DRB1 polymorphisms in Japanese patients with rheumatoid arthritis. Arthritis Rheum 2000; 43:753-7.
27. Jawaheer D, Li W, Graham RR et al. Dissecting the genetic complexity of the association between human leukocyte antigens and rheumatoid arthritis. Am J Hum Genet 2002; 71:585-594.
28. Nelson JL, Lambert NC, Brautbar C et al. The 13th International Histocompatibility Working Group For Rheumatoid Arthritis Joint Report. In: Hansen J, Dupont B, eds. HLA 2004: Immunobiology of the Human MHC. Proceedings of the 13th International Histocompatibility Workshop and Conference. Seattle, WA: IHWG Press, in press.
29. Hillarby MC, Hopkins J, Grennan DM. A reanalysis of the association between rheumatoid arthritis with and without extra-articular features, HLA-DR4, and DR4 subtypes. Tissue Antigens 1991; 37:39-41.
30. Fischer SA, Lanchbury JS, Lewis CM. Meta-analysis of four rheumatoid arthritis genome-wide linkage studies. Arthritis Rheum 2003; 48:1200-6.
31. Cornelis F, Faure S, Martinez M et al. New susceptibility locus for rheumatoid arthritis suggested by a genome-wide linkage study. Proc Natl Acad Sci USA 1998; 95:10746-50.
32. Mackay K, Eyre S, Myerscough A et al. Whole-genome linkage analysis of rheumatoid arthritis susceptibility loci in 252 affected sibling pairs in the United Kingdom. Arthritis Rheum 2002; 46:632-9.
33. Jawaheer D, Seldin MF, Amos CI et al. A genomewide screen in multiplex rheumatoid arthritis families suggests genetic overlap with other autoimmune diseases. Am J Hum Gen 2001; 68:927-36.
34. Shiozawa S, Hayashi S, Tsukamoto Y et al. Identification of the gene loci that predispose to rheumatoid arthritis. Internat Immunol 1998; 10:1891-5.
35. Suzuki A, Yamada R, Chang X et al. Functional haplotypes of PADI4, encoding citrullinating enzyme peptidylarginine deiminase 4, are associated with rheumatoid arthritis. Nat Genet 2003; 34:395-402.
36. Englert H, Small-McMahon J, Chambers P et al. Familial risk estimation on systemic sclerosis. Aus NZ J Med 1999; 29:36-41.
37. Johnson RW, Tew MB, Arnett FC. The genetics of systemic sclerosis. Curr Rheumatol Rep 2002; 4:99-107.

38. Takeuchi F, Nakano K, Yamada H et al. Association of HLA-DR with progressive systemic sclerosis in Japanese. J Rheum 1994; 21:857-863.
39. Arnett FC, Howard RF, Tan F et al. Increased prevalence of systemic sclerosis in a Native American tribe in Oklahoma. Association with an Amerindian HLA haplotype. Arthritis Rheum 1996; 39:1362-1370.
40. Lambert N, Distler O, Muller-Ladner U et al. HLA DQA1*0501 is associated with diffuse systemic sclerosis in men. Arthritis Rheum 2000; 43:2005-10.
41. Gilchrist FC, Bunn C, Foley PJ et al. Class II HLA associations with autoantibodies in scleroderma: A highly significant role for HLA-DP. Genes Immunity 2001; 2:76-81.
42. Fanning GC, Welsh KI, Bunn C et al. HLA associations in three mutually exclusive autoantibody subgroups in UK systemic sclerosis patients. Br J Rheumatol 1998; 37:201-7.
43. Reveille JD, Durban E, MacLeod-St.Clair M et al. Association of amino acid sequences in the HLA-DQB1 first domain with the antitopoisomerase I autoantibody response in scleroderma (progressive systemic sclerosis). J Clin Invest 1992; 90:973-980. (c)
44. Kuwana M, Kaburaki J, Okano Y et al. The HLA-DR and DQ genes control the autoimmune response to DNA topoisomerase I in systemic sclerosis (scleroderma). J Clin Invest 1993; 92:1296-1301.
45. Morel PA, Chang HJ, Wilson JW et al. Severe systemic sclerosis with anti-topoisomerase I antibodies is associated with an HLA-DRw11 allele. Hum Immunol 1994; 40:101-110.
46. Kuwana M, Okano Y, Kaburaki J et al. HLA class II genes associated with anticentromere antibody in Japanese patients with systemic sclerosis (scleroderma). Ann Rheum Dis 1995; 54:983-987.
47. Morel PA, Chang HJ, Wilson JW et al. HLA and ethnic associations among systemic sclerosis patients with anticentromere antibodies. Hum Immunol 1995; 42:35-42.
48. Reveille JD, Owerbach D, Goldstein R et al. Association of polar amino acids at position 26 of the HLA-DQB1 first domain with the anticentromere autoantibody response in systemic sclerosis (scleroderma). J Clin Invest 1992; 89:1208-1213.
49. Tan FK, Stivers DN, Foster MW et al. Association of microsatellite markers near the fibrillin 1 gene on human chromosome 15q with scleroderma in a Native American population. Arthritis Rheum 1998; 41:1729-1737.
50. Zhou X, Tan FK, Wang N et al. Genome-wide association study for regions of systemic sclerosis susceptibility in a Choctaw Indian population with high disease prevalence. Arthritis Rheum 2003; 48:2585-2592.
51. Hochberg MC. Updating the American College of Rheumatology revised criteria for the classification of systemic lupus erythematosus. Arthritis Rheum 1997; 40:1725-34.
52. Kelly JA et al. The genetics of systemic lupus erythematosus: Putting the pieces together. Genes and Immunity 2002; 3:S71-S85.
53. Tsao BP. The genetics of human systemic lupus erythematosus. Trends in Immunology 2003; 24(11):595-602.
54. Reisertson JL, Klippel JH, Johnson AH et al. B lymphocyte alloantigens associated with systemic lupus erythematosus. N Eng J Med 1978; 299:515-8.
55. Kachru RB, Sequire W, Mittal KK et al. A significant increase of HLA-DR3 and DR2 in SLE among blacks. J Rheumatol 1984; 11:471-4.
56. Howard PF, Hochberg MC, Bias WB et al. Relationship between C4A null genes, HLA-D region antigens and genetic susceptibility to SLE in Caucasian and Black Americans. Am J Med 1986; 81:187-93.
57. Skarsväg S, Hansen KE, Holst A et al. Distribution of HLA class II alleles among Scandinavian patients with systemic lupus erythematosus (SLE): An increase risk of SLE among non [DRB1*03,DQA1*0501,DQB1*0201] Class II homozygotes? Tissue Antigens 1992; 40:128-33.
58. Hashimoto H, Nishimura Y, Dong RP et al. HLA antigens in Japanese patients with systemic lupus erythematosus. Scan J Rheumatol 1994; 23:191-6.
59. Topaloglu R, Bakkaloglu A, Slingsby JH et al. Survey of Turkish systemic lupus erythematosus patients for a particular mutation of C1Q deficiency. Clin Exp Rheumatol 2000; 18:75-77.
60. Salmon JE, Edberg JC, Brogle NL et al. Allelic polymorphisms of human Fcγ.
61. Salmon JE, Ng S, Yoo DH et al. Altered distribution of Fc gamma receptor IIIA alleles in a cohort of Korean patients with lupus nephritis. Arthritis Rheum 1999; 42:818-819.
62. Hatta Y, Tsuchiya N, Ohashi J et al. Association of Fc gamma receptor IIIB, but not Fc gamma receptor IIA and IIIA, polymorphisms with systemic lupus erythematosus in Japanese. Genes Immun 1999; 1:53-60.
63. Kyogoku C et al. Fcγ receptor gene polymorphisms in Japanese patients with systemic lupus erythematosus: Contribution of FCGR2B to genetic susceptibility. Arthritis Rheum 2002; 46:1242-1254.
64. Prokunina L et al. A regulatory polymorphism in PDCD1 is associated with susceptibility to systemic lupus erythematosus in humans. Nat Get 2002; 32:666-9.

Chapter 7

Gastroenterologic and Hepatic Diseases

Marcela K. Tello-Ruiz, Emily C. Walsh and John D. Rioux

Overview and Introduction

Genes and Disease Risk

Celiac disease, autoimmune hepatitis (AIH), and the inflammatory bowel diseases (IBDs), Crohn's disease and ulcerative colitis (UC), are chronic inflammatory diseases of unknown etiology. They are considered complex genetic diseases because both inherited and environmental influences appear to be important in determining risk. Complex genetic diseases are more common than Mendelian diseases in the population. Prevalence ranges for AIH, IBD and celiac disease are given in Table 1. Generally, accepted average prevalences are 1 in 1,000 persons for Crohn's disease and UC, and 3 in 1,000 for celiac disease. However, the prevalence rate of Crohn's, UC and celiac disease are much lower in some populations (e.g., 1.25 in 100,000 for Crohn's disease in Hong Kong[1]). The average prevalence of AIH is 10-fold lower at 1 in 10,000.

Some effort has been devoted to understanding the relative contribution of environmental and genetic factors to disease risk. One method for ascertaining the genetic component of a disease is to compute the risk to siblings divided by the population risk (λs). Mendelian genetic diseases have extremely high λs values (λs = 500 for cystic fibrosis), while diseases with weaker genetic components have lower values (λs = 2 for hypertension). Crohn's disease, UC, and celiac disease have sibling relative risks that are higher than most complex traits (shown in Table 1). The risk to any first-degree family member for Crohn's disease is 10-32 fold higher than in the general population; for UC it is 5-12 fold, and for celiac disease it is 20-53 fold.[2,3] Familial risk has not been reported in AIH, perhaps due to its lower prevalence. Notably, both celiac disease and AIH more commonly affect women (Table 1), suggesting that sex steroids or other female-specific factors may play a role in the etiology of these diseases.

In this chapter, we address the etiology of each disease by first providing a summary of the known environmental influences, and then reviewing the genetic studies aimed at the identification of susceptibility loci. One of the genetic loci we will give attention to is the major histocompatibility complex (MHC). The MHC is home to over 140 genes, including the eight highly variable classical human leukocyte antigen (HLA) loci. HLA genes encode cell surface molecules that present antigenic peptides to T cells, thereby initiating acquired immune response to invading pathogens and other foreign antigens. T cells determine whether antigens are "self" or "nonself" based on the specific antigenic peptide sequence as well as the HLA variant that presents the peptide. Given their central role in self/nonself distinction, associations between autoimmune diseases and variation in the classical HLA genes are among the most consistent findings in human genetics.[4] The relative contribution of the MHC to disease risk for celiac disease, Crohn's disease, and UC can be determined by assessing the sibling risk based on MHC haplotype sharing (MHC λs). The ratio of the MHC λs value to the λs implies the

Immunogenetics of Autoimmune Disease, edited by Jorge Oksenberg and David Brassat.

Table 1. Epidemiologic and genetic data for IBD, celiac disease and AIH

Disease	Prevalence (per 100,000)	Sibling Risk (λs)	MHC λs	Sex Ratio (Female:Male)	References
Crohn's disease	1-199	16-32	1.3	1:1	1, 2, 5, 6
UC	5-268	12	8.3	1:1	1, 2, 5, 6
Celiac disease	147-3,000*	20-53	2.3-4.6	2:1	7-10
AIH	4-43	ND	ND	2-11:1	11-14

λs = prevalence in siblings/prevalence in the general population; MHC λs = prevalence in MHC identical siblings/prevalence in the general population.[15] ND, not determined. *Includes only those studies where the initial diagnosis was confirmed by biopsy.

degree to which non-MHC genes are involved in the risk to disease. We see that the non-MHC component is larger for Crohn's disease and UC risk is associated more with the MHC.

Complex Trait Genetics

Genetic studies fall into two main categories: linkage studies and association tests. Linkage studies, which are most often performed on a genomewide scale, seek to identify genomic regions (linkage peaks) with increased allele sharing between affected family members. These peaks may be interpreted as large regions where causal variation may lie. Association testing aims to determine whether statistically significant correlation exists between a particular allele and a given phenotype.

Genomewide linkage studies have the benefit of assessing the entire genome in an unbiased manner. A linkage peak is considered suggestive evidence when it is expected to occur by chance about once per genome scan, and becomes significant when this expectation decreases to once per 20 scans.[16] Confirmed linkage is only achieved after significant linkage in one study is replicated in a second independent study. Because replication involves one or a small number of tests, and is derived from prior evidence of linkage in a genomic scan, a modest threshold is sufficient (e.g., $p < 0.05$ for a single test). However, extremely large study sizes and dense coverage are required for linkage studies to obtain the statistical power necessary for identifying loci of modest effect. One approach to increase statistical power is through meta-analyses of multiple linkage studies. We will review the meta-analyses that have recently been performed for Crohn's and celiac disease later in the chapter.

Association studies are more powerful than linkage studies at assessing the role of a particular genomic region in disease. It is difficult to perform association studies in a genomewide manner due to the current costs of genotyping. However, the recent finding that the human genome is organized in "haplotype blocks" of relatively low diversity[17,18] is reducing the effort required to thoroughly test large regions for association to disease. Haplotype blocks are regions in the human genome (extending from 1-2 to > 100 kb) within which the underlying genetic variation exists in linkage disequilibrium and little recombination has occurred.[17-19] Approximately 90% of the genetic variation observed in human chromosomes can be parsed into only 3-5 common patterns of variation, or haplotypes, per block. As a result of this genomic structure, the common haplotypes within a block can be identified with a subset of variants or haplotype tagging SNPs (htSNPs).[18] Consequently, these haplotype frameworks offer a reduction in genotyping costs and an increase in statistical power of association studies because not every SNP in a particular haplotype block needs to be tested. Instead, a few haplotype-identifying SNPs can be employed to test all the variation at any given block for association to disease.

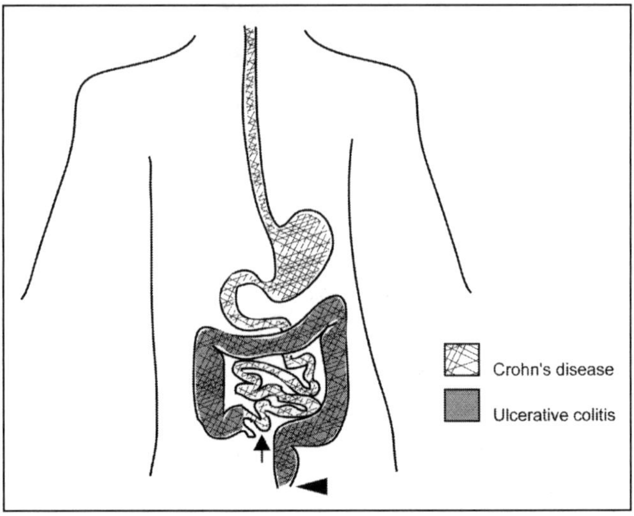

Figure 1. Localization of Crohn's disease and ulcerative colitis in the gastrointestinal tract. Ulcerative colitis tissue damage usually begins at the rectum (arrowhead) and continues proximally in a continuous fashion throughout the colon (indicated in gray). The discontinuous tissue damage found in Crohn's patients can involve any part of the gastrointestinal tract from mouth to anus (indicated by hatches). However, damage is frequently localized to the terminal ileum (arrow) and colon (gray).

An international effort—the International HapMap Project—aims to identify the haplotype structure of the entire human genome (http://www.hapmap.org).[20] The completion of this haplotype map holds great promise for future genetic studies of human complex traits. After we discuss the current state of the field for IBD, celiac disease and AIH, we will return to the role that the HapMap Project and other genetic advances will play in the future of these diseases.

Inflammatory Bowel Diseases

Definition, Classification and Symptoms

Inflammatory bowel diseases are characterized by chronic relapsing inflammation of the gastrointestinal tract. Crohn's disease (MIM 266600) and ulcerative colitis (MIM 191390) are the two main subtypes of IBD. Crohn's disease most frequently manifests itself with abdominal pain and diarrhea and is often complicated by intestinal fistulization (an abnormal passage between an injured organ and a healthy organ), intestinal obstruction or both. Tissue damage in Crohn's patients may involve any part of the gastrointestinal tract but is frequently localized to the terminal ileum and/or colon (Fig. 1); inflammation is transmural and discontinuous and may contain granulomas.[21] The major symptoms of ulcerative colitis (UC) include diarrhea, rectal bleeding, the passage of mucus and abdominal pain. Inflammation in UC patients is continuous and limited to the rectal and colonic mucosal layers (Fig. 1); no fistulas and granulomas are observed.[22] Approximately 5-10% of IBD cases cannot be unequivocally assigned to Crohn's disease or UC and so are diagnosed with indeterminate colitis (IC). IC is often a temporary classification until a final diagnosis can be made. In two independent prospective studies, 32-50% of IC patients were classified as having either Crohn's disease or UC at follow-up that ranged from 1 month to 26 years after the diagnosis of IC.[23,24]

Autoimmune Features

Whether Crohn's disease and UC are true autoimmune disorders is an open question, although production of autoantibodies is observed in IBD patients. Sources of the targeted autoantigens include the colon, DNA, thyroglobulin, tropomyosin, smooth muscle, gastric parietal cell, erythrocyte, pancreas, and neutrophil cytoplasm (i.e., anti-neutrophil cytoplasmic antibodies or ANCA).[25] Production of anti-colonic, anti-tropomyosin and ANCA is observed more often in UC than in Crohn's disease; however, not all patients are seropositive. Moreover, none of these autoantibodies has been shown to directly cause gut inflammation. Therefore, whether they are central to disease pathogenesis remains to be established. An alternate hypothesis is that IBD is an immune reaction to antigens in the intestinal microflora. We will revisit this possibility when we discuss the association between Crohn's disease and the *caspase recruitment domain-15* (*CARD15*) gene below.

Epidemiology: Inheritance and Environment

The combined prevalence of all IBD diseases is estimated to affect about 1 per 1,000 individuals. The incidence of IBD has been suggested to be highest in developed industrialized countries, but few studies have been done in developing countries. IBDs are most prevalent in Ashkenazi Jews and are rare in Asian and Hispano-American populations.[1,5] Despite conflicting data on the prevalence of IBD among African-Americans, there has been a steady increase in reported cases among this ethnic group.[5] Overall, the prevalence and incidence of IBD, and Crohn's disease in particular, seem to have increased significantly in the last few decades.[5]

Genetic determinants are important in both UC and Crohn's disease. The range for the estimated familial recurrence among patients with IBD is 5-30%, and the risk to first-degree relatives of affected individuals is estimated to be 5-32 fold.[2,26] Moreover, the concordance rate in monozygotic twins compared with dizygotic twins is significantly greater for both Crohn's disease (58-63% vs 0-4%) and UC (18-19% vs 0-5%),[27,28] establishing a stronger genetic influence in Crohn's than in UC.

The environmental factor most convincingly associated with IBD is smoking. Smoking increases the risk for Crohn's disease by a factor of 2-5 fold and decreases the risk for UC by a similar magnitude.[29,30] Nicotine is speculated to be the principal component responsible for this effect, possibly via the dysregulation of the T-helper (Th) immune response pathways. Th1 cells activate cellular immunity to fight viruses and other intracellular pathogens, eliminate cancerous cells, and stimulate delayed-type hypersensitivity skin reactions, resulting in inflammatory response. In contrast, Th2 cells induce humoral and allergic responses, up-regulate antibody production to fight extracellular organisms, and suppress inflammation. In vivo, nicotine inhibits Th2 in nonadherent mononuclear cells of healthy nonsmokers undergoing nicotine patch treatment, perhaps explaining the increased Crohn's disease risk as Crohn's phenotypes are thought to be Th1 mediated.[31] Conversely, UC protection may result from a mucin deficiency that smoking acts to reverse.[32] Studies showed that nicotine significantly increased mucin synthesis in colonic cultured epithelial biopsies from both UC patients and control individuals,[33] and inhibited the synthesis of the pro-inflammatory cytokines IL-1β and TNFα in the mouse colonic mucosa.[34] In addition, nicotine was found to reduce circular colonic smooth muscle activity, which appears to be up-regulated in active UC.[35] Finally, clinical trials have shown nicotine to be of some benefit in UC;[36] however, further research is required to establish its therapeutic role and the mechanisms responsible for its action.

There is little correlation of dietary habits with IBD, in contrast with celiac disease (discussed later). High consumption of refined sugar and little dietary fiber seems to increase the risk for IBD;[37,38] similarly, zinc deficiency in Crohn's disease patients is associated with an increased absorption dysfunction.[39] Diet may affect disease susceptibility by modulating the intestinal permeability or the intestinal flora milieu, and this possibility is the underlying principle for prebiotics therapy. Prebiotics are nondigestible edibles that are proposed to selectively stimulate the growth and activity of beneficial gut bacteria. Prebiotics currently under study for treatment of IBD include lactosucrose, oligofructose, inulin, bran, psyllium, and germinated barley.[40]

Table 2. Summary of IBD susceptibility loci

Locus	Chromosomal Region	Disease Specificity	Variation Identified	References
IBD1	16q12	Crohn's specific	*CARD15* gene	41,42,59,60
IBD2	12p	Possibly UC-specific	No	43
IBD3	6p	IBD	Potential HLA alleles	46,48
IBD4	14q11-12	Possibly Crohn's specific	No	61
IBD5	5q31	IBD	250-kb haplotype allele	48,62
IBD6	19p13	IBD	No	48
IBD7	1p36	IBD	No	44
IBD8	16p	IBD	No	46

Genetics

Linkage Studies

Seven genomewide scans and several targeted scans in families with Crohn's disease and/or UC have identified eight regions potentially conferring susceptibility to IBD (Table 2). The first genomewide search in Crohn's disease reported a potential locus in the pericentromeric region of chromosome 16 (LOD score = 5.79).[41] This locus (*IBD1*) was also the first replicated through pooling genotype data from over 600 families collected by 11 centers distributed throughout North America, Europe, and Australia.[42] This supports the hypothesis that common diseases can be explained by genetic risk factors that are common to many populations, but exist at different frequencies.

Potential IBD susceptibility loci identified through genome scans are localized on chromosomes 3p, 7 and 12;[43] 5q35, 14q11, and 17q21;[45] 1, 6, 10, 22, and X;[46] 14q11;[47] and 3p, 6p, 5q31, and 19p13.[48] Some of the reported loci were replicated in follow-up studies, but no one locus was identified in every study.[49-57] This apparent lack of consistency can be explained by the modest effect of most genetic loci in complex human traits and by the modest power and significant effect of sampling variance on linkage results in a single cohort. Nonetheless, a recent meta-analysis of data from nearly 500 Crohn's families and five genomewide scans identified five top-ranking Crohn's loci: *IBD1* (16q12), *IBD5* (5q31), *IBD3* (MHC), *IBD2* (12p), and *IBD6* (19p13).[58]

While causal variation was identified under the *IBD1* and *IBD5* linkage peaks (discussed below), the etiological alleles underlying the other loci have yet to be identified. This is likely because many of the remaining linkage peaks have not yet experienced the same level of scrutiny as *IBD1* and *IBD5*. Extensive analysis of the MHC locus on 6p has been performed, but no consistent association with disease has been found, in spite of the fact that the attention given to the MHC is similar to that in other diseases where clear associations have been defined (e.g., multiple sclerosis, systemic lupus, type 1 diabetes).

Association: MHC Genes

The interest in the MHC region of 6p resulted in ~100 association studies that examined the role of specific MHC variation in UC and Crohn's disease. Yet, with the exception of studies in Japanese UC patients, no single gene or allele has emerged as consistently associated with disease (ECW, personal communication and ref. 68). All five Japanese studies found statistically significant positive associations between UC and either DRB1*1502 or the DR2 serotype that includes this variant.[63-67] However, the DRB1*1502 allele is not found in high frequency in Caucasians. This observation may suggest genetic heterogeneity between Caucasian and Japanese populations. Another possibility is that DRB1 is not causal and that the association reflects a common causal variant that is in linkage disequilibrium with different alleles in these two populations.

Association: Non-MHC Genes

CARD15

Parallel studies using positional mapping[59] and candidate gene analysis[60] allowed the identification of the underlying genetic variation associated with Crohn's disease at the *IBD1* (16q12) locus. Strong association of three variants in *CARD15* (previously known as *NOD2*) is observed in Crohn's patients of European descent.[59,60,69-72] Two of the three variants are missense mutations (Arg702Trp and Gly908Arg) and one is a frameshift mutation resulting in early truncation of the CARD15 protein (Leu1007fsinsC). The genotype relative risk (GRR) for heterozygotes of any of the three variants is ~2-6 fold, while homozygotes and compound heterozygotes have a GRR of >20 fold.[73] These mutations are found at an appreciable frequency in European-derived Crohn's cohorts where between 30-40% of all individuals have at least one copy of one of these three variants compared with 1-7% of control individuals.[74] Interestingly, these variants are very rare in the Japanese, Chinese and Korean populations, possibly explaining the decreased disease prevalence in these populations.[72,75-78]

CARD15 belongs to a large family of genes involved in the innate immune response.[79] Members of this family are also orthologues of defense genes found in a wealth of species, including plants. Specifically, CARD proteins bear sequence similarity to plant disease resistance proteins (R proteins) that detect pathogens and initiate defense mechanisms, including MAP kinase activation, oxygen radical formation, salicylate production, induced transcription of kinases and transcription factors, and rapid cell death.[80] One potential function of *CARD15* is as a similar interface between pathogens and the human immune system, thus raising the possibility that Crohn's is not autoimmune per se, but rather the result of an abnormal immune response triggered by gut pathogens.

In addition to its expression in peripheral blood monocytes, *CARD15* mRNA is found in primary intestinal cells,[81] and specifically detected in terminal ileum Paneth cells.[82] Overexpression of wild-type *CARD15* in intestinal epithelial cells reduces bacterial survival, possibly serving as a key component of the innate mucosal responses to luminal bacteria, while the *3020insC* truncation variant fails to exhibit such antibacterial properties.[81] Interestingly, both *CARD15* mRNA and protein are up-regulated by TNFα in colonic epithelial cell lines.[81] Further understanding of *CARD15* function may help reveal an aspect of the underlying etiology of Crohn's disease and clarify whether this disease is the result of a pathogenic immune reaction to antigens derived from the intestinal microflora.

IBD5

Substantial effort was invested in the identification of causal variation at the *IBD5* locus.[62] This effort represents the first successful mapping of a susceptibility locus for a complex genetic disease based on haplotype analysis. Reiterative mapping with a large number of microsatellite markers allowed the definition of a 500-kb critical region. Thorough mutation screening of the genes in the region revealed no likely causal sequence variants, so a comprehensive sequence analysis of the entire critical region was performed (eight individuals sequenced for 470 kb). In this study, 301 of the 651 single nucleotide polymorphisms (SNPs) discovered were typed in Crohn's simplex families. Analysis of these data led to the discovery of a block-like haplotype structure of the genome that was reviewed in the introduction of this chapter.[17,18] A single risk haplotype (transmission ratio = 2.5:1) was identified with a frequency of 37% in controls and 75% in Crohn's patients. Current simulations show that the disease locus has a 90% probability of being within a 250-kb region where the relative risk to developing Crohn's disease is ~2.[82a] SNPs that are unique to this overtransmitted haplotype have been shown to be associated with disease in four independent studies.[83-86] Once this finding has been confirmed extensively through replication, the challenge is to demonstrate the functionality that is relevant for IBD pathogenesis and is perturbed in individuals bearing the mutated haplotype.

Candidate Genes

Additional association studies have examined gene candidates that were chosen based on their relevant immunological function. A small number of variants in these genes have been examined in multiple studies. For example, positive association was observed for identical variants of the *DNA mismatch repair* (*MLH1*) gene by two independent groups.[87,88] Conversely, seemingly significant disease associations have been challenged by subsequent studies, including those with the *CD11* gene cluster,[89,90] *interleukin 1 receptor antagonist* (*IL-1RN*),[91-104] *IL-1B*,[92,96,98,103] *IL-4R*,[90,105,106] *IL-10*,[107,108] *immunoglobulin* (*Ig*) *G1 heavy chain* (*Gm*),[109,110] *vitamin D receptor* (*VDR*),[111,112] and *intercellular adhesion molecule-1* (*ICAM-1*).[113-116]

The association with the C3435T polymorphism in the *multi-drug resistance-1* (*MDR1*) gene identifies important caveats for the interpretation of genetic association results, therefore we discuss it in some detail. *MDR1* is an interesting candidate gene since *MDR1* knockout mice spontaneously develop colitis due to an intestinal epithelial barrier dysfunction[117] (Table 3). The C3435T polymorphism was first associated with UC in a German cohort,[118] but four independent cohorts of German, English, Greek or North American origin[119-121] could not replicate the finding (the significance of the association seen in a fifth Caucasian cohort depended on the choice of control group[122]). C3435T is in strong linkage disequilibrium with a second polymorphism (Ala893Ser/Thr),[123] which was associated with IBD in a North American cohort.[120] Therefore, some of the controversy may reflect population differences in haplotype structure at the *MDR1* locus. Further studies are necessary to fully delineate the *MDR1* haplotype structure and whether any variation at this locus influences risk to IBD.

Preliminary associations to IBD, for which replication has not yet been reported, include *NRAMP-1*,[124] *IL-4*,[106] *IL-11*,[125] *IL-16*,[126] *Factor V* (Leiden mutation),[127] *microsomal epoxide hydrolase*,[128] *kinin receptor* β*1*,[129] *manose-binding lectin* (*MBL*),[130] *mucin-3*,[131] *epidermal growth factor receptor* (*EGFR*),[112] and *NF*κ*B*.[132] Preliminary studies for other genes show no association with IBD risk, including *Ig superfamily 6*,[133] *prothrombin G20210A*,[134] *IL-12*β,[135] *IL-25*,[136] *interferon-*γ,[137] *chemokine receptor 5*,[103,138] *NRAMP-2*,[96] β*7 integrin*,[139] *CTLA-4*,[140] *CARD4/NOD1*,[141] and *STAT6*.[90] However, only after the existing variation has been thoroughly sampled should a gene be confidently excluded as a susceptibility candidate.

Genotype-Phenotype and Genotype-Genotype Interactions

The identification of causal variation is by no means the end of the genetic investigation. Subsequent studies are necessary to determine whether specific variants preferentially influence discrete disease subphenotypes. In the case of IBD, *CARD15* variants are associated with ileal disease localization,[42,69,71,73,74,142-145] fibrostenosis,[146,147] and fistulization.[147] In addition, *CARD15* variation may explain the opposite effects of smoking—which promotes Crohn's disease but prevents UC[29,30]—since the risk for ileal disease was found to be increased in Crohn's disease patients with a smoking history.[144]

Moreover, as complex genetic diseases are thought to be the synthesis of positively and negatively acting variation, one must determine whether a causal variant influences disease independently or synergistically. For example, once identified, *IBD5* and *CARD15* variation could be assessed for interaction. In multiple studies, these variants seem to independently influence risk for Crohn's disease.[83-86] Linkage analyses stratified on genotype have provided additional insight into genotype-genotype interactions. *CARD15*-stratified genomewide scans identified suggestive linkage at 6p and 10p,[56] implicating specific interaction between these loci. Similarly, stratification by *CARD15* and *IBD5* variation together demonstrated linkage to chromosomes 3 and X.[57] However, much more analysis is needed to fully understand the relationship between these two variants and disease.

Table 3. Animal models for IBD

	Organism	Notes on Phenotype	Refs.
Spontaneous Mutations			
Cotton top tamarin	Monkey	Spontaneous colitis	156
C3H/HeJBir substrain	Mouse	Spontaneous colitis	157
SAMP1/Yit	Mouse	Th1-mediated spontaneous ileitis	158,159
Chemical Induction (Intramural Injection/Enema)			
TNBS or DNBS	Rat and mouse	Colitis	160
Oxazolone	Mouse	Th2-mediated spontaneous ileitis	161
Acetic acid	Rat	Diffuse colitis	162
Peptidoglycan polysaccharide	Rat	Colitis	163
Immune complex	Rabbit	Colitis	164
Chemical Induction (Oral Administration)			
Carrageenan	Guinea pig	UC-like phenotype	165
DSS	Mouse	UC-like phenotype	166
Indomethacin	Dog	UC-like phenotype	167
Cyclosporin A	Mouse	Colitis with autoimmune features	168
Iodoacetamide	Rat	CD-like phenotype	169
Microbial Infection			
Chlamydia trachomatis	Monkey	Lymphogranuloma venereum-induced proctitis	170
Helicobacter bilis	Mouse	Immune-mediated and intestinal flora-dependent colitis	171
H. hepaticus	Mouse	Immune-mediated and intestinal flora-dependent colitis	172
Genetically Engineered (Transgenic)			
HLA-B27/β2-microglobulin	Rat	Spontaneous and systemic inflammation	173
IL-7 with SR promoter	Mouse	Increased effector T-cell responses	174
N-cadherin dominant negative	Mouse	Intestinal epithelial barrier dysfunction	175
Gp39 overexpression	Mouse	Thymus dysfunction-mediated tissue inflammation	176
HSV-thymidine kinase (astroglial GFAP-specific promoter)	Mouse	Fulminant and fatal jejuno-ileitis	177
TGF-RII dominant negative (epithelium-specific promoter)	Mouse	Regulatory T-cell defects	178

Table continued on next page

Animal Models

Numerous animal models of colitis have been examined, however none precisely recapitulates the chronic and relapsing expression of IBD. These models can be classified by five categories: spontaneously occurring, induced by microbial infection, cell transfer, chemically induced, and genetically engineered models (Table 3). Each of these models gives special insight into the specific pathways that may play roles in human disease. On one hand, evidence from cell

Table 3. Continued

	Organism	Notes on Phenotype	Refs.
Genetically Engineered (Knockout)			
TGFβ-1	Mouse	Regulatory T-cell defects	179
Stat3	Mouse	Th1-mediated enterocolitis	180
Stat4	Mouse	Increased effector T-cell responses	181
ITF	Mouse	Intestinal epithelial barrier dysfunction	182
IL-2	Mouse	Regulatory T-cell defects	183
IL-2R	Mouse	Regulatory T-cell defects	184
IL-10	Mouse	Regulatory T-cell defects	185
TNF^{ARE}	Mouse	Increased effector T-cell responses	186
NFκB	Mouse	Increased effector T-cell responses	187
TCRα	Mouse	Increased effector T-cell responses	152
TCRβ	Mouse	Spontaneous UC-like colitis	152
TCRβ x TCRδ	Mouse	Spontaneous UC-like colitis	152
MHCII	Mouse	Spontaneous UC-like colitis	152
Gαi2	Mouse	Increased effector T-cell responses	188
Keratin-8	Mouse	Colorectal hyperpasia and intestinal inflammation	189
Mdr1α	Mouse	Intestinal epithelial barrier dysfunction	117
CRF2-4	Mouse	Regulatory T-cell defects	190
WASP	Mouse	Defects in T-cell responses	191
Cell Transfer			
CD45RB-high cells into SCID mice	Mouse	Defective induction of regulatory T-cells	192
CD45RB cells transfer into Tgε26	Mouse	Defective induction of regulatory T-cells	193
Hsp60-reactive CD8+ T-cells	Mouse	Increased effector T-cell responses	194

DNBS: 2,4-trinitrobenzensulfonic acid; TNBS: 2,4,6-trinitrobenzensulfonic acid; DSS: dextran sodium sulphate

transfer models suggests that the observed inflammatory response is actively inhibited by CD4+ regulatory T-cells and immunosuppressive cytokines such as *IL-10* and *TGFβ1*.[148] Chemically induced models, on the other hand, have identified cytokines that may lessen disease symptoms. Specifically, DNBS-induced colitis can be prevented by *IL-10* gene transfer[149] and TNBS-induced colitis can be ameliorated by *IL-4*[150] or anti-*IL-12* antibodies.[151] Lastly, genetically engineered models have demonstrated that while disruption of both the Th1 and Th2 pathways induces colitis, there are differences in the inflammatory response that mimic the differences observed between Crohn's and UC. By example, *TCRα* knockout mice exhibit colitis that shares many features with UC, including dominant Th2 response in the colonic inflammation.[152] Intriguingly, in many of these genetic models, inflammation did not develop if the mice were maintained in germ-free conditions, suggesting that the disease symptoms are an abnormal inflammatory response to components of the intestinal flora.

It is worth mentioning that, despite the association of *CARD15* variants and human disease, mice bearing a targeted deletion of the CARD domains of this gene showed no signs of intestinal pathology.[153] One possible explanation for this lack of phenotype is functional overlap with another murine CARD domain protein (NOD1) also involved in bacterial recognition.[154,155] Regardless, the lack of intestinal phenotype in the *CARD15*-deficient mice

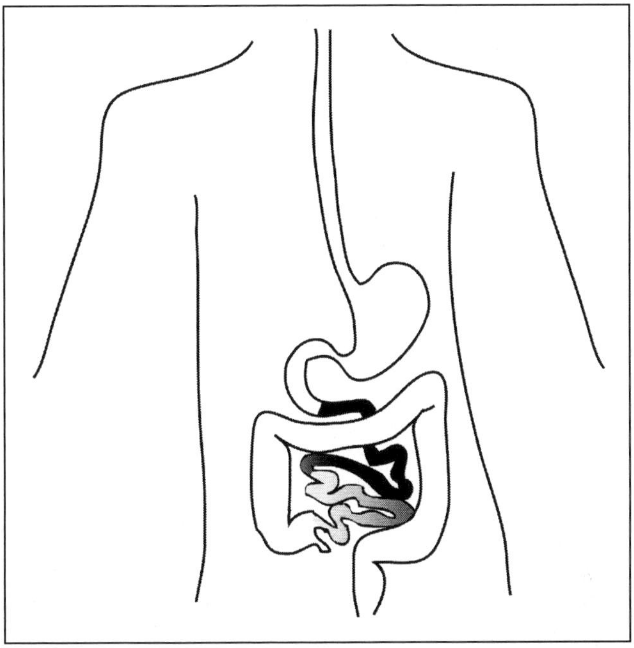

Figure 2. Localization of celiac disease in the gastrointestinal tract. Tissue damage in celiac disease affects the mucosa of the proximal small intestine with damage gradually decreasing in severity distally (indicated by decreasing grayscale). In severe cases, damage continues to the terminal ileum.

illustrates that IBD is a complex disease resulting from a combinatorial effect of multiple genetic variants and environmental factors.

Celiac Disease

Definition, Classification and Symptoms

Celiac disease (also known as celiac sprue or gluten-sensitive enteropathy; MIM 212750) is a chronic gastrointestinal disease in which exposure to proteins from wheat, rye, barley and possibly oats leads to villous atrophy in the small intestine and consequent nutrient malabsorption. In wheat, such proteins are collectively known as gliadins and constitute the toxic component of gluten. Symptoms include diarrhea, general weakness, anemia and weight loss. The disease affects the mucosa of the proximal small intestine with damage gradually decreasing in severity distally (Fig. 2). However, in severe cases, the lesions extend to the ileum. Diagnosis of the disease is ultimately confirmed by small intestinal biopsy showing a flat mucosa that is reversed on a gluten-free diet.[195]

Autoimmune Features

In the past 6 years, valuable discoveries were made with respect to celiac disease mechanism; however, many questions remain. Deamidation of the gliadin component of gluten[196] and its resultant aggregation in the gut is thought to be an important disease trigger.[197,198] Deamidation is required for HLA-DQ2 and HLA-DQ8 presentation.[199-201] Recognition of the gliadin/HLA complex by T-cells leads to, among other consequences, the production of anti-gliadin antibodies. These anti-gliadin antibodies are indicators of the disease; however, they are not detected in all celiac cases.[198] Rather, the presence of autoantibodies targeting various submucosal connective tissue (endomysium) antigens is the most accurate serological marker for celiac disease.[198] Recently, antibodies to tissue transglutaminase (tTG) were identified as a major component of these anti-endomysial antibodies.[202] Presence of these anti-tTG specific antibodies is also an accurate diagnostic measure of disease (95-100% sensitivity; 94-97% specificity).[203-205]

Normally an intracellular enzyme, it appears tTG is released by cells upon wounding. Intriguingly, such extracellular calcium-dependent tTG was shown to be sufficient to catalyze gluten deamidation.[200] Moreover, it was shown through immunoprecipitation that tTG is more abundant in gliadin complexes in the duodenal mucosa of celiac patients compared with controls.[198] While unlikely to be coincidental given the serological characteristics of celiac disease, a direct connection between these observations has not yet been defined. It remains to be determined whether anti-tTG antibodies are actually causal in the flattening of the intestinal mucosa (i.e., whether celiac disease is truly autoimmune). Future studies should aim to dissect the mechanism by which gluten, tTG, and the immune system conspire to cause celiac disease.

Epidemiology: Inheritance and Environment

Using data from post-biopsy confirmed celiac cases, the estimated prevalence for celiac disease ranges from 147-3,000 per 100,000 individuals, including reports in North and South American, European, Indian, Arab, and South Asian populations (Table 1). There is a slight predominance of celiac disease in females. The risk for first-degree relatives to manifest the disease ranges from 5-20%.[3] The concordance rate for HLA-identical siblings is 30%[206] while that of monozygous twins is 70-86%,[207] suggesting that the contribution of nonHLA risk factors in the etiology of this disease is substantial. As mentioned above, the main environmental etiological factor for celiac disease is wheat gluten.

Genetics

Linkage Studies

Genomewide searches for genetic risk factors have identified numerous putative loci (Table 4). Confirmed linkage of the MHC region (*CELIAC 1*) in celiac disease exists).[10,208-214] In addition, significant linkage was shown for four non-MHC regions: 5q31-33 (*CELIAC 2*),[213] 2q23-33 (*CELIAC 3*),[214] 19p13 (*CELIAC 4*),[10] and 15q12.[215] These findings need to be confirmed by replication in independent data sets. Unlike for IBD, no genes have been identified for linkage studies for celiac disease.

Association: MHC Genes

Consistent with their ability to present epitopes from deamidated gluten molecules, susceptibility to celiac disease is associated primarily with HLA-DQ2 and HLA-DQ8.[228] Association has also been reported with various DR serotypes, including DR3, DR5, and DR7,[229-233] as well as variation in *tumor necrosis factor-α* (*TNFα*),[234-238] *heat-shock protein 70* (*HSP70-1* and *HSP70-2*),[239,240] *inhibitor of κB-like* (*IKBL*),[241] and the *MHC class I chain-related* (*MICA*) genes.[242,243] However, recent studies suggest that these variants are simply in linkage disequilibrium with the causal variation.[244]

Association: Non-MHC Genes

The power of a study to definitively exclude a locus of a particular strength of effect depends on two things: sample size and marker coverage. Thus, negative association studies must be interpreted cautiously since it is difficult to exclude a locus absolutely. For celiac disease, a number of genes have been reported as unassociated at various levels of statistical significance: T-cell receptors genes *TCRα, TCRβ, TCRγ, TCRδ*,[245] *nitride oxide synthase* (*NOS*),[246] matrix metalloproteinase genes *MMP-1* and *MMP-3*,[247] *IL-12B*,[248,249] *interferon regulatory factor 1* (*IRF1*),[249] *insulin* (*INS*),[250] and *tissue transglutaminase* (*TGM2*).[251,252] However, positive evidence for association has been observed for genes encoding Ig Gm allotypes,[253] *cytotoxic*

Table 4. Summary of celiac disease genetic linkage studies

Genetic Study	Suggestive Linkage*	Significant Linkage*	References
Genomewide scan	6p21,6p23, 11p11	NS	208
Genomewide scan	5qter	6p21	209
Genomewide scan	NS	NS	216
Genomewide scan	NS	6p	210
Genomewide scan	4p15	6p21	212
Genomewide scan	NS	15q12	215
Genomewide scan	NS	NS	217
Genomewide scan	3p26, 5p21, 18q23	NS	218
Genomewide scan	6q21-22	6p, 19p13	10
Genomewide scan	10p	2q23-32, 6p	214
Meta and pooled linkage analysis	NS	5q31-33, 6p21	213
Targeted scan	NS	NS	219
Targeted scan	CTLA-4/CD28	NS	220
Targeted scan	NS	NS	221
Targeted scan	NS	NS	222
Targeted scan	NS	NS	223
Targeted scan	5q32	NS	224
Targeted scan	11p11, 6p12	NS	225
Targeted scan	NS	6p	211
Targeted scan	NS	NS	226
Targeted scan (pooled)	CTLA-4/CD28	NS	227

* Suggestive and significant linkage established according to criteria proposed in ref. 16; NS indicates that the indicated genomewide threshold was not reached.

T-lymphocyte associated antigen 4 (*CTLA-4*; D2S2216,[220] D2S2214,[226] CT-60,[254] and +49*A/G see below), *MBL2*,[257] *inducible costimulator* (*ICOS*),[255] and for microsatellite markers at locus 19p13.[10] Only the +49*A/G dimorphism of *CTLA-4* has been examined in numerous studies. Therefore we will restrict our discussion to this variant.

The evidence for association with *+49*A* is not consistent across studies,[220-222,226,227,256-260] but a meta-analysis shows modest association for *CTLA-4+49*A* in celiac disease.[214] Importantly, variation contained in the *CTLA-4* gene has been reported to confer susceptibility to many autoimmune genetic diseases, including insulin-dependent diabetes mellitus (IDDM), Grave's disease, and Hashimoto's hypothyroidism.[261] However, a recent positional mapping association study of 109 polymorphisms in the 330-kb region surrounding the *CTLA-4* gene strongly suggests that a yet unidentified common variant in the 6.1-kb region 3' of *CTLA-4* is responsible for the association with IDDM, Grave's and autoimmune hypothyrodism.[262] Moreover, these data firmly rejected +49A/G as IDDM's causal SNP,[262] a result which raises the possibility that *+49*A* is simply linked to the causal variant in celiac disease as well.

Animal Models

Presently, there are no adequate animal models for the systemic complications of celiac disease. A model of gluten-sensitive enteropathy occurs spontaneously in a strain of Irish setter dogs.[263] Few studies have used this model system to address the etiopathology of celiac disease in the past. One possible reason for this is that no linkage was seen between the enteropathy of these dogs and the canine MHC.[264] Moreover, there is limited interest in developing animal models for celiac disease, which may be in part due to the fact that biological samples derived from celiac patients, such as blood and small intestine T-cells, constitute an advantageous experimental

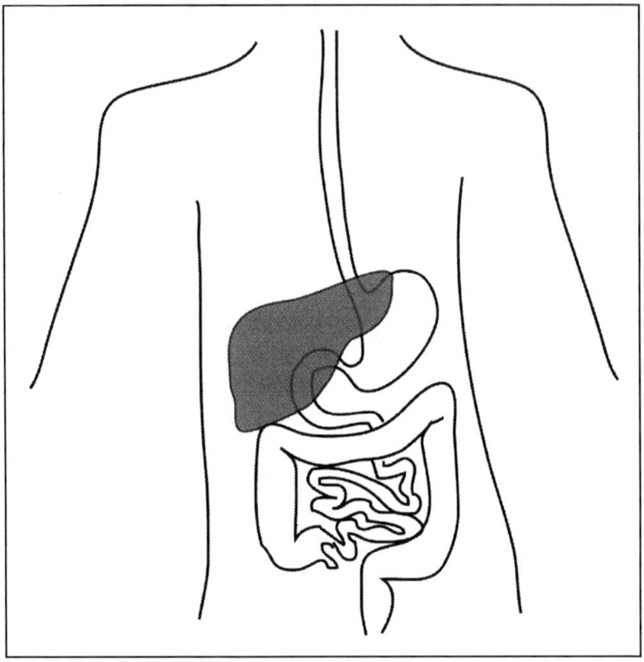

Figure 3. Localization of autoimmune hepatitis. Inflammation in autoimmune hepatitis is observed throughout the liver (gray). Compared to primary biliary cirrhosis and primary sclerosing cholangitis, which affect the bile ducts, autoimmune hepatitis affects hepatocytes.

system where the major environmental component (i.e., gluten and related proteins) can be easily controlled through dieting. Nonetheless, it is most likely that gene knock-out models will be engineered as disease susceptibility-conferring gene variants are revealed, allowing for the exploration of in vivo factors that modulate intestinal permeability, mechanisms for extraintestinal alterations, interactions between gluten and other metabolic, nutritional and environmental factors involved in the disease, as well as genetically-based (i.e., pharmacogenomic) therapies.

Autoimmune Hepatitis

Definition, Classification and Symptoms

Autoimmune hepatitis (AIH) is a chronic inflammation of the liver (Fig. 3) for which early symptoms are fatigue, jaundice and anorexia.[265] AIH accounts for 10-20% of chronic hepatitis cases in North America, but less than 4% of patients in India.[266,267] AIH is diagnosed based on criteria defined by the International Autoimmune Hepatitis Group.[268] A scoring system for these criteria allows the classification of cases as definite AIH or probable AIH. These criteria include the absence of infection with hepatitis viruses (i.e., exclusion of viral nucleic acids, antigens and antibodies), the presence of circulating autoantibodies (see below), hypergammaglobulinemia, and being of the female sex.

Autoimmune Features

The loss of tolerance to autologous liver tissue is the likely cause of inflammation in AIH, but the autoantibodies present in AIH patients have yet to be functionally implicated in the pathogenesis of AIH.[269] In the absence of this functional knowledge, two distinct forms of AIH have been identified based on the patient's particular autoantibody set: AIH type 1 (AIH-1) and AIH type 2 (AIH-2).

AIH-1 is characterized by anti-nuclear (ANA) and anti-smooth muscle (SMA) antibodies. These patients account for 70-80% of AIH patients. Although the frequency of AIH-2 is lower (3-4%), autoimmune characteristics are better characterized for this subtype. For instance, the target of anti-liver/kidney microsome type 1 (LKM1) antibodies, which are the hallmark of AIH-2, is cytochrome P450-2D6.[270] AIH-2 patients also experience an earlier onset and more aggressive course of disease, a higher prevalence of autoimmunity directed against other organs, and progress to cirrhosis more frequently.[271] In addition, the serum of about 10% of these patients contains autoantibodies that detect specific UDP-glucuronosyltransferases (UGTs). A third form, AIH-3, which is clinically indistinguishable from AIH-1, was proposed based on the presence of antibodies against cytosolic liver or liver-pancreas antigens.[272]

Epidemiology: Inheritance and Environment

There are few epidemiological studies for AIH. Prevalence of the disease is estimated to be 4, 16.9 and 42.9 per 100,000 individuals in populations from Singapore, Norway and Alaska, respectively.[11-13] The AIH-2 subtype is much less common than AIH-1 and is more frequent in southern Europe than in northern Europe, the United States or Japan.[14]

Various drugs and viral infections are environmental factors associated with the onset of hepatitis with autoimmune involvement (see, for example, refs. 273, 274). However, no infectious agent, metabolic defect or toxin has been determined to be a risk factor for AIH.

Genetics

Linkage Studies

Given the limited number of families with multiple members affected with AIH, no whole-genome linkage scans have been performed to date, and all genetic studies for AIH are based on case-control association analysis of candidate genes with known immunoregulatory functions.

Association: MHC Locus

Larger cohorts and more complete analysis of the variation at the MHC locus will be required to precisely identify the genetic variation that influences risk for AIH. However, some studies provide preliminary insight into the search for susceptibility loci.

MHC variants that have been associated with risk to AIH-1 include HLA-DR3, HLA-DR4, and *DRB1*1301*.[275,276] Interestingly, the particular DR4 suballeles associated with AIH-1 appear to differ in different populations, suggesting that risk is associated with the larger DR4 superclass and not a particular allele. Genetic studies in AIH-2 are limited by its rarity and regional occurrence. However, the *DRB1*07*, *DRB1*15*, *DQB1*06*, and *DRB1*03* alleles have been shown to be associated with risk for disease.[275]

Association: Non-MHC Loci

Among the potential non-MHC susceptibility factors (Table 5) are the *CTLA-4 +49G* allele,[277,278] the *VDR Fok* polymorphism,[279] and the *CD45 tyrosine phosphatase +77C/G* mutation.[280] In addition, genetic variants for the heavy chain constant regions of both *TCRβ*[281] and IgG1[282] were reportedly associated with AIH. Interestingly, the association with *TCRβ* was strongest in patients without HLA-DR3 and DR4, and is significantly decreased in early onset cases.[281] These associations remain to be confirmed in larger samples. Other studies of candidate genes, such as *IL-1B*, *IL-1RN*, and *IL-10*,[283,284] and the autoimmune regulator *AIRE*,[285] failed to identify an association with disease susceptibility. Caveats for the apparent lack of association in negative studies might be the limited number of samples available for study and the heterogeneity of the sample population (e.g., in the *AIRE* study of 85 AIH cases, 14% of individuals were seropositive for AIH-2, while the remaining 86% were diagnosed as AIH-1).

Table 5. AIH non-MHC association studies

Locus	Gene (Polymorphisms)	Association	References
1q32	*IL-10* (-1082, -819, -592)	NS	283, 284
2q13	*IL-1β* (IL-1B*1, IL-1B*2)	NS	283, 284
2q13	*IL-1RN* (IL-1RN*1, *2, *3, *4, *R5)	NS	283, 284
2q33	*CTLA-4* (+49 A/G, (AT)8)	+	278, 286, 287
7q34	*TCRβ* (BglI)	+	281
11q13	*CD45* (+77C/G)	+	280
12q13	*VDR* (Fok, BsmI, TaqI, ApaI)	+	279
19q13	*IgG1, Gm* (serotype)	+	282
21q22	*AIRE* (808C/T, 844C/T, R257X, G305S, 1324T/C)	NS	285

+: statistically significant; NS: not significant.

Animal Models

Most experimental models for AIH result from the immunization of rodents or rabbits with liver antigens in complete Freund's adjuvant (CFA), and have been recently reviewed.[288-290] No model recapitulates all the features of the disease, and hepatic lesions are also observed in control animals injected with CFA. However, adoptive transfer of the disease into syngeneic recipients by splenocytes and lymph node cells from immunized animals (see, for example, ref. 291) support the autoimmune causal nature of the disease in these models. There are no published reports of experimental induction of AIH with purified cytochrome P450 IID6 or any other AIH-related autoantigen. Transgenic models allow examination of liver-specific immune responses, with the disadvantage that most develop tolerance for the transgene (reviewed in ref. 288). Proposed knockout models include *TGFβ*- and *IL-2*-deficient mice; however, although these mice develop spontaneous hepatitis with autoimmune features, various additional complications are not specific to AIH, and this phenotype is absolutely dependent on the genetic background of the BALB/c murine strain.[292,293]

Conclusions

Association Studies

Association studies are a powerful approach for identifying common loci of modest effect. However, positive association studies are often not replicated in subsequent data sets. This is seen for some of the studies presented in this chapter, for example, the UC association to *IL-1RN* for which an initial positive result failed to replicate. While it is possible that this reflects a lack of association, it is also possible that the replication studies were not appropriately powered to detect an association. Careful attention to original and replication study designs can help increase the reproducibility of results. Specific steps to improve the reliability of data include fully assessing variation at a locus, obtaining appropriate sample size given the estimated frequency and effect of the target variant, and evaluating cohort stratification, for example, by comparing allele frequencies of randomly chosen markers in suspected subpopulations. These steps will provide higher confidence in positively associated variation as well as allow unassociated loci to be more definitively excluded.

An additional challenge to association studies is extended linkage disequilibrium. This is acutely illustrated in the case of MHC studies.[294-296] To surmount this obstacle it is particularly important to fully assess all variation for association with disease. Historically, the MHC has been studied by typing a handful of genes (usually the classical HLA loci, *TNFα* and *C4*).

However, as seen for IBD, celiac disease and AIH, association studies using these methods generally implicate more than one allele as influencing disease susceptibility. While this may indicate a multi-gene or multi-allelic disease etiology, it may simply reflect an inability to discriminate between causal alleles and variation that is merely in linkage disequilibrium. For instance, preliminary data suggest that celiac disease associations to DR types are in fact secondary due to linkage disequilibrium with DQ.[244]

Recently, a preliminary integrated map of the SNP, HLA, and microsatellite variation in the MHC was reported.[296] Analysis of these data showed that the haplotype structure of the MHC is no different than that of the genome as a whole, and, also, that a higher density of markers would provide a powerful resource for disease studies. In combination with larger cohort sizes, this map may help narrow associated regions through mapping ancestral recombination events. Such efforts may permit the definitive identification of causal variation in many diseases, including IBD, AIH, and celiac disease.

Functional Studies

Once a susceptibility-conferring haplotype is identified, the specific variation responsible for the association needs to be determined. As mentioned, a major obstacle in this regard is linkage disequilibrium, which makes it difficult to isolate the effect of causal variation from that of one which is simply linked. However, determination of causality is the end goal of any human complex genetic disease study. Therefore, researchers turn to functional studies to provide definitive proof.

Candidate genes should be expressed in cells that may play roles in disease etiology. For instance, IBD researchers hope to see expression in immune tissues or the gut—or in both, as is the case for *CARD15*. Depending on the location of the hypothesized causal variation (promoter, intronic, coding), distinct approaches are taken. If the variant is located in the gene's promoter or in a splice junction, expression levels or tissue localization patterns of specific isoforms may differ in individuals bearing the putative causal variant. If the variation is in the coding sequence, one might turn to in vitro biochemistry to determine whether the associated protein variant had different properties.

These experiments only determine that the variant of interest causes changes in gene expression or protein function; they do not elucidate the mechanism by which disease results. Animal models and in vitro disease models can be useful to bridge the gap between function and disease mechanism. For instance, if researchers can replicate disease phenotypes by "knocking-in" the human variant into a mouse model, they can be fairly certain that the variation plays a role in disease mechanism. However, an inability to show involvement in a model system may simply reflect the limitations of the model. Such a result does not rule out that the variant contributes to human disease. This is perfectly illustrated in the case of *CARD15*.[153] The targeted disruption in the mouse homologue of the *CARD15* gene shows no intestinal pathology, however the human genetic evidence (three independent mutations with compound heterozygotes conferring similar risk to homozygotes[73]) is conclusive. While the challenges of identifying disease-causing variation are great, determining function of those variants and establishing definitive roles in disease will likely prove even more difficult.

Future Directions

As detailed in this chapter, significant progress has been made in recent years toward understanding the etiology of IBD, celiac disease and AIH. Yet, the genetic variation that influences each disease is not fully understood. Recent accomplishments have provided the community a greater understanding of the genetics of complex disease; however, well-powered, well-phenotyped cohorts are required to further improve our knowledge of disease mechanism. These studies will likely require multi-center collaborative efforts such as those that have already begun to benefit our insight into IBD and celiac disease.

Acknowledgements

We thank Cisca Wijmenga, Leslie Gaffney, Philip De Jager, Lisa Farwell and Tracey Petryshen for critical reading of this manuscript. ECW is supported by a Cancer Research Institute Fellowship. This work was supported by NIH-R01#DK64869 (JDR).

References

1. Yang SK, Loftus Jr EV, Sandborn WJ. Epidemiology of inflammatory bowel disease in Asia. Inflamm Bowel Dis 2001; 7(3):260-270.
2. Yang H, Taylor KD, Rotter JI. Inflammatory bowel disease. I. Genetic epidemiology. Mol Genet Metab 2001; 74(1-2):1-21.
3. Book L, Zone JJ, Neuhausen SL. Prevalence of celiac disease among relatives of sib pairs with celiac disease in U.S. families. Am J Gastroenterol 2003; 98(2):377-381.
4. Beck S, Trowsdale J. The human major histocompatability complex: Lessons from the DNA sequence. Annu Rev Genomics Hum Genet 2000; 1:117-137.
5. Farrokhyar F, Swarbrick ET, Irvine EJ. A critical review of epidemiological studies in inflammatory bowel disease. Scand J Gastroenterol 2001; 36(1):2-15.
6. Vyse TJ, Todd JA. Genetic analysis of autoimmune disease. Cell 1996; 85(3):311-318.
7. AGA. AGA technical review on celiac sprue. Gastroenterology 2001; 120(6):1526-1540.
8. Fasano A, Catassi C. Current approaches to diagnosis and treatment of celiac disease: An evolving spectrum. Gastroenterology 2001; 120(3):636-651.
9. Bevan S, Popat S, Braegger CP et al. Contribution of the MHC region to the familial risk of coeliac disease. J Med Genet 1999; 36(9):687-690.
10. Van Belzen MJ, Meijer JW, Sandkuijl LA et al. A major nonHLA locus in celiac disease maps to chromosome 19. Gastroenterology 2003; 125(4):1032-1041.
11. Boberg KM. Prevalence and epidemiology of autoimmune hepatitis. Clin Liver Dis 2002; 6(3):347-359.
12. Hurlburt KJ, McMahon BJ, Deubner H et al. Prevalence of autoimmune liver disease in Alaska natives. Am J Gastroenterol 2002; 97(9):2402-2407.
13. Lee YM, Teo EK, Ng TM et al. Autoimmune hepatitis in Singapore: A rare syndrome affecting middle-aged women. J Gastroenterol Hepatol 2001; 16(12):1384-1389.
14. Feld JJ, Heathcote EJ. Epidemiology of autoimmune liver disease. J Gastroenterol Hepatol 2003; 18(10):1118-1128.
15. Risch N. Assessing the role of HLA-linked and unlinked determinants of disease. Am J Hum Genet 1987; 40(1):1-14.
16. Lander E, Kruglyak L. Genetic dissection of complex traits: Guidelines for interpreting and reporting linkage results. Nat Genet 1995; 11(3):241-247.
17. Daly MJ, Rioux JD, Schaffner SF et al. High-resolution haplotype structure in the human genome. Nat Genet 2001; 29(2):229-232.
18. Gabriel SB, Schaffner SF, Nguyen H et al. The structure of haplotype blocks in the human genome. Science 2002; 296(5576):2225-2229.
19. Jeffreys AJ, Kauppi L, Neumann R. Intensely punctate meiotic recombination in the class II region of the major histocompatibility complex. Nat Genet 2001; 29(2):217-222.
20. Gibbs RA, Belmont JW, Hardenbol P et al. The international HapMap project. Nature 2003; 426(6968):789-796.
21. Kornbluth A, Sachar DB, Salomon P. Crohn's disease. In: Feldman M, Friedman LS, Sleisenger MH, eds. Sleisenger and Fordtran's Gastrointestinal and Liver Disease. 6th ed. Philadelphia: WB Saunders, 1998; 2:1708-1734.
22. Jewell DP. Ulcerative colitis. In: Feldman M, Friedman LS, Sleisenger MH, eds. Sleisenger and Fordtran's Gastrointestinal and Liver Disease. 6th ed. Philadelphia: WB Saunders, 1998; 2:1735-1761.
23. Joossens S, Reinisch W, Vermeire S et al. The value of serologic markers in indeterminate colitis: A prospective follow-up study. Gastroenterology 2002; 122(5):1242-1247.
24. Moum B, Ekbom A, Vatn MH et al. Inflammatory bowel disease: Reevaluation of the diagnosis in a prospective population based study in south eastern Norway. Gut 1997; 40(3):328-332.
25. Reumaux D, Sendid B, Poulain D et al. Serological markers in inflammatory bowel diseases. Best Pract Res Clin Gastroenterol 2003; 17(1):19-35.
26. Binder V. Genetic epidemiology in inflammatory bowel disease. Dig Dis 1998; 16(6):351-355.
27. Orholm M, Binder V, Sorensen TI et al. Concordance of inflammatory bowel disease among Danish twins. Results of a nationwide study. Scand J Gastroenterol 2000; 35(10):1075-1081.

28. Halfvarson J, Bodin L, Tysk C et al. Inflammatory bowel disease in a Swedish twin cohort: A long-term follow-up of concordance and clinical characteristics. Gastroenterology 2003; 124(7):1767-1773.
29. Cottone M, Rosselli M, Orlando A et al. Smoking habits and recurrence in Crohn's disease. Gastroenterology 1994; 106(3):643-648.
30. Reif S, Lavy A, Keter D et al. Lack of association between smoking and Crohn's disease but the usual association with ulcerative colitis in Jewish patients in Israel: A multicenter study. Am J Gastroenterol 2000; 95(2):474-478.
31. Madretsma S, Wolters LM, van Dijk JP et al. In-vivo effect of nicotine on cytokine production by human nonadherent mononuclear cells. Eur J Gastroenterol Hepatol 1996; 8(10):1017-1020.
32. Pullan RD. Colonic mucus, smoking and ulcerative colitis. Ann R Coll Surg Engl 1996; 78(2):85-91.
33. Finnie IA, Campbell BJ, Taylor BA et al. Stimulation of colonic mucin synthesis by corticosteroids and nicotine. Clin Sci (Lond) 1996; 91(3):359-364.
34. Van Dijk JP, Madretsma GS, Keuskamp ZJ et al. Nicotine inhibits cytokine synthesis by mouse colonic mucosa. Eur J Pharmacol 1995; 278(1):R11-12.
35. Green JT, Richardson C, Marshall RW et al. Nitric oxide mediates a therapeutic effect of nicotine in ulcerative colitis. Aliment Pharmacol Ther 2000; 14(11):1429-1434.
36. Wolf JM, Lashner BA. Inflammatory bowel disease: Sorting out the treatment options. Cleve Clin J Med 2002; 69(8):621-626, 629-631.
37. Katschinski B, Logan RF, Edmond M et al. Smoking and sugar intake are separate but interactive risk factors in Crohn's disease. Gut 1988; 29(9):1202-1206.
38. Persson PG, Ahlbom A, Hellers G. Diet and inflammatory bowel disease: A case-control study. Epidemiology 1992; 3(1):47-52.
39. Ainley C, Cason J, Slavin BM et al. The influence of zinc status and malnutrition on immunological function in Crohn's disease. Gastroenterology 1991; 100(6):1616-1625.
40. Kanauchi O, Mitsuyama K, Araki Y et al. Modification of intestinal flora in the treatment of inflammatory bowel disease. Curr Pharm Des 2003; 9(4):333-346.
41. Hugot JP, Laurent-Puig P, Gower-Rousseau C et al. Mapping of a susceptibility locus for Crohn's disease on chromosome 16. Nature 1996; 379(6568):821-823.
42. Cavanaugh J. International collaboration provides convincing linkage replication in complex disease through analysis of a large pooled data set: Crohn disease and chromosome 16. Am J Hum Genet 2001; 68(5):1165-1171.
43. Satsangi J, Parkes M, Louis E et al. Two stage genome-wide search in inflammatory bowel disease provides evidence for susceptibility loci on chromosomes 3, 7 and 12. Nat Genet 1996; 14(2):199-202.
44. Cho JH, Nicolae DL, Gold LH et al. Identification of novel susceptibility loci for inflammatory bowel disease on chromosomes 1p, 3q, and 4q: Evidence for epistasis between 1p and IBD1. Proc Natl Acad Sci USA 1998; 95(13):7502-7507.
45. Ma Y, Ohmen JD, Li Z et al. A genome-wide search identifies potential new susceptibility loci for Crohn's disease. Inflamm Bowel Dis 1999; 5(4):271-278.
46. Hampe J, Schreiber S, Shaw SH et al. A genomewide analysis provides evidence for novel linkages in inflammatory bowel disease in a large European cohort. Am J Hum Genet 1999; 64(3):808-816.
47. Duerr RH, Barmada MM, Zhang L et al. Linkage and association between inflammatory bowel disease and a locus on chromosome 12. Am J Hum Genet 1998; 63(1):95-100.
48. Rioux JD, Silverberg MS, Daly MJ et al. Genomewide search in Canadian families with inflammatory bowel disease reveals two novel susceptibility loci. Am J Hum Genet 2000; 66:1863-1870.
49. Cavanaugh JA, Callen DF, Wilson SR et al. Analysis of Australian Crohn's disease pedigrees refines the localization for susceptibility to inflammatory bowel disease on chromosome 16. Ann Hum Genet 1998; 62(Pt 4):291-298.
50. Brant SR, Fu Y, Fields CT et al. American families with Crohn's disease have strong evidence for linkage to chromosome 16 but not chromosome 12. Gastroenterology 1998; 115(5):1056-1061.
51. Rioux JD, Daly MJ, Green T et al. Absence of linkage between inflammatory bowel disease and selected loci on chromosomes 3, 7, 12, and 16. Gastroenterology 1998; 115(5):1062-1065.
52. Annese V, Latiano A, Bovio P et al. Genetic analysis in Italian families with inflammatory bowel disease supports linkage to the IBD1 locus—a GISC study. Eur J Hum Genet 1999; 7(5):567-573.
53. Vermeire S, Peeters M, Vlietinck R et al. Exclusion of linkage of Crohn's disease to previously reported regions on chromosomes 12, 7, and 3 in the Belgian population indicates genetic heterogeneity. Inflamm Bowel Dis 2000; 6(3):165-170.

54. Hampe J, Lynch NJ, Daniels S et al. Fine mapping of the chromosome 3p susceptibility locus in inflammatory bowel disease. Gut 2001; 48(2):191-197.
55. Paavola P, Helio T, Kiuru M et al. Genetic analysis in Finnish families with inflammatory bowel disease supports linkage to chromosome 3p21. Eur J Hum Genet 2001; 9(5):328-334.
56. Shaw SH, Hampe J, White R et al. Stratification by CARD15 variant genotype in a genome-wide search for inflammatory bowel disease susceptibility loci. Hum Genet 2003; 113(6):514-521.
57. Van Heel DA, Dechairo BM, Dawson G et al. The IBD6 Crohn's disease locus demonstrates complex interactions with CARD15 and IBD5 disease-associated variants. Hum Mol Genet 2003; 12(20):2569-2575.
58. Williams CN, Kocher K, Lander ES et al. Using a genome-wide scan and meta-analysis to identify a novel IBD locus and confirm previously identified IBD loci. Inflamm Bowel Dis 2002; 8(6):375-381.
59. Hugot JP, Chamaillard M, Zouali H et al. Association of NOD2 leucine-rich repeat variants with susceptibility to Crohn's disease. Nature 2001; 411(6837):599-603.
60. Ogura Y, Bonen DK, Inohara N et al. A frameshift mutation in NOD2 associated with susceptibility to Crohn's disease. Nature 2001; 411(6837):603-606.
61. Duerr RH, Barmada MM, Zhang L et al. High-density genome scan in Crohn disease shows confirmed linkage to chromosome 14q11-12. Am J Hum Genet 2000; 66(6):1857-1862.
62. Rioux JD, Daly MJ, Silverberg MS et al. Genetic variation in the 5q31 cytokine gene cluster confers susceptibility to Crohn disease. Nat Genet 2001; 29(2):223-228.
63. Kobayashi K, Atoh M, Konoeda Y et al. HLA-DR, DQ and T cell antigen receptor constant beta genes in Japanese patients with ulcerative colitis. Clin Exp Immunol 1990; 80(3):400-403.
64. Asakura H, Tsuchiya M, Aiso S et al. Association of the human lymphocyte-DR2 antigen with Japanese ulcerative colitis. Gastroenterology 1982; 82(3):413-418.
65. Sugimura K, Asakura H, Mizuki N et al. Analysis of genes within the HLA region affecting susceptibility to ulcerative colitis. Hum Immunol 1993; 36(2):112-118.
66. Futami S, Aoyama N, Honsako Y et al. HLA-DRB1*1502 allele, subtype of DR15, is associated with susceptibility to ulcerative colitis and its progression. Dig Dis Sci 1995; 40(4):814-818.
67. Yoshitake S, Kimura A, Okada M et al. HLA class II alleles in Japanese patients with inflammatory bowel disease. Tissue Antigens 1999; 53(4 Pt 1):350-358.
68. Stokkers PC, Reitsma PH, Tytgat GN et al. HLA-DR and -DQ phenotypes in inflammatory bowel disease: A meta-analysis. Gut 1999; 45(3):395-401.
69. Hampe J, Cuthbert A, Croucher PJ et al. Association between insertion mutation in NOD2 gene and Crohn's disease in German and British populations. Lancet 2001; 357(9272):1925-1928.
70. Lesage S, Zouali H, Cezard JP et al. CARD15/NOD2 mutational analysis and genotype-phenotype correlation in 612 patients with inflammatory bowel disease. Am J Hum Genet 2002; 70(4):845-857.
71. Vermeire S, Wild G, Kocher K et al. CARD15 genetic variation in a Quebec population: Prevalence, genotype-phenotype relationship, and haplotype structure. Am J Hum Genet 2002; 71(1):74-83.
72. Croucher PJ, Mascheretti S, Hampe J et al. Haplotype structure and association to Crohn's disease of CARD15 mutations in two ethnically divergent populations. Eur J Hum Genet 2003; 11(1):6-16.
73. Cuthbert AP, Fisher SA, Mirza MM et al. The contribution of NOD2 gene mutations to the risk and site of disease in inflammatory bowel disease. Gastroenterology 2002; 122(4):867-874.
74. Helio T, Halme L, Lappalainen M et al. CARD15/NOD2 gene variants are associated with familially occurring and complicated forms of Crohn's disease. Gut 2003; 52(4):558-562.
75. Inoue N, Tamura K, Kinouchi Y et al. Lack of common NOD2 variants in Japanese patients with Crohn's disease. Gastroenterology 2002; 123(1):86-91.
76. Yamazaki K, Takazoe M, Tanaka T et al. Absence of mutation in the NOD2/CARD15 gene among 483 Japanese patients with Crohn's disease. J Hum Genet 2002; 47(9):469-472.
77. Marsh S, McLeod HL. Crohn's disease: Ethnic variation in CARD15 genotypes. Gut 2003; 52(5):770.
78. Leong RW, Armuzzi A, Ahmad T et al. NOD2/CARD15 gene polymorphisms and Crohn's disease in the Chinese population. Aliment Pharmacol Ther 2003; 17(12):1465-1470.
79. Inohara N, Nunez G. NODs: Intracellular proteins involved in inflammation and apoptosis. Nat Rev Immunol 2003; 3(5):371-382.
80. Dangl JL, Jones JD. Plant pathogens and integrated defence responses to infection. Nature 2001; 411(6839):826-833.
81. Hisamatsu T, Suzuki M, Reinecker HC et al. CARD15/NOD2 functions as an antibacterial factor in human intestinal epithelial cells. Gastroenterology 2003; 124(4):993-1000.
82. Ogura Y, Lala S, Xin W et al. Expression of NOD2 in Paneth cells: A possible link to Crohn's ileitis. Gut 2003; 52(11):1591-1597.

82a. Daly MJ, Rioux JD. New approaches to gene hunting in IBD. Inflamm Bowel Dis 2004; 10(3):312-317.
83. Giallourakis C, Stoll M, Miller K et al. IBD5 is a general risk factor for inflammatory bowel disease: Replication of association with Crohn disease and identification of a novel association with ulcerative colitis. Am J Hum Genet 2003; 73(1):205-211.
84. Negoro K, McGovern DP, Kinouchi Y et al. Analysis of the IBD5 locus and potential gene-gene interactions in Crohn's disease. Gut 2003; 52(4):541-546.
85. Mirza MM, Fisher SA, King K et al. Genetic evidence for interaction of the 5q31 cytokine locus and the CARD15 gene in Crohn disease. Am J Hum Genet 2003; 72(4):1018-1022.
86. Armuzzi A, Ahmad T, Ling KL et al. Genotype-phenotype analysis of the Crohn's disease susceptibility haplotype on chromosome 5q31. Gut 2003; 52(8):1133-1139.
87. Pokorny RM, Hofmeister A, Galandiuk S et al. Crohn's disease and ulcerative colitis are associated with the DNA repair gene MLH1. Ann Surg 1997; 225(6):718-723, discussion 723-715.
88. Annese V, Piepoli A, Andriulli A et al. Association of Crohn's disease and ulcerative colitis with haplotypes of the MLH1 gene in Italian inflammatory bowel disease patients. J Med Genet 2002; 39(5):332-334.
89. Frenzel H, Hampe J, Huse K et al. Mutation detection and physical mapping of the CD11 gene cluster in association with inflammatory bowel disease. Immunogenetics 2002; 53(10-11):835-842.
90. de Jong DJ, Franke B, Naber AH et al. No evidence for involvement of IL-4R and CD11B from the IBD1 region and STAT6 in the IBD2 region in Crohn's disease. Eur J Hum Genet 2003; 11(11):884-887.
91. Mansfield JC, Holden H, Tarlow JK et al. Novel genetic association between ulcerative colitis and the anti-inflammatory cytokine interleukin-1 receptor antagonist. Gastroenterology 1994; 106(3):637-642.
92. Bioque G, Crusius JB, Koutroubakis I et al. Allelic polymorphism in IL-1 beta and IL-1 receptor antagonist (IL-1Ra) genes in inflammatory bowel disease. Clin Exp Immunol 1995; 102(2):379-383.
93. Roussomoustakaki M, Satsangi J, Welsh K et al. Genetic markers may predict disease behavior in patients with ulcerative colitis. Gastroenterology 1997; 112(6):1845-1853.
94. Heresbach D, Alizadeh M, Dabadie A et al. Significance of interleukin-1beta and interleukin-1 receptor antagonist genetic polymorphism in inflammatory bowel diseases. Am J Gastroenterol 1997; 92(7):1164-1169.
95. Hacker UT, Bidlingmaier C, Gomolka M et al. Inflammatory bowel disease: No association between allele combinations of the interleukin (IL) I beta and IL-I receptor antagonist gene polymorphisms. Eur J Clin Invest 1998; 28(3):214-219.
96. Stokkers PC, van Aken BE, Basoski N et al. Five genetic markers in the interleukin 1 family in relation to inflammatory bowel disease. Gut 1998; 43(1):33-39.
97. Gonzalez Sarmiento R, Araoz P, Rodriguez R et al. Polymorphism of the IL1RN gene in Spanish patients with ulcerative colitis. Med Clin (Barc) 1999; 112(20):778-779.
98. Nemetz A, Kope A, Molnar T et al. Significant differences in the interleukin-1beta and interleukin-1 receptor antagonist gene polymorphisms in a Hungarian population with inflammatory bowel disease. Scand J Gastroenterol 1999; 34(2):175-179.
99. Bouma G, Crusius JB, Garcia-Gonzalez MA et al. Genetic markers in clinically well defined patients with ulcerative colitis (UC). Clin Exp Immunol 1999; 115(2):294-300.
100. Tountas NA, Casini-Raggi V, Yang H et al. Functional and ethnic association of allele 2 of the interleukin-1 receptor antagonist gene in ulcerative colitis. Gastroenterology 1999; 117(4):806-813.
101. Papo M, Quer JC, Gutierrez C et al. Genetic heterogeneity within ulcerative colitis determined by an interleukin-1 receptor antagonist gene polymorphism and antineutrophil cytoplasmic antibodies. Eur J Gastroenterol Hepatol 1999; 11(4):413-420.
102. Carter MJ, di Giovine FS, Jones S et al. Association of the interleukin 1 receptor antagonist gene with ulcerative colitis in Northern European Caucasians. Gut 2001; 48(4):461-467.
103. Craggs A, Welfare M, Donaldson PT et al. The CC chemokine receptor 5 delta32 mutation is not associated with inflammatory bowel disease (IBD) in NE England. Genes Immun 2001; 2(2):114-116.
104. Nohara H, Saito Y, Higaki S et al. Polymorphisms of the IL-1beta and IL-1beta-inducible genes in ulcerative colitis. J Gastroenterol 2002; 37(Suppl 14):107-110.
105. Olavesen MG, Hampe J, Mirza MM et al. Analysis of single-nucleotide polymorphisms in the interleukin-4 receptor gene for association with inflammatory bowel disease. Immunogenetics 2000; 51(1):1-7.

106. Aithal GP, Day CP, Leathart J et al. Association of single nucleotide polymorphisms in the interleukin-4 gene and interleukin-4 receptor gene with Crohn's disease in a British population. Genes Immun 2001; 2(1):44-47.
107. Tagore A, Gonsalkorale WM, Pravica V et al. Interleukin-10 (IL-10) genotypes in inflammatory bowel disease. Tissue Antigens 1999; 54(4):386-390.
108. Mitchell SA, Grove J, Spurkland A et al. Association of the tumour necrosis factor alpha -308 but not the interleukin 10 -627 promoter polymorphism with genetic susceptibility to primary sclerosing cholangitis. Gut 2001; 49(2):288-294.
109. Kagnoff MF, Brown RJ, Schanfield MS. Association between Crohn's disease and immunoglobulin heavy chain (Gm) allotypes. Gastroenterology 1983; 85(5):1044-1047.
110. Gudjonsson H, Schanfield MS, Albertini RJ et al. Association and linkage studies of immunoglobulin heavy chain allotypes in inflammatory bowel disease. Tissue Antigens 1988; 31(5):243-249.
111. Simmons JD, Mullighan C, Welsh KI et al. Vitamin D receptor gene polymorphism: Association with Crohn's disease susceptibility. Gut 2000; 47(2):211-214.
112. Martin K, Radlmayr M, Borchers R et al. Candidate genes colocalized to linkage regions in inflammatory bowel disease. Digestion 2002; 66(2):121-126.
113. Yang H, Vora DK, Targan SR et al. Intercellular adhesion molecule 1 gene associations with immunologic subsets of inflammatory bowel disease. Gastroenterology 1995; 109(2):440-448.
114. Braun C, Zahn R, Martin K et al. Polymorphisms of the ICAM-1 gene are associated with inflammatory bowel disease, regardless of the p-ANCA status. Clin Immunol 2001; 101(3):357-360.
115. Matsuzawa J, Sugimura K, Matsuda Y et al. Association between K469E allele of intercellular adhesion molecule 1 gene and inflammatory bowel disease in a Japanese population. Gut 2003; 52(1):75-78.
116. Papa A, Danese S, Armuzzi A et al. Association between K469E allele of intercellular adhesion molecule 1 gene and inflammatory bowel disease in different populations. Gut 2003; 52(8):1227-1228, author reply 1228.
117. Panwala CM, Jones JC, Viney JL. A novel model of inflammatory bowel disease: Mice deficient for the multiple drug resistance gene, mdr1a, spontaneously develop colitis. J Immunol 1998; 161(10):5733-5744.
118. Schwab M, Schaeffeler E, Marx C et al. Association between the C3435T MDR1 gene polymorphism and susceptibility for ulcerative colitis. Gastroenterology 2003; 124(1):26-33.
119. Croucher PJ, Mascheretti S, Foelsch UR et al. Lack of association between the C3435T MDR1 gene polymorphism and inflammatory bowel disease in two independent Northern European populations. Gastroenterology 2003; 125(6):1919-1920, author reply 1920-1921.
120. Brant SR, Panhuysen CI, Nicolae D et al. MDR1 Ala893 polymorphism is associated with inflammatory bowel disease. Am J Hum Genet 2003; 73(6):1282-1292.
121. Gazouli M, Zacharatos P, Gorgoulis P. The C3435T MDR1gene polymorphism is not associated with susceptibility for ulcerative colitis in a Greek population. Gastroenterology 2004; 126(1):367-369.
122. Glas J, Torok HP, Schiemann U et al. MDR1 gene polymorphism in ulcerative colitis. Gastroenterology 2004; 126(1):367.
123. Kim RB, Leake BF, Choo EF et al. Identification of functionally variant MDR1 alleles among European Americans and African Americans. Clin Pharmacol Ther 2001; 70(2):189-199.
124. Hofmeister A, Neibergs HL, Pokorny RM et al. The natural resistance-associated macrophage protein gene is associated with Crohn's disease. Surgery 1997; 122(2):173-178, discussion 178-179.
125. Klein W, Tromm A, Griga T et al. A polymorphism in the IL11 gene is associated with ulcerative colitis. Genes Immun 2002; 3(8):494-496.
126. Glas J, Torok HP, Unterhuber H et al. The -295T-to-C promoter polymorphism of the IL-16 gene is associated with Crohn's disease. Clin Immunol 2003; 106(3):197-200.
127. Haslam N, Standen GR, Probert CS. An investigation of the association of the factor V Leiden mutation and inflammatory bowel disease. Eur J Gastroenterol Hepatol 1999; 11(11):1289-1291.
128. de Jong DJ, van der Logt EM, van Schaik A et al. Genetic polymorphisms in biotransformation enzymes in Crohn's disease: Association with microsomal epoxide hydrolase. Gut 2003; 52(4):547-551.
129. Bachvarov DR, Landry M, Houle S et al. Altered frequency of a promoter polymorphic allele of the kinin B1 receptor gene in inflammatory bowel disease. Gastroenterology 1998; 115(5):1045-1048.
130. Rector A, Lemey P, Laffut W et al. Mannan-binding lectin (MBL) gene polymorphisms in ulcerative colitis and Crohn's disease. Genes Immun 2001; 2(6):323-328.
131. Kyo K, Muto T, Nagawa H et al. Associations of distinct variants of the intestinal mucin gene MUC3A with ulcerative colitis and Crohn's disease. J Hum Genet 2001; 46(1):5-20.
132. Karban AS, Okazaki T, Panhuysen CI et al. Functional annotation of a novel NFKB1 promoter polymorphism that increases risk for ulcerative colitis. Hum Mol Genet 2004; 13(1):35-45.

133. King K, Moody A, Fisher SA et al. Genetic variation in the IGSF6 gene and lack of association with inflammatory bowel disease. Eur J Immunogenet 2003; 30(3):187-190.
134. Haslam N, Standen GR, Probert CS. An investigation of the association of the prothrombin G20210A gene mutation and inflammatory bowel disease: Factor II and IBD. Inflamm Bowel Dis 2001; 7(2):133-135.
135. Seegers D, Zwiers A, Strober W et al. A TaqI polymorphism in the 3'UTR of the s gene correlates with increased IL-12 secretion. Genes Immun 2002; 3(7):419-423.
136. Buning C, Genschel J, Weltrich R et al. The interleukin-25 gene located in the inflammatory bowel disease (IBD) 4 region: No association with inflammatory bowel disease. Eur J Immunogenet 2003; 30(5):329-333.
137. Hampe J, Hermann B, Bridger S et al. The interferon-gamma gene as a positional and functional candidate gene for inflammatory bowel disease. Int J Colorectal Dis 1998; 13(5-6):260-263.
138. Rector A, Vermeire S, Thoelen I et al. Analysis of the CC chemokine receptor 5 (CCR5) delta-32 polymorphism in inflammatory bowel disease. Hum Genet 2001; 108(3):190-193.
139. Van Heel DA, Carey AH, Jewell DP. Identification of novel polymorphisms in the beta7 integrin gene: Family-based association studies in inflammatory bowel disease. Genes Immun 2001; 2(8):455-460.
140. Xia B, Crusius JB, Wu J et al. CTLA4 gene polymorphisms in Dutch and Chinese patients with inflammatory bowel disease. Scand J Gastroenterol 2002; 37(11):1296-1300.
141. Zouali H, Lesage S, Merlin F et al. CARD4/NOD1 is not involved in inflammatory bowel disease. Gut 2003; 52(1):71-74.
142. Murillo L, Crusius JB, van Bodegraven AA et al. CARD15 gene and the classification of Crohn's disease. Immunogenetics 2002; 54(1):59-61.
143. Bairead E, Harmon DL, Curtis AM et al. Association of NOD2 with Crohn's disease in a homogenous Irish population. Eur J Hum Genet 2003; 11(3):237-244.
144. Brant SR, Picco MF, Achkar JP et al. Defining complex contributions of NOD2/CARD15 gene mutations, age at onset, and tobacco use on Crohn's disease phenotypes. Inflamm Bowel Dis 2003; 9(5):281-289.
145. Tomer G, Ceballos C, Concepcion E et al. NOD2/CARD15 variants are associated with lower weight at diagnosis in children with Crohn's disease. Am J Gastroenterol 2003; 98(11):2479-2484.
146. Abreu MT, Taylor KD, Lin YC et al. Mutations in NOD2 are associated with fibrostenosing disease in patients with Crohn's disease. Gastroenterology 2002; 123(3):679-688.
147. Radlmayr M, Torok HP, Martin K et al. The c-insertion mutation of the NOD2 gene is associated with fistulizing and fibrostenotic phenotypes in Crohn's disease. Gastroenterology 2002; 122(7):2091-2092.
148. Strober W, Fuss IJ, Blumberg RS. The immunology of mucosal models of inflammation. Annu Rev Immunol 2002; 20:495-549.
149. Barbara G, Xing Z, Hogaboam CM et al. Interleukin 10 gene transfer prevents experimental colitis in rats. Gut 2000; 46(3):344-349.
150. Hogaboam CM, Vallance BA, Kumar A et al. Therapeutic effects of interleukin-4 gene transfer in experimental inflammatory bowel disease. J Clin Invest 1997; 100(11):2766-2776.
151. Neurath MF, Fuss I, Kelsall BL et al. Antibodies to interleukin 12 abrogate established experimental colitis in mice. J Exp Med 1995; 182(5):1281-1290.
152. Mombaerts P, Mizoguchi E, Grusby MJ et al. Spontaneous development of inflammatory bowel disease in T cell receptor mutant mice. Cell 1993; 75(2):274-282.
153. Pauleau AL, Murray PJ. Role of nod2 in the response of macrophages to toll-like receptor agonists. Mol Cell Biol 2003; 23(21):7531-7539.
154. Chamaillard M, Hashimoto M, Horie Y et al. An essential role for NOD1 in host recognition of bacterial peptidoglycan containing diaminopimelic acid. Nat Immunol 2003; 4(7):702-707.
155. Girardin SE, Boneca IG, Carneiro LA et al. Nod1 detects a unique muropeptide from gram-negative bacterial peptidoglycan. Science 2003; 300(5625):1584-1587.
156. Madara JL, Podolsky DK, King NW et al. Characterization of spontaneous colitis in cotton-top tamarins (Saguinus oedipus) and its response to sulfasalazine. Gastroenterology 1985; 88(1 Pt 1):13-19.
157. Sundberg JP, Elson CO, Bedigian H et al. Spontaneous, heritable colitis in a new substrain of C3H/HeJ mice. Gastroenterology 1994; 107(6):1726-1735.
158. Matsumoto S, Okabe Y, Setoyama H et al. Inflammatory bowel disease-like enteritis and caecitis in a senescence accelerated mouse P1/Yit strain. Gut 1998; 43(1):71-78.
159. Kosiewicz MM, Nast CC, Krishnan A et al. Th1-type responses mediate spontaneous ileitis in a novel murine model of Crohn's disease. J Clin Invest 2001; 107(6):695-702.
160. Morris GP, Beck PL, Herridge MS et al. Hapten-induced model of chronic inflammation and ulceration in the rat colon. Gastroenterology 1989; 96(3):795-803.

161. Boirivant M, Fuss IJ, Chu A et al. Oxazolone colitis: A murine model of T helper cell type 2 colitis treatable with antibodies to interleukin 4. J Exp Med 1998; 188(10):1929-1939.
162. MacPherson BR, Pfeiffer CJ. Experimental production of diffuse colitis in rats. Digestion 1978; 17(2):135-150.
163. Yamada T, Sartor RB, Marshall S et al. Mucosal injury and inflammation in a model of chronic granulomatous colitis in rats. Gastroenterology 1993; 104(3):759-771.
164. Hodgson HJ, Potter BJ, Skinner J et al. Immune-complex mediated colitis in rabbits. An experimental model. Gut 1978; 19(3):225-232.
165. Watt J, Marcus R. Ulcerative colitis in the guinea-pig caused by seaweed extract. J Pharm Pharmacol 1969; 21(Suppl):187S+.
166. Okayasu I, Hatakeyama S, Yamada M et al. A novel method in the induction of reliable experimental acute and chronic ulcerative colitis in mice. Gastroenterology 1990; 98(3):694-702.
167. Stewart TH, Hetenyi C, Rowsell H et al. Ulcerative enterocolitis in dogs induced by drugs. J Pathol 1980; 131(4):363-378.
168. Bucy RP, Xu XY, Li J et al. Cyclosporin A-induced autoimmune disease in mice. J Immunol 1993; 151(2):1039-1050.
169. Rachmilewitz D, Okon E, Karmeli F. Sulphydryl blocker induced small intestinal inflammation in rats: A new model mimicking Crohn's disease. Gut 1997; 41(3):358-365.
170. Quinn TC, Taylor HR, Schachter J. Experimental proctitis due to rectal infection with Chlamydia trachomatis in nonhuman primates. J Infect Dis 1986; 154(5):833-841.
171. Shomer NH, Dangler CA, Schrenzel MD et al. Helicobacter bilis-induced inflammatory bowel disease in scid mice with defined flora. Infect Immun 1997; 65(11):4858-4864.
172. Cahill RJ, Foltz CJ, Fox JG et al. Inflammatory bowel disease: An immunity-mediated condition triggered by bacterial infection with Helicobacter hepaticus. Infect Immun 1997; 65(8):3126-3131.
173. Hammer RE, Maika SD, Richardson JA et al. Spontaneous inflammatory disease in transgenic rats expressing HLA-B27 and human beta 2m: An animal model of HLA-B27-associated human disorders. Cell 1990; 63(5):1099-1112.
174. Watanabe M, Ueno Y, Yajima T et al. Interleukin 7 transgenic mice develop chronic colitis with decreased interleukin 7 protein accumulation in the colonic mucosa. J Exp Med 1998; 187(3):389-402.
175. Hermiston ML, Gordon JI. Inflammatory bowel disease and adenomas in mice expressing a dominant negative N-cadherin. Science 1995; 270(5239):1203-1207.
176. Clegg CH, Rulffes JT, Haugen HS et al. Thymus dysfunction and chronic inflammatory disease in gp39 transgenic mice. Int Immunol 1997; 9(8):1111-1122.
177. Bush TG, Savidge TC, Freeman TC et al. Fulminant jejuno-ileitis following ablation of enteric glia in adult transgenic mice. Cell 1998; 93(2):189-201.
178. Hahm KB, Im YH, Parks TW et al. Loss of transforming growth factor beta signalling in the intestine contributes to tissue injury in inflammatory bowel disease. Gut 2001; 49(2):190-198.
179. Shull MM, Ormsby I, Kier AB et al. Targeted disruption of the mouse transforming growth factor-beta 1 gene results in multifocal inflammatory disease. Nature 1992; 359(6397):693-699.
180. Takeda K, Clausen BE, Kaisho T et al. Enhanced Th1 activity and development of chronic enterocolitis in mice devoid of Stat3 in macrophages and neutrophils. Immunity 1999; 10(1):39-49.
181. Wirtz S, Finotto S, Kanzler S et al. Cutting edge: Chronic intestinal inflammation in STAT-4 transgenic mice: Characterization of disease and adoptive transfer by TNF- plus IFN-gamma-producing CD4+ T cells that respond to bacterial antigens. J Immunol 1999; 162(4):1884-1888.
182. Mashimo H, Wu DC, Podolsky DK et al. Impaired defense of intestinal mucosa in mice lacking intestinal trefoil factor. Science 1996; 274(5285):262-265.
183. Sadlack B, Merz H, Schorle H et al. Ulcerative colitis-like disease in mice with a disrupted interleukin-2 gene. Cell 1993; 75(2):253-261.
184. Willerford DM, Chen J, Ferry JA et al. Interleukin-2 receptor alpha chain regulates the size and content of the peripheral lymphoid compartment. Immunity 1995; 3(4):521-530.
185. Kuhn R, Lohler J, Rennick D et al. Interleukin-10-deficient mice develop chronic enterocolitis. Cell 1993; 75(2):263-274.
186. Kontoyiannis D, Pasparakis M, Pizarro TT et al. Impaired on/off regulation of TNF biosynthesis in mice lacking TNF AU-rich elements: Implications for joint and gut-associated immunopathologies. Immunity 1999; 10(3):387-398.
187. Fox JG, Rogers AB, Whary MT et al. Gastroenteritis in NF-kappaB-deficient mice is produced with wild-type Campylobacter jejuni but not with C. jejuni lacking cytolethal distending toxin despite persistent colonization with both strains. Infect Immun 2004; 72(2):1116-1125.
188. Rudolph U, Finegold MJ, Rich SS et al. Gi2 alpha protein deficiency: A model of inflammatory bowel disease. J Clin Immunol 1995; 15(6 Suppl):101S-105S.

189. Baribault H, Penner J, Iozzo RV et al. Colorectal hyperplasia and inflammation in keratin 8-deficient FVB/N mice. Genes Dev 1994; 8(24):2964-2973.
190. Spencer SD, Di Marco F, Hooley J et al. The orphan receptor CRF2-4 is an essential subunit of the interleukin 10 receptor. J Exp Med 1998; 187(4):571-578.
191. Snapper SB, Rosen FS, Mizoguchi E et al. Wiskott-Aldrich syndrome protein-deficient mice reveal a role for WASP in T but not B cell activation. Immunity 1998; 9(1):81-91.
192. Morrissey PJ, Charrier K, Braddy S et al. CD4+ T cells that express high levels of CD45RB induce wasting disease when transferred into congenic severe combined immunodeficient mice. Disease development is prevented by cotransfer of purified CD4+ T cells. J Exp Med 1993; 178(1):237-244.
193. Hollander GA, Simpson SJ, Mizoguchi E et al. Severe colitis in mice with aberrant thymic selection. Immunity 1995; 3(1):27-38.
194. Steinhoff U, Brinkmann V, Klemm U et al. Autoimmune intestinal pathology induced by hsp60-specific CD8 T cells. Immunity 1999; 11(3):349-358.
195. AGA. AGA technical review on celiac sprue. Gastroenterology 2001; 120(6):1526-1540.
196. Shan L, Molberg O, Parrot I et al. Structural basis for gluten intolerance in celiac sprue. Science 2002; 297(5590):2275-2279.
197. Teshigawara K, Kannagi R, Noro N et al. Possible involvement of transglutaminase in endocytosis and antigen presentation. Microbiol Immunol 1985; 29(8):737-750.
198. Ciccocioppo R, Di Sabatino A, Ara C et al. Gliadin and tissue transglutaminase complexes in normal and coeliac duodenal mucosa. Clin Exp Immunol 2003; 134(3):516-524.
199. Lundin KE, Scott H, Hansen T et al. Gliadin-specific, HLA-DQ(alpha 1*0501,beta 1*0201) restricted T cells isolated from the small intestinal mucosa of celiac disease patients. J Exp Med 1993; 178(1):187-196.
200. Molberg O, McAdam SN, Korner R et al. Tissue transglutaminase selectively modifies gliadin peptides that are recognized by gut-derived T cells in celiac disease. Nat Med 1998; 4(6):713-717.
201. Molberg O, McAdam S, Lundin KE et al. T cells from celiac disease lesions recognize gliadin epitopes deamidated in situ by endogenous tissue transglutaminase. Eur J Immunol 2001; 31(5):1317-1323.
202. Dieterich W, Ehnis T, Bauer M et al. Identification of tissue transglutaminase as the autoantigen of celiac disease. Nat Med 1997; 3(7):797-801.
203. Sulkanen S, Halttunen T, Laurila K et al. Tissue transglutaminase autoantibody enzyme-linked immunosorbent assay in detecting celiac disease. Gastroenterology 1998; 115(6):1322-1328.
204. Dieterich W, Laag E, Schopper H et al. Autoantibodies to tissue transglutaminase as predictors of celiac disease. Gastroenterology 1998; 115(6):1317-1321.
205. Llorente MJ, Sebastian M, Fernandez-Acenero MJ et al. IgA antibodies against tissue transglutaminase in the diagnosis of celiac disease: Concordance with intestinal biopsy in children and adults. Clin Chem 2004; 50(2):451-453.
206. Sollid LM, Thorsby E. HLA susceptibility genes in celiac disease: Genetic mapping and role in pathogenesis. Gastroenterology 1993; 105(3):910-922.
207. Greco L, Romino R, Coto I et al. The first large population based twin study of coeliac disease. Gut 2002; 50(5):624-628.
208. Zhong F, McCombs CC, Olson JM et al. An autosomal screen for genes that predispose to celiac disease in the western counties of Ireland. Nat Genet 1996; 14(3):329-333.
209. Greco L, Corazza G, Babron MC et al. Genome search in celiac disease. Am J Hum Genet 1998; 62(3):669-675.
210. Naluai AT, Nilsson S, Gudjonsdottir AH et al. Genome-wide linkage analysis of Scandinavian affected sib-pairs supports presence of susceptibility loci for celiac disease on chromosomes 5 and 11. Eur J Hum Genet 2001; 9(12):938-944.
211. Neuhausen SL, Feolo M, Farnham J et al. Linkage analysis of HLA and candidate genes for celiac disease in a North American family-based study. BMC Med Genet 2001; 2(1):12.
212. Liu J, Juo SH, Holopainen P et al. Genomewide linkage analysis of celiac disease in Finnish families. Am J Hum Genet 2002; 70(1):51-59.
213. Babron MC, Nilsson S, Adamovic S et al. Meta and pooled analysis of European coeliac disease data. Eur J Hum Genet 2003; 11(11):828-834.
214. Rioux JD, Karinen H, Kocher K et al. Genomewide search and association studies in a Finnish celiac disease population: Identification of a novel locus and replication of the HLA and CTLA4 loci. Am J Med Genet epub ahead of print Sep 22, 2004.
215. Woolley N, Holopainen P, Ollikainen V et al. A new locus for coeliac disease mapped to chromosome 15 in a population isolate. Hum Genet 2002; 111(1):40-45.
216. King AL, Yiannakou JY, Brett PM et al. A genome-wide family-based linkage study of coeliac disease. Ann Hum Genet 2000; 64(Pt 6):479-490.

217. Popat S, Bevan S, Braegger CP et al. Genome screening of coeliac disease. J Med Genet 2002; 39(5):328-331.
218. Neuhausen SL, Feolo M, Camp NJ et al. Genome-wide linkage analysis for celiac disease in North American families. Am J Med Genet 2002; 111(1):1-9.
219. Houlston RS, Tomlinson IP, Ford D et al. Linkage analysis of candidate regions for coeliac disease genes. Hum Mol Genet 1997; 6(8):1335-1339.
220. Holopainen P, Arvas M, Sistonen P et al. CD28/CTLA4 gene region on chromosome 2q33 confers genetic susceptibility to celiac disease. A linkage and family-based association study. Tissue Antigens 1999; 53(5):470-475.
221. Clot F, Fulchignoni-Lataud MC, Renoux C et al. Linkage and association study of the CTLA-4 region in coeliac disease for Italian and Tunisian populations. Tissue Antigens 1999; 54(5):527-530.
222. Naluai AT, Nilsson S, Samuelsson L et al. The CTLA4/CD28 gene region on chromosome 2q33 confers susceptibility to celiac disease in a way possibly distinct from that of type 1 diabetes and other chronic inflammatory disorders. Tissue Antigens 2000; 56(4):350-355.
223. Holopainen P, Mustalahti K, Uimari P et al. Candidate gene regions and genetic heterogeneity in gluten sensitivity. Gut 2001; 48(5):696-701.
224. Greco L, Babron MC, Corazza GR et al. Existence of a genetic risk factor on chromosome 5q in Italian coeliac disease families. Ann Hum Genet 2001; 65(Pt 1):35-41.
225. King AL, Fraser JS, Moodie SJ et al. Coeliac disease: Follow-up linkage study provides further support for existence of a susceptibility locus on chromosome 11p11. Ann Hum Genet 2001; 65(Pt 4):377-386.
226. King AL, Moodie SJ, Fraser JS et al. CTLA-4/CD28 gene region is associated with genetic susceptibility to coeliac disease in UK families. J Med Genet 2002; 39(1):51-54.
227. Popat S, Hearle N, Hogberg L et al. Variation in the CTLA4/CD28 gene region confers an increased risk of coeliac disease. Ann Hum Genet 2002; 66(Pt 2):125-137.
228. Louka AS, Sollid LM. HLA in coeliac disease: Unravelling the complex genetics of a complex disorder. Tissue Antigens 2003; 61(2):105-117.
229. Keuning JJ, Pena AS, van Leeuwen A et al. HLA-DW3 associated with coeliac disease. Lancet 1976; 1(7958):506-508.
230. Ek J, Albrechtsen D, Solheim BG et al. Strong association between the HLA-Dw3-related B cell alloantigen -DRw3 and coeliac disease. Scand J Gastroenterol 1978; 13(2):229-233.
231. Mearin ML, Biemond I, Pena AS et al. HLA-DR phenotypes in Spanish coeliac children: Their contribution to the understanding of the genetics of the disease. Gut 1983; 24(6):532-537.
232. Tosi R, Vismara D, Tanigaki N et al. Evidence that celiac disease is primarily associated with a DC locus allelic specificity. Clin Immunol Immunopathol 1983; 28(3):395-404.
233. Trabace S, Giunta A, Rosso M et al. HLA-ABC and DR antigens in celiac disease. A study in a pediatric Italian population. Vox Sang 1984; 46(2):102-106.
234. McManus R, Wilson AG, Mansfield J et al. TNF2, a polymorphism of the tumour necrosis-alpha gene promoter, is a component of the celiac disease major histocompatibility complex haplotype. Eur J Immunol 1996; 26(9):2113-2118.
235. Polvi A, Maki M, Collin P et al. TNF microsatellite alleles a2 and b3 are not primarily associated with celiac disease in the Finnish population. Tissue Antigens 1998; 51(5):553-555.
236. de la Concha EG, Fernandez-Arquero M, Vigil P et al. Celiac disease and TNF promoter polymorphisms. Hum Immunol 2000; 61(5):513-517.
237. Hahn-Zoric M, Hytonen AM, Hanson LA et al. Association of -1087 IL10 and -308 TNFA gene polymorphisms with serological markers of coeliac disease. J Clin Immunol 2003; 23(4):291-296.
238. Louka AS, Lie BA, Talseth B et al. Coeliac disease patients carry conserved HLA-DR3-DQ2 haplotypes revealed by association of TNF alleles. Immunogenetics 2003; 55(5):339-343.
239. Partanen J, Milner C, Campbell RD et al. HLA-linked heat-shock protein 70 (HSP70-2) gene polymorphism and celiac disease. Tissue Antigens 1993; 41(1):15-19.
240. Ramos-Arroyo MA, Feijoo E, Sanchez-Valverde F et al. Heat-shock protein 70-1 and HLA class II gene polymorphisms associated with celiac disease susceptibility in Navarra (Spain). Hum Immunol 2001; 62(8):821-825.
241. de la Concha EG, Fernandez-Arquero M, Lopez-Nava G et al. Susceptibility to severe ulcerative colitis is associated with polymorphism in the central MHC gene IKBL. Gastroenterology 2000; 119(6):1491-1495.
242. Fernandez L, Fernandez-Arquero M, Gual L et al. Triplet repeat polymorphism in the transmembrane region of the MICA gene in celiac disease. Tissue Antigens 2002; 59(3):219-222.
243. Rueda B, Pascual M, Lopez-Nevot MA et al. Association of MICA-A5.1 allele with susceptibility to celiac disease in a family study. Am J Gastroenterol 2003; 98(2):359-362.

244. Van Belzen MJ, Koeleman BP, Crusius JB et al. Defining the contribution of the HLA region to DQ2-positive coeliac disease patients. Genes Immun 2004; 5(3):215-220.
245. Roschmann E, Wienker TF, Volk BA. Role of T cell receptor delta gene in susceptibility to celiac disease. J Mol Med 1996; 74(2):93-98.
246. Rueda B, Lopez-Nevot MA, Pascual M et al. Polymorphism of the inducible nitric oxide synthase gene in celiac disease. Hum Immunol 2002; 63(11):1062-1065.
247. Louka AS, Stensby EK, Ek J et al. Coeliac disease candidate genes: No association with functional polymorphisms in matrix metalloproteinase 1 and 3 gene promoters. Scand J Gastroenterol 2002; 37(8):931-935.
248. Louka AS, Torinsson Naluai A, D'Alfonso S et al. The IL12B gene does not confer susceptibility to coeliac disease. Tissue Antigens 2002; 59(1):70-72.
249. Seegers D, Borm ME, van Belzen MJ et al. IL12B and IRF1 gene polymorphisms and susceptibility to celiac disease. Eur J Immunogenet 2003; 30(6):421-425.
250. Perez De Nanclares G, Bilbao JR, Calvo B et al. 5'-Insulin gene VNTR polymorphism is specific for type 1 diabetes: No association with celiac or Addison's disease. Ann NY Acad Sci 2003; 1005:319-323.
251. Aldersley MA, Hamlin PJ, Jones PF et al. No polymorphism in the tissue transglutaminase gene detected in coeliac disease patients. Scand J Gastroenterol 2000; 35(1):61-63.
252. Van Belzen MJ, Mulder CJ, Pearson PL et al. The tissue transglutaminase gene is not a primary factor predisposing to celiac disease. Am J Gastroenterol 2001; 96(12):3337-3340.
253. Bouguerra F, Dugoujon JM, Babron MC et al. Susceptibility to coeliac disease in Tunisian children and GM immunoglobulin allotypes. Eur J Immunogenet 1999; 26(4):293-297.
254. Van Belzen MJ, Mulder CJJ, Zhernakova A et al. CTLA4 +49A/G and CT60 polymorphisms in Dutch coeliac disease patients. Eur J Hum Genet 2004; 12(9):782-785.
255. Boniotto M, Braida L, Spano A et al. Variant mannose-binding lectin alleles are associated with celiac disease. Immunogenetics 2002; 54(8):596-598.
256. Haimila K, Smedberg T, Mustalahti K et al. Genetic association of coeliac disease susceptibility to polymorphisms in the ICOS gene on chromosome 2q33. Genes Immun 2004; 5(2):85-92.
257. Djilali-Saiah I, Schmitz J, Harfouch-Hammoud E et al. CTLA-4 gene polymorphism is associated with predisposition to coeliac disease. Gut 1998; 43(2):187-189.
258. Popat S, Hearle N, Wixey J et al. Analysis of the CTLA4 gene in Swedish coeliac disease patients. Scand J Gastroenterol 2002; 37(1):28-31.
259. Mora B, Bonamico M, Indovina P et al. CTLA-4 +49 A/G dimorphism in Italian patients with celiac disease. Hum Immunol 2003; 64(2):297-301.
260. King AL, Moodie SJ, Fraser JS et al. Coeliac disease: Investigation of proposed causal variants in the CTLA4 gene region. Eur J Immunogenet 2003; 30(6):427-432.
261. Kristiansen OP, Larsen ZM, Pociot F. CTLA-4 in autoimmune diseases—a general susceptibility gene to autoimmunity? Genes Immun 2000; 1(3):170-184.
262. Ueda H, Howson JM, Esposito L et al. Association of the T-cell regulatory gene CTLA4 with susceptibility to autoimmune disease. Nature 2003; 423(6939):506-511.
263. Batt RM, McLean L, Carter MW. Sequential morphologic and biochemical studies of naturally occurring wheat-sensitive enteropathy in Irish setter dogs. Dig Dis Sci 1987; 32(2):184-194.
264. Polvi A, Garden OA, Houlston RS et al. Genetic susceptibility to gluten sensitive enteropathy in Irish setter dogs is not linked to the major histocompatibility complex. Tissue Antigens 1998; 52(6):543-549.
265. Manns MP, Luttig B, Obermayer-Straub P. Autoimmune diseases: The liver. In: Rose NR, McKay IR, eds. The Autoimmune Diseases. 3rd ed. New York: Academic Press, 1998:511-544.
266. Gupta R, Agarwal SR, Jain M et al. Autoimmune hepatitis in the Indian subcontinent: 7 years experience. J Gastroenterol Hepatol 2001; 16(10):1144-1148.
267. Yachha SK, Srivastava A, Chetri K et al. Autoimmune liver disease in children. J Gastroenterol Hepatol 2001; 16(6):674-677.
268. Johnson PJ, McFarlane IG. Meeting report: International Autoimmune Hepatitis Group. Hepatology 1993; 18(4):998-1005.
269. Manns MP, Obermayer-Straub P. Cytochromes P450 and uridine triphosphate-glucuronosyltransferases: Model autoantigens to study drug-induced, virus-induced, and autoimmune liver disease. Hepatology 1997; 26(4):1054-1066.
270. Zanger UM, Hauri HP, Loeper J et al. Antibodies against human cytochrome P-450db1 in autoimmune hepatitis type II. Proc Natl Acad Sci USA 1988; 85(21):8256-8260.
271. Czaja AJ, Manns MP. The validity and importance of subtypes in autoimmune hepatitis: A point of view. Am J Gastroenterol 1995; 90(8):1206-1211.

272. Manns M, Gerken G, Kyriatsoulis A et al. Characterisation of a new subgroup of autoimmune chronic active hepatitis by autoantibodies against a soluble liver antigen. Lancet 1987; 1(8528):292-294.
273. Strassburg CP, Obermayer-Straub P, Manns MP. Autoimmunity in hepatitis C and D virus infection. J Viral Hepat 1996; 3(2):49-59.
274. Goldstein NS, Bayati N, Silverman AL et al. Minocycline as a cause of drug-induced autoimmune hepatitis. Report of four cases and comparison with autoimmune hepatitis. Am J Clin Pathol 2000; 114(4):591-598.
275. Czaja AJ, Donaldson PT. Genetic susceptibilities for immune expression and liver cell injury in autoimmune hepatitis. Immunol Rev 2000; 174:250-259.
276. Czaja AJ, Souto EO, Bittencourt PL et al. Clinical distinctions and pathogenic implications of type 1 autoimmune hepatitis in Brazil and the United States. J Hepatol 2002; 37(3):302-308.
277. Agarwal K, Jones DE, Daly AK et al. CTLA-4 gene polymorphism confers susceptibility to primary biliary cirrhosis. J Hepatol 2000; 32(4):538-541.
278. Djilali-Saiah I, Ouellette P, Caillat-Zucman S et al. CTLA-4/CD 28 region polymorphisms in children from families with autoimmune hepatitis. Hum Immunol 2001; 62(12):1356-1362.
279. Vogel A, Strassburg CP, Manns MP. Genetic association of vitamin D receptor polymorphisms with primary biliary cirrhosis and autoimmune hepatitis. Hepatology 2002; 35(1):126-131.
280. Vogel A, Strassburg CP, Manns MP. 77 C/G mutation in the tyrosine phosphatase CD45 gene and autoimmune hepatitis: Evidence for a genetic link. Genes Immun 2003; 4(1):79-81.
281. Manabe K, Hibberd ML, Donaldson PT et al. T-cell receptor constant beta germline gene polymorphisms and susceptibility to autoimmune hepatitis. Gastroenterology 1994; 106(5):1321-1325.
282. Whittingham S, Mathews JD, Schanfield MS et al. Interaction of HLA and Gm in autoimmune chronic active hepatitis. Clin Exp Immunol 1981; 43(1):80-86.
283. Cookson S, Constantini PK, Clare M et al. Frequency and nature of cytokine gene polymorphisms in type 1 autoimmune hepatitis. Hepatology 1999; 30(4):851-856.
284. Czaja AJ, Cookson S, Constantini PK et al. Cytokine polymorphisms associated with clinical features and treatment outcome in type 1 autoimmune hepatitis. Gastroenterology 1999; 117(3):645-652.
285. Vogel A, Liermann H, Harms A et al. Autoimmune regulator AIRE: Evidence for genetic differences between autoimmune hepatitis and hepatitis as part of the autoimmune polyglandular syndrome type 1. Hepatology 2001; 33(5):1047-1052.
286. Agarwal K, Czaja AJ, Jones DE et al. Cytotoxic T lymphocyte antigen-4 (CTLA-4) gene polymorphisms and susceptibility to type 1 autoimmune hepatitis. Hepatology 2000; 31(1):49-53.
287. Bittencourt PL, Palacios SA, Cancado EL et al. Cytotoxic T lymphocyte antigen-4 gene polymorphisms do not confer susceptibility to autoimmune hepatitis types 1 and 2 in Brazil. Am J Gastroenterol 2003; 98(7):1616-1620.
288. Jaeckel E. Animal models of autoimmune hepatitis. Semin Liver Dis 2002; 22(4):325-338.
289. Peters MG. Animal models of autoimmune liver disease. Immunol Cell Biol 2002; 80(1):113-116.
290. Howell CD. Animal models of autoimmunity. Clin Liver Dis 2002; 6(3):487-495.
291. Lohse AW, Brunner S, Kyriatsoulis A et al. Autoantibodies in experimental autoimmune hepatitis. J Hepatol 1992; 14(1):48-53.
292. Sadlack B, Lohler J, Schorle H et al. Generalized autoimmune disease in interleukin-2-deficient mice is triggered by an uncontrolled activation and proliferation of CD4+ T cells. Eur J Immunol 1995; 25(11):3053-3059.
293. Gorham JD, Lin JT, Sung JL et al. Genetic regulation of autoimmune disease: BALB/c background TGF-beta 1-deficient mice develop necroinflammatory IFN-gamma-dependent hepatitis. J Immunol 2001; 166(10):6413-6422.
294. Alper CA, Awdeh Z, Yunis EJ. Conserved, extended MHC haplotypes. Exp Clin Immunogenet 1992; 9(2):58-71.
295. Cullen M, Perfetto SP, Klitz W et al. High-resolution patterns of meiotic recombination across the human major histocompatibility complex. Am J Hum Genet 2002; 71(4):759-776.
296. Walsh EC, Mather KA, Schaffner SF et al. An integrated haplotype map of the human major histocompatibility complex. Am J Hum Genet 2003; 73(3):580-590.

Chapter 8

Inflammatory Myopathies:
Dermatomyositis, Polymyositis and Inclusion Body Myositis

Renato Mantegazza and Pia Bernasconi

Abstract

Dermatomyositis (DM), polymyositis (PM) and inclusion body myositis (IBM) belong to the heterogeneous group of the inflammatory myopathies and are characterized by muscle cell infiltrations and specific alterations of the muscle fibers. In DM it is evident a perifascicular atrophy of muscle tissue due to the activation and deposition of complement on capillaries; in PM and IBM there is a prominent endomysial infiltration of clonally expanded $CD8^+$ T lymphocytes that surround and eventually invade single nonnecrotic muscle fibers, positive for MHC class I molecules. Muscle fibers in PM/IBM die for the action of cytotoxic enzymes (perforin and granzymes) released by the invading $CD8^+$ T lymphocytes. In IBM, beside the autoimmune attack, there is an abnormal accumulation of proteins in vacuoles within muscle fibers. Triggering factors of myositis as well as the processes by which the immunological attack induces muscle weakness are still unknown. Upregulation of adhesion molecules, cytokines, chemokines contribute to recruit cells of the immune system and to maintain a chronic inflamed area. In vivo and in vitro studies on muscle cells have assessed their functions as target cells or antigen presenting cells. Combined studies on gene profiles and cellular immunology of disease-associated muscle biopsies will be of great help in clarifying the pathogenetic mechanisms underlying these inflammatory myopathies.

Introduction

The idiopathic inflammatory myopathies (IIM) are a heterogeneous group of diseases characterized by muscle inflammation.[1,2] The principal clinical variants of IIM are: dermatomyositis (DM), polymyositis (PM), and inclusion body myositis (IBM).[1,2] The latter is divided into: sporadic-IBM (s-IBM), the most common muscle disease that starts after age 50 years and leads to severe disability, and hereditary inclusion body myopathies (h-IBM), characterized by pathologic features that strikingly resemble those of s-IBM except for lack of lymphocyte inflammation (hence the term "myopathy" instead of "myositis").[3] Inflammatory myopathies are included in the clinicopathological interest of different medical specialties (e.g., neurology, rheumatology, dermatology, etc.) resulting in different diagnostic evaluation and treatment work-up. A recent meeting, under the auspices of the ENMC (European Neuromuscular Centre) in which European and American neurologists and rheumatologists convened, put a tremendous effort in establishing common diagnostic criteria and measuring outcomes in the perspective of international randomized clinical trials.[4]

DM is a humorally mediated microangiopathy, while PM is a T-cell mediated disorder in which a cytotoxic attack against single nonnecrotic muscle fibers occurs. The pathogenesis of IBM is unknown.[3] DM and PM are considered to be responsive to immunosuppressive and immunomodulating therapies, in contrast to IBM, which is refractory to all treatment.[4] The

Immunogenetics of Autoimmune Disease, edited by Jorge Oksenberg and David Brassat.

triggering factors of IIM are still unknown; a growing body of evidence suggests that genetically susceptible individuals probably develop an idiopathic inflammatory myopathy in response to particular environment stimuli.

Clinical Aspects

Dermatomyositis

DM is a rare multisystemic autoimmune disease that affects children and adults of both genders and all ethnic groups (Table 1). It primarily involves skin and skeletal muscle. Cutaneous manifestations may precede the onset of myositis by several months or up to 2 years and more; Gottron's papules, heliotrope rash, and macular erythemas are the most typical manifestations.[5] Skin lesions can be worsened by UVA and UVB light; this increased photosensitivity may be due to a polymorphism in tumor necrosis factor-α (TNF-α)-308A allele, detected with high frequency in adult and juvenile DM Caucasian patients (reviewed in ref. 5). Muscle weakness can vary from mild to severe (quadriparesis). Clinical manifestations other than those involving muscle tissue can occur: subcutaneous calcifications, joint contractures, dysphagia, fever, malaise, weight loss, arthralgia, Raynaud's phenomenon, tumor.[1,2] DM diagnosis is confirmed by muscle biopsy (see paragraph regarding histopathology).

Polymyositis

PM, as a difference with DM, has less distinguished clinical features (Table 1).[1,2] However, PM can be suspected in all cases presenting as a subacute proximal myopathy without evidence of inherited transmission. Incidence and prevalence are reported to be similar to those of DM, but PM is extremely rare in infancy. Female to male ratio is 3:1. The clinical course of PM is usually subacute. In the typical affected adult patient anamnesis is negative for: cutaneous symptoms, involvement of ocular and facial muscles, presence of hereditary muscular diseases and exposure to myotoxic drugs or toxins. Onset of the disease can be difficult to ascertain because a subclinical disease may persist over months before the patients refer to the physician. Apart from cutaneous alterations, the degree of severity and distribution of muscle weakness and wasting are similar to those described for DM, except for myalgia and muscle tenderness, which are less frequent than in DM.

Inclusion Body Myositis

IBM has clinical-pathological features well differentiated from PM or DM (Table 1).[1,3] IBM is tipically a chronic evolutive muscle disorders whose onset is usually after the age of 50. Because onset is extremely insidious and disease course so slow, the time of beginning and the incidence of the disease is very difficult to establish. IBM is more frequent in males (male to female ratio 3:1) and in whites than in blacks. Muscle weakness and atrophy affect more frequently distal muscles: deficit of the foot extensors might be evident in more than 50% of the cases and represent the clue of early diagnosis. Selective involvement of triceps, biceps, ileopsoas and quadriceps is frequently evident and responsible for sudden falls of these patients. A noticeable evidence of asymmetric involvement of muscles is a typical feature of IBM. Tendon reflexes are usually lost and because of distal atrophy and weakness a neurogenic disease can be misdiagnosed. Though IBM is considered an acquired IM, familial cases have been described, some associated with leukoencephalopathy. An empyrical criterion to suspect IBM is the unresponsiveness to immunosuppressive therapy of suspected PM patients.

Histopathology

PM and s-IBM are characterized by an endomysial mononuclear cell infiltrate, mainly composed of cytotoxic $CD8^+$ T lymphocytes and macrophages, which surrounds and eventually invades single nonnecrotic muscle fibers. $CD8^+$ T cells are activated ($HLA\text{-}DR,^+$ $LFA\text{-}1^+$), have a memory phenotype ($CD45RO^+$) and released perforin when in close contact with muscle fiber.[1,2] Besides inflammation, in s-IBM muscle fibers abnormally accumulated

Table 1. Idiopathic inflammatory myopathies: clinical features

Clinical Features	Dermatomyositis	Polymyositis	Inclusion Body Myositis
Age at onset	Children/adults	Adults (> 18 years)	Adults (> 80 years)
Sex	F = M	F > M	M > F
Ethnic group	All	All, HLA restriction according to race	Whites > blacks, ethnic clusters
Familial association	No	No	Yes
Other disorders	Neoplasm, CTD, autoimm. dis.	Autoimm. dis., viral infections	CTD, viral infections
Main clinical manifestations	Cutaneous* and muscle weakness: symmetrical prox. legs > arms neck flexors > neck extensors, myalgia	Muscle weakness: symmetrical prox. legs > arms neck flexors > neck extensors	Muscle weakness: asymmetric prox./distal leg and arm muscle, wrist/fingers flexors ≥ deltoids
EMG	Myopathic	Myopathic	Myopathic or neurogenic
Muscle enzymes	High or normal	High	Normal or high
Muscle biopsy	Perifascicular atrophy perifascicular, perimysial infiltrates, capillary alterations	Endomysial inflammatory cell infiltrates surrounding and invading non-necrotic muscle fibers	Endomysial inflammatory cell infiltrates surrounding and invading non-necrotic muscle fibers, vacuolated m. fibers
Response to immunosuppression	Yes	Yes	No

*Gottron's papules, heliotrope rash, and macular erythemas. F: female; M: male; HLA: human leukocyte antigen; CTD: connective tissue disease.

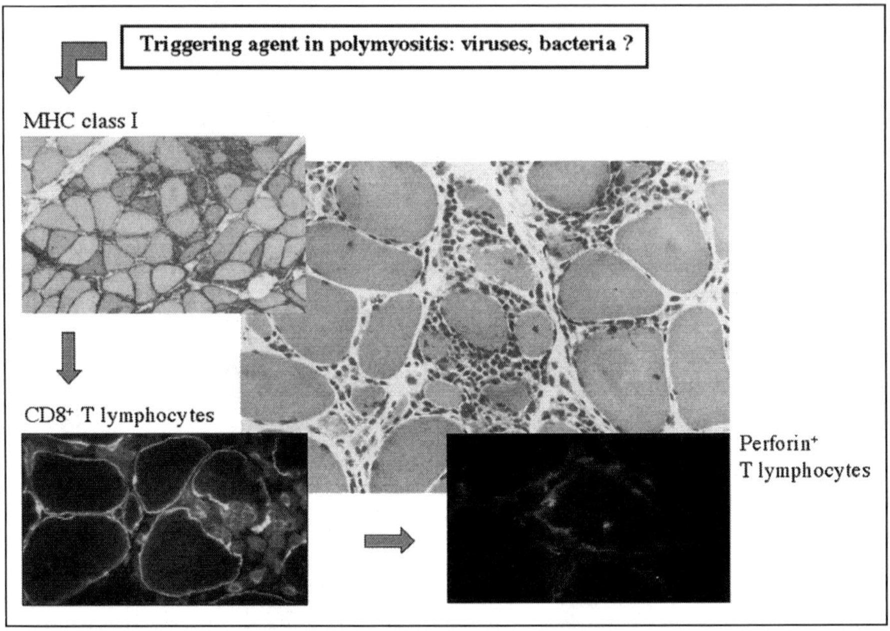

Figure 1. Polymyositis (PM) muscle biopsy is characterized by perimysial and endomysial mononuclear cell infiltrates, necrobiosis, variation in myofiber diameter and increased perimysial and endomysial connective tissue (hematoxylin-eosin staining). Nonnecrotic muscle fibers, positive for major histocompatibility complex class I and II molecules, are surrounded and invaded by mononuclear cells, mainly cytotoxic T lymphocytes, strongly positive for CD8 staining (red fluorescence). Some of the endomysial $CD8^+$ T lymphocytes are perforin positive. As in DM the triggering factor is still unknown; it is clear that there is an active interaction between the MHC^+ muscle fibers and T lymphocytes, it remains to be elucidated whether muscle fibers are able to activate naïve T cells or their immune capacity is secondary to inflammation.

proteins are observed (Figs. 1, 2).[6] In DM the most prominent cells are $CD4^+$ T lymphocytes localized in the perivascular site which might provide help to B cells to produce antibodies that, fixing complement, induce a vascular damage. The deposition of the lytic membrane attack complex (MAC) on capillaries induces perivascular inflammation, capillary depletion, muscle fiber necrosis and perifascicular atrophy, diagnostic for DM even in the absence of inflammation (Fig. 3).[1,2]

Immunopathogenesis

We will focus on the genetic characteristics of inflammatory myopathy patients and the phenotypes of effector and target cells involved in the immune response. All the information are summarized in Tables 2-4.

Major Histocompatibility Complex (MHC)

As for other autoimmune diseases, a strong association between human leukocyte antigen (HLA) genes and all clinical forms of IIM has been found (Table 2). At first the genetic marker associated with IIM was HLA B8 (studied in patients with juvenile DM), then the studies were extended including a large number of patients and the major genetic risk factors for the development of myositis were identified in HLA DRB1*0301 and DQA1*0501 in whites.[7] DRB1*0301 is a common genetic risk factor for familial and sporadic IIM, but

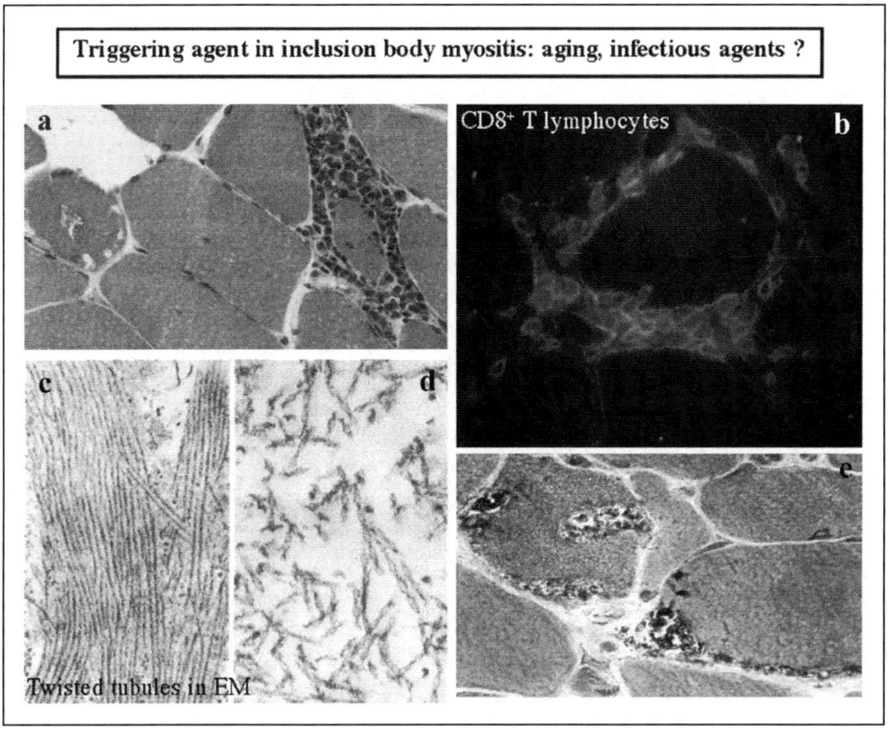

Figure 2. Inclusion body myositis (IBM): a) rimmed vacuoles can be observed (hematoxylin-eosin staining); b) a mononuclear cell infiltrate, mainly composed by CD8$^+$T lymphocytes, surrounds a nonnecrotic muscle fiber. e) Modified Gomori trichrome staining shows typical vacuoles with basophilic red granular material in the muscle cell cytoplasm. Electron microscopy (EM) analysis demonstrates the presence (within muscle fibers) of c) cytoplasmic twisted tubulofilaments and d) amyloid-like fibrils. As for the other IIM forms, the activating factor is unknown. It has been proposed that factors, related to muscle aging or to environment (for sporadic-IBM) or of genetic origin (for hereditary-IBM), lead to a defect in the protein processing machinery that in turn causes abnormal protein accumulation within muscle fibers. This accumulation might lead to oxidative stress and other alterations, responsible for muscle fiber degeneration and death.

contributes in a lesser extent in the familial IIM; while, the unique genetic risk factor to familial IIM is homozygosity at the HLA-DQA1 locus.[8] Hausmanowa-Petrusewicz et al[9] reported that the HLA-DRB1*0301; DQA1*0501 haplotype was found to be significantly increased in Polish IIM population as a whole and in those IIM patients positive for anti-synthetase, anti-PM-Scl, and anti-Ku autoantibodies. Other groups observed that HLA-DRB1*0301 (DR3), DQA1*0501, and DQB1*0201 (DQ2) alleles were each increased in white patients with myositis, especially those with PM, and most strikingly in those with myositis-specific autoantibodies. In other ethnic groups, except the Japanese, only frequencies of HLA-DQA1*0501 and the structurally similar DQA1*0401 alleles were significantly increased and most significantly associated with anti-Jo-1, anti-PL-12, and other autoantibodies, compared with IIM patients without autoantibodies. HLA-DQA1*0102 and *0103 alleles predominated in those IIM patients, including Japanese, positive for myositis-specific antibodies but negative for HLA-DQA1*0501 and *0401. A negative association of the HLA-DR2 alleles (DRB1*1501 and *1503) with PM but not with DM was found.[10]

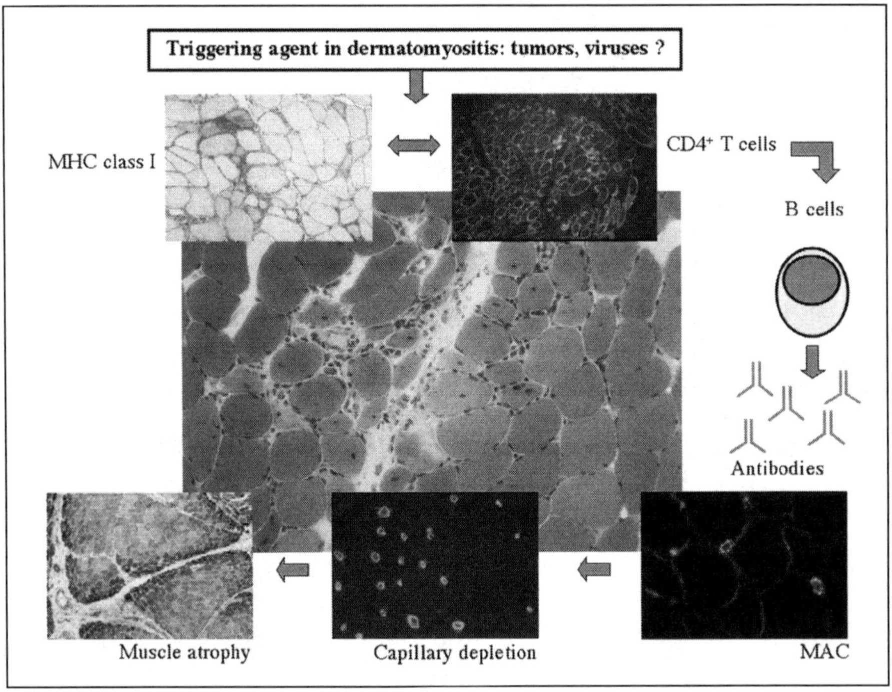

Figure 3. The histopathological features of dermatomyositis (DM) muscle biopsy are shown. A still unknown triggering factor activates $CD4^+$ T lymphocytes, which in turn might provide help to B cells to produce antibodies. The antibodies activate the complement cascade that ends with membranolytic attack complex (MAC) deposition on capillaries. This induces capillary depletion (capillaries are stained with fluorescent *Ulex europaeus* agglutinin lectin) and eventually perifascicular atrophy (outlined as intense NADH-stained fibers), due to the endofascicular hypoperfusion of muscle tissue. Muscle fibers are positive for major histocompatibility complex (MHC) class I molecule expression.

Table 2. Association between human leukocyte antigen genes and idiopathic inflammatory myopathies

Clinical Group	Haplotype	Clinical Features
IIM (Caucasian)	DRB1*0301/DQA1*0501	Sporadic IIM; mild association with familial IIM
	DQA1 homozygosity	Familial IIM (particular in patients positive for autoantibodies)
	DRB1*0301/DQA1*0501/DQB1*0201	IIM, especially in PM and in those patients positive for MSA
IIM (except Japanese)	DQA1*0501/DQA1*0401	IIM positive for anti-Jo-1, anti-PL-12 autoantibodies
IIM (including Japanese)	DQA1*0102 and *0103	IIM positive for MSA, but negative for DQA1*0501 and *0401

IIM: idiopathic inflammatory myopathies; PM: polymyositis; MSA: myositis-specific antibodies.

Table 3. Phenotypes of effector cells in inflammatory myopathies (updated 9-1-2004)

	DM[a]	PM[a]	s-IBM[a]
T lymphocytes[b]			
endomysial	+	+++	++
perimysial	++	++	+
perivascular	+/++	+	+
B lymphocytes[b]			
endomysial	+	+/-	+/-
perimysial	++	+	+
perivascular	+++	+	+/-
Macrophages[b]	+	+/++	+/++
NK cells[b]	+/-	+	+
T cell receptor			
α/β heterodimer	present	present	present
γ/δ heterodimer	rare	rare	rare
α/β repertoire[c]	polyclonal	oligoclonal	oligoclonal
CDR3	random	conserved	conserved
Cytokines[b]			
IL-1α	PA[d]	in EC and IC[d]	in EC and IC[d]
IL-1β	in MC[e]	in MC[e]	in MC[e]
TNF-α	+/-	+/-	++
IL-2/IL-2R	+	+	-
IFN-γ	+/-	+	+
IL-4/5/6/10/13	-	+/-	+/-
TGF-β1	++	+	+
Chemokines[b]			
CCL2	++	+	+
CCL3	+	++	++
CCL4	+	+	+
CCL5	+	+	+
CXCL8	-	-	-
CXCL9	+	+	+
CXCL10	+	+	+
CXCL11	-	-	-
Cytotoxic enzymes			
Perforin	absent	present	present
Granzyme	absent	present	present
Apoptotic signals[b]			
Fas	-/+	+	+
FasL	-/+	++	++
FLIP	not investigated	+	+
Stimulatory signals[b]			
CD28/CTLA4	-	T cells invading BB-1$^+$ muscle fibers	T cells invading BB-1$^+$ muscle fibers
ICOS	+	+	+

[a] DM: dermatomyositis; PM: polymyositis; s-IBM: sporadic inclusion body myositis. [b] +++: strong signal; ++: medium signal; +: weak signal; -/+: very weak signal; -: no signal. [c] Polyclonal or oligoclonal TCR repertoire expressed as number of Vα or Vβ rearrangements detected. [d] EC: endothelial cells; IC: infiltrating cells; PA: perifascicular arterioles. [e] MC: mononuclear cells.

Recently, HLA I and II haplotypes have been analyzed in a cohort of s-IBM patients:[11] the previously mentioned association with B8 and DR3[7,8,10] was detected and a new HLA association, A*03, DQ5/DQB1*05, was observed.[12] Three hypothesis about the cause of HLA association with s-IBM were put forward by the authors: (1) s-IBM is caused by a viral infection

Table 4. Immunobiological features of muscle cells in inflammatory myopathies (updated 9-1-2004)

	DM[a]	PM[a]	s-IBM[a]
MHC[b]			
Class I	+++	+++	++
Class II	++	++	+
HLA-G	+	+	+
Adhesion molecules[b]			
ICAM-1	-	+++	+++
VCAM-1	-	-	-
LFA-1	-	-	-
LFA-3	-	+	+
Co-stimulatory molecules[b]			
B7.1	-	-	-
B7.2	-	-	-
BB-1	++ (only on regenerating N-CAM$^+$ fibers)	+++	+++
B7-H1	++	+++	++
ICOSL	++ (on endothelial cells)	+++	++
Chemokines[b]			
CCL2	+[c]	+[c]	+[c]
CCL3	-	-	-
CCL5	+[c]	+[c]	+[c]
CXCL8	+[c]	+[c]	+[c]
CXCL9	+	+	+
CXCL10	+[c]	+[c]	+[c]
CXCL11	-	-	-
Apoptotic signals			
Fas	-/+	+	+
FasL	+[d]	+[d]	+[d]
Bcl-2	+	+	+
FLIP	not investigated	+	+
hILP	+	+	+

[a] DM: dermatomyositis; PM: polymyositis; s-IBM: sporadic inclusion body myositis. [b] +++: strong signal; ++: medium signal; +: weak signal; -/+: very weak signal; -: no signal. [c] mRNA and protein seen only on muscle cells in vitro as constitutive expression or after IFN-γ stimulus. [d] Observed on regenerating muscle fibers.

(even if in s-IBM it appears unlikely); (2) s-IBM is an autoimmune disease (putative antigens can be auto and viral antigens); (3) s-IBM is due to genes, so far unidentified, in linkage disequilibrium with HLA alleles (for example, in MHC locus are located genes for TNF-α and β, the complement factors 2 and 4, heat shock protein 70).[11]

The importance of HLA molecules in the pathogenesis of IIM is strongly supported by the observation that, while normal muscle fibers do not express MHC class I molecules on their surface, IIM muscle fibers are strongly positive for MHC class I and class II expression, even in cells apparently distant from cell infiltrates.[1,12,13] It remains to be elucidated whether MHC molecule expression is induced by infectious agents or by proinflammatory cytokines[14,15] or by a nonspecific response to tissue injury and regeneration. Lundberg et al[16] observed that in chronic PM and DM clinical symptoms persist even in the absence of inflammatory infiltrates together with an increased expression of IL-1α in the capillaries and MHC class I on muscle fibers, mainly confined to type II muscle fibers.[17] The authors hypothesized that infiltrating cells might not be the primary factors of muscle damage. As observed in an animal model,[18] overexpression of IL-1α and MHC class I might be sufficient to induce clinical myositis, muscle damage and eventually muscle inflammation.

In vitro myoblasts and myotubes constitutively express low levels of MHC class I and adhesion molecules such as LFA-3. After myoblast stimulation with IFN-γ or IFN-γ and TNF-α increased expression of MHC class I and de novo synthesis of MHC class II and ICAM-1 has been observed.[19-25] When myoblasts are allowed to fuse into myotubes and these cells are innervated MHC class II molecules disappear on cell surface even after IFN-γ stimulation, suggesting that MHC class II synthesis is developmentally regulated during myogenesis and that overexpression of this molecule on pathological muscle fibers might be independent by proinflammatory cytokine production.[22]

In the last years, it is emerging the role of non classic MHC class I molecules, in particular of HLA-G, in IIM pathogenesis. This molecule is similar to the MHC class I (β2-microglobulin association, CD8 binding, presentation of a restricted peptide repertoire) but with peculiar characteristics: less polymorphic, highly restricted tissue distribution, seven different isoforms (membrane-associated, HLA-G1, -G2, -G3, -G4, and soluble, HLA-G5, -G6, -G7).[26] HLA-G is a key molecule in fetal-maternal tolerance and in the adult life protects target cells from cytotoxic T and natural killer cell attack.[27] Normally muscle fibers do not express HLA-G, while a highly positive signal has been observed on IIM muscle fibers, also positive for MHC class I molecules, and on many inflammatory cells.[28] Moreover, the authors demonstrated that in vitro IFN-γ was able to up regulate mRNA transcripts corresponding to different isoforms of HLA-G and their surface expression in cultured myoblasts isolated from control subjects and patients.[28] Transfection of myoblasts or muscle cell line (TE671) with HLA-G molecules (HLA-G1 and -G5) rendered these cells resistant to alloreactive lysis, reduced alloproliferation, interfered with priming of antigen-specific cytotoxic T cells or inhibited antigen-specific effector lysis.[29] In inflammatory myopathies and in other conditions of inflamed muscles (e.g., myoblast transplantation, vaccination) HLA-G might be a muscle cell effort to protect themselves from immune cell-mediated attack.[30]

Besides MHC class I and II molecules, costimulatory molecules are necessary to stimulate T lymphocytes. Three different costimulatory pathways have been discovered: the B7-1/B7-2 (CD80/CD86) and their receptors CD28/CTLA-4, the best characterized; the inducible costimulatory ligand (ICOSL) and its receptor ICOS (a T cell specific costimulatory molecule homologous to CD28/CTLA4); the receptor PD-1 (programmed death gene 1), which interacts with two novel B7 family members, PD-L1 (B7-H1) and PD-L2 (B7-DC). All these coreceptors can enhance or attenuate T cell activation.[31]

Muscle fibers do not express constitutively or under pro-inflammatory stimuli, detectable levels of CD80/CD86 molecules both in vivo and in vitro.[32-35] Nevertheless, they are able to activate antigen-specific T cell response.[36] It is not yet clear whether they are able to prime naïve T cells. Other molecules have been postulated to be expressed on muscle fibers such as a yet unidentified B7-related protein (BB-1) that interacts with CD28/CTLA4 and stimulates T lymphocytes.[34,35] Recently, important advances in the field of muscle capacity to stimulate an immune response have been obtained by analyzing the costimulatory pathways alternative to CD80/CD86-CD28/CTLA4 pathway. ICOSL was expressed at low levels on muscle fibers and to be up regulated in IIM muscle tissue, in particular in PM, on the muscle fibers surrounded and invaded by T lymphocytes $ICOS^+$ [37] (a marker of T cell activation).[38] In DM a strong positivity for ICOSL was observed on endothelial cells of blood vessels.[37] Furthermore, ICOSL was observed on cultured myoblasts in basal condition and enhanced after TNF-α stimulation. Cocultures of MHC class II^+ myoblasts with $CD4^+$ T cells together with superantigen demonstrated that ICOSL is active since it modulates Th1 and Th2 cytokine synthesis by activated T cells.[37] These observations paralleled those of B7-H1 molecule. This protein was expressed in IIM muscle biopsies and not in normal or nonmyopathic muscle tissues; it was localized to areas of strong inflammation either on muscle and mononuclear cells.[39] In vitro myoblasts became positive for B7-H1 only after IFN-γ stimulation. Anti-B7-H1 monoclonal antibody strongly augmented the Th1 and Th2 cytokines in cocultures of IFN-γ stimulated myoblasts, CD4+ or CD8+ T cells and superantigens.[39] The authors speculate that B7-H1 could interfere with the activity of cytotoxic T cells and, hence, this expression is another effort of muscle fiber to protect itself from the autoimmune attack.[39]

T Cell Receptor (TCR)

T lymphocytes recognize the antigen, presented by the MHC class I or II, via T cell receptor (TCR), a heterodimer composed by two chains, α/β or γ/δ (less frequent), encoded by different gene families combined to form the variable (V), diversity (D), joining (J) and constant (C) regions.[40,41] The contact point between TCR and the antigen-MHC complex lies in the complementarity-determining region 3 (CDR3), composed by the V-(D)-J combination. If TCR recognizes an antigen the amino acid sequence of the CDR3 region should be conserved in the recruited T cells.[40,41] In PM and s-IBM patients, but not in DM, T lymphocytes with a restricted TCR repertoire are recruited from the blood stream to the muscle tissue. Sequence analysis of the TCR families revealed a restricted use of Jβ genes and a CDR3 consensus motif. These data are suggestive of the presence of a conventional antigen on muscle fibers, which attracts specifically CD8+ T cells.[42-50] In selected s-IBM patients the TCR repertoire has been analyzed in sequential muscle biopsies during a period of 19-22 months.[51] A persistent clonal expansion of CD8+ T cells with the same TCRBV families and a persistent CDR3 amino acid sequence were observed, supporting the hypothesis that endomysial T cells are recruited by a continuous presentation by muscle fibers of the same antigen(s), even in the late stages of the disease.[51] Analysis of peripheral T cells from IIM patients and age-matched controls showed in the patients a more frequent CD8+ T cell clonal expansion than CD4+ T cells. The expanded T cells persisted as large populations over time and some of the expanded clones were found in the affected muscles from the same patients.[52] These results provide the evidence that a local autoimmune reaction can directly influence the periphery. Moreover, to have the possibility to isolate pathological T cell clones from the periphery will be of great help in understanding the evolution of the disease and the efficacy of specific therapeutic treatments. Benveniste et al[53] demonstrated that TCR repertoire was perturbated in the peripheral blood of PM patients but not of DM patients. Analysis of TCR repertoire in the periphery might be useful in differential diagnosis between PM and DM. However, a study like this does not allow proving that clonally expanded T cells are those that invade the single nonnecrotic muscle fibers. The use of a laser microdissector has overcome this problem. Hofbauer et al[54] combined CDR3 spectratyping analysis with single cell PCR performed on cells localized in direct contact with the muscle fiber and isolated by laser microdissector. With this approach they were able to identify and track autoaggressive T lymphocytes. It is accepted that in PM/IBM specific antigens, presented by muscle fibers, recruit T cells, what is the antigen remains a mistery.

Myositis-Specific Autoantibodies

Most of IIM patients' sera, approximately 50%, are positive for myositis-specific autoantibodies (MSAs). The targeted antigens are not specific for muscle tissue, the majority of them are aminoacyl-tRNA synthetases, components of the signal recognition particle, translation factors, components of a nucleosome remodelling complex (for a comprehensive review see ref. 55). MSAs are associated with specific clinical characteristics, for example anti-Jo-1 (anti-histidyl tRNA synthetase, HisRS) antibodies and the antisynthetase syndrome (DM or PM, idiopathic interstitial lung disease, arthritis and Raynaud phenomenon).[55] The exact role of MSAs in IIM immunopathogenesis is still unknown. Nagaraju et al[18] demonstrated that conditional overexpression of MHC class I molecules in the skeletal muscles of young mice was able to induce an inflammatory disease, limited to skeletal muscles, self-sustaining, more severe in females, and often accompanied by autoantibodies, including, in some mice, anti-Jo-1 autoantibodies (the most frequent antibodies in IIM patients, 15-25% of cases). The authors suggested that an apparently non specific event, such as the up-regulation of MHC class I in a tissue, might generate a highly specific autoimmune disease and that specific autoantibodies derive not from the specificity of the stimulus, but from the context, location, and probably the duration of the stimulus.

The majority of autoantigens, including the aminoacyl-tRNA synthetases, targets of the immune attack in different systemic autoimmune diseases, have in their sequence the cleavage site recognized by granzyme B, a highly specific protease released by activated immune cells that cuts target molecule after aspartate residues.[56-58] Nonautoantigens are refractory to granzyme B cleavage.[57] The HisRS is cleaved by granzyme B in the N-terminal domain and the presence of anti-Jo-1 antibodies inhibited the granzyme B cleavage, suggesting that the immunodominant epitope and the cleavage site are very close.[58] HisRS and asparaginyl-tRNA synthetase (AsnRS) have chemoattractant properties versus CCR3- and CCR5-expressing cells, and can recruit immature dendritic cells.[59] Moreover, T cells isolated from peripheral blood of PM patients, positive for anti-Jo-1 antibodies, and from control subjects proliferated in response to Jo-1 full-length, or peptides, in the presence of dendritic cells with a predominant response versus the N-terminal domain (the dominant B cell epitope). This response was MHC class II dependent.[60] Altogether these results suggest an active role of aminoacyl-tRNA synthetase in initiating and perpetuating the immune response within IIM muscle tissue. A still unknown event (e.g., viral infection) in the appropriate host might damage muscle tissue, aminoacyl-tRNA synthetases might undergo conformational changes becoming susceptible to granzyme B cleavage and be released in the microenvironment. The fragmented aminoacyl-tRNA synthetase might recruit mononuclear cells initiating a cascade of immune events such as antigen presentation to T lymphocytes, production of B cell stimulating cytokines that results in autoantibody synthesis, further muscle damage via release of cytotoxic enzymes.[58,59]

Cytokines and Chemokines

Cytokines play a crucial role in inflammatory reaction. These molecules are soluble, short-lived proteins produced, constitutively or under proper stimulation, by several cell types.[61] In muscle biopsies of patients with IIM several cytokines can be amplified or immunolocalized: interleukin (IL)-1α and 1β, IL-2, IL-6, IL-10, TNF-α, IFN-γ, TGF-β and GM-CSF.[62-67] Some of them might play an important role in the pathogenesis of IIM, in particular IL-1α, TNF-α and TGF-β. IL-1α was mainly expressed in endomysial capillaries, in perifascicular arterioles and venules, even in the absence of inflammation,[16] and in in vitro experiments it influenced MHC expression on cultured human myoblasts and myotubes, suggesting that an altered muscle metabolism can cause an eventually immune response.[68] TNF-α, an important mediator of inflammation and cellular immune responses, was occasionally expressed in mononuclear cells and on muscle fibre membranes.[66,67,69] A proportion of TNF-α positive fibers were also positive for the developmental form of myosin heavy chain, indicating that TNF-α might implicated also in the regenerative process and that muscle fibers can be the target of infiltrating cells, but also an active player in the immune response.[69] In muscle fibers of juvenile DM (JDM) patients TNF-α was higher expressed in those patients positive for TNF-α-308A allele than in JDM patients negative for the allele. It has been hypothesized that TNF-α-308A allele influencing the overproduction of the cytokine in response to the stimulus, contributes to the chronicity of the disease and, if not treated, to the formation of calcifications (for a comprehensive review, see ref. 70). TGF-β1 was immunolocalized in extracellular matrix of IIM muscle biopsies and never in correspondence of mononuclear cell infiltrates.[71] TGF-β1, linked to the extracellular matrix, might contribute to the recruitment of mononuclear cells within the muscle, since it increases the adhesiveness of endothelial cells for leukocytes, inhibits E-selectin expression in endothelial cells[72] and induces the chemokine monocyte chemoattractant protein (MCP)-1/CCL2 synthesis.[73]

Chemokines are chemotactic cytokines that regulate leukocyte migration into inflamed area, as well as homeostatic trafficking of lymphocytes and dendritic cells. Their primary structure is characterized by the presence of four conserved cysteine residues. The largest and best-characterized families are the α-chemokines (CXCL) and the β-chemokines (CCL).[74] Several chemokines (CCL2, CCL3, CCL5, CCL9, CXCL8, CXCL9, CXCL10) have been detected in IIM muscle tissue localized in correspondence of infiltrating inflammatory cells and in the extracellular matrix with a pattern of distribution related to the different pathogenetic processes underlying the three IIM forms.[75-77] Chemokine synthesis and storage in the extracellular matrix can act as a microenviromental factor amplifying lymphocyte activation and migration, thereby maintaining the autoimmune attack and tissue degeneration.

Muscle cells might be actively involved in chemokine synthesis and release in the inflamed area. It has been demonstrated that CXCL8, CCL5 were constitutively expressed by cultured myoblasts and enhanced after pro-inflammatory stimulus;[78] CCL2, CXCL9, CXCL10 were induced by IFN-γ or TNF-α stimulus.[77,78] These data further support the hypothesis that muscle cells are not only the target of the immune-mediated attack but that they may directly release cytokines/chemokines necessary to initiate and perpetuate immunocompetent cell recruitment.

Mechanisms of Muscle Cell Damage

Degeneration and necrosis of muscle fibers by $CD8^+$ T lymphocytes in PM and s-IBM is predominantly mediated by release of cytotoxic enzymes: perforin and granzymes.

When cytotoxic T cells recognize the antigen via TCR, the lytic granules polarise towards the interface with the target cell (the immunological synapse), fuse with the target cell plasma membrane, and focally release soluble lytic proteins (including perforin and granzymes) to induce target cell death.[79] In DM and PM perforin and granzyme transcripts were expressed at similar levels and either $CD3^+$ $CD4^+$ and $CD3^+$ $CD8^+$ T cells were perforin positive.[62,80] By confocal microscopy, in DM perforin was distributed randomly in the cytoplasm of the inflammatory T cells, while in PM the cytotoxic T cells that contacted a muscle fiber showed perforin located vectorially towards the target muscle cell. This suggests that in DM perforin distribution reflects a nonspecific T cell activation, while in PM the oriented perforin distribution reflects a specific T cell activation by an antigen present on muscle fibers.[80]

The Fas-FasL process does not seem to be involved in IIM muscle degeneration. IIM muscle fibers and T lymphocytes, but not the control muscles, are Fas positive and FasL has been observed on some degenerating/regenerating fibers and on most of infiltrating $CD8^+$ T cells, however, apoptotic signs are absent.[81-86] The resistance to Fas-mediated cell death seems to be due to the expression of anti-apoptotic molecules heterogeneously expressed in muscle fibers: Bcl-2, Fas-associated death domain-like IL-1-converting enzyme inhibitory protein (FLIP), which inhibits Fas-mediated death signaling, and human inhibitor of apoptosis (IAP)-like protein (hILP), which inhibits the activity of caspases, all proteins that play an important role in initiating and maintaining the apoptotic process.[81,83,87]

Gene Expression Profiles

As yet a limited experience on gene expression profile of IIM muscle biopsies by microarray technology has been reported. The study from Greenberg et al[88] showed that muscle tissues from IIM patients expressed genes different from the normal muscles and that these gene profiles were diverse among the different IIM forms. With this approach the authors had the possibility to make diagnosis in two patients for whom the muscle biopsy did not show the classical pathological alterations. Several genes (MHC class I and II, cytokines, chemokines, granzyme proteases, adhesion molecules, matrix metalloproteinases) are overexpressed confirming previous data obtained with other approaches (PCR and/or immunohistochemistry). On the other hand, the molecular approach revealed some unexpected results: for example, keeping in mind the histopathology of the single IIM forms, a number of immunoglobulin genes were more abundantly expressed in PM/IBM than in DM, while IFN-inducible genes were more expressed in DM than PM/IBM, the latter result resembles that observed in JDM, where a viral antigen as triggering factor has been hypothesized;[89] genes reported as relevant for IBM pathogenesis are also significantly overexpressed in PM and DM, suggesting that in IBM the abnormal accumulation of different proteins might be due to post-transcriptional defects.

IBM-Specific Genetics

A characteristic feature of IBM muscle is the abnormal accumulation, aggregation, and misfolding of several proteins, a scenario similar to that observed in Alzheimer disease brain.[3,6] The major accumulated proteins include: amyloid-β precursor protein (AβPP) and amyloid-β; phosphorylated tau in the form of paired helical filaments (PHFs); presenilin-1. Since in s-IBM the disease onset is usually after age 50 years, it has been hypothesized that the abnormal protein accumulation might be due to a defective processing related to muscle fiber aging. The abnormally processed proteins might then make the muscle fiber a "foreign" to be attacked by the immune system. For h-IBM, in which no signs of inflammation are observed, responsible for protein accumulations might be a genetic defect. Candidate genes are: UDP-N-acetylglucosamine-2 epimerase/N-acetylmannosamine kinase (GNE) gene, myosin heavy chain IIa gene, transthyterin (for a comprehensive review see refs. 3,6). GNE is a bifunctional enzyme catalyzing the first two steps in the synthesis of N-acetylneuraminic (sialic) acid. Any dysregulation of sialic acid biosynthesis and distribution could lead to severe abnormalities of glycoconjugate biosynthesis. Missense mutations were identified in h-IBM Iranian Jews, Japanese and few other ethnic groups. The mutations might induce an uncorrect sialation/glycation of one or several muscle proteins, causing their misfolding and eventually abnormal processing. A missense mutation in the myosin heavy chain IIa gene has been reported in Swedish h-IBM; the observation of an overexpression of myosin heavy chain IIa protein in the IBM vacuoles suggests that mutations in myosin heavy chain IIa gene might influence the formation of vacuoles. Transthyterin binds β-amyloid preventing its fibrillar amyloidogenesis; a transthyterin mutation (Val122Ile), found in a patient with h-IBM and cardiac amyloidosis, might cause the abnormal β-amyloid deposits and amyloidogenesis.[6]

Acknowledgements

The authors wish to thank their research and clinical colleagues, and particularly Dr. Paolo Confalonieri, for their participation in various aspects of these studies and in the preparation of the present manuscript.

References

1. Mantegazza R, Bernasconi P, Confalonieri P et al. Inflammatory myopathies and systemic disorder: A review of immunopathogenetic mechanisms and clinical features. J Neurol 1997; 244:277-287.
2. Dalakas MC, Hohlfeld R. Polymyositis and dermatomyositis. Lancet 2003; 362:971-982.
3. Askanas V, Engel WK. Inclusion-body myositis and myopathies: Different etiologies, possibly similar pathogenic mechanisms. Curr Opin Neurol 2002; 15:525-531.
4. Hoogendijk JE, Amato AA, Lecky BR et al. 119th ENMC International Workshop: Trial design in adult idiopathic inflammatory myopathies, with the exception of inclusion body myositis. Neuromuscul Disord 2004; 14:337-345.
5. Santmyire-Rosenberger B, Dugan EM. Skin involvement in dermatomyositis. Curr Opin Rheumatol 2003; 15:714-722.
6. Askanas V, Engel WK. Proposed pathogenetic cascade of inclusion-body myositis: Importance of amyloid-β, misfolded proteins, predisposing genes, and aging. Curr Opin Rheumatol 2003; 15:737-744.
7. Shamin EA, Rider LG, Miller FW. Update on the genetics of the idiopathic inflammatory myopathies. Curr Opin Rheumatol 2000; 12:482-491.
8. Rider LG, Gurley RC, Pandey JP et al. Clinical, serologic, and immunogenetic features of familial idiopathic inflammatory myopathy. Arthritis Rheum 1998; 41:710-719.
9. Hausmanowa-Petrusewicz I, Kowalska-Oledzka E, Miller FW et al. Clinical, serologic, and immunogenetic features in polish patients with idiopathic inflammatory myopathies. Arthritis Rheum 1997; 40:1257-1266.
10. Arnett FC, Targoff IN, Mimori T et al. Interrelationship of major histocompatibility complex class II alleles and autoantibodies in four ethnic groups with various forms of myositis. Arthritis Rheum 1996; 39:1507-1518.
11. Lampe JB, Gossrau G, Kempe A et al. Analysis of HLA class I and II alleles in sporadic inclusion-body myositis. J Neurol 2003; 250:1313-1317.
12. Karpati G, Pouiliot Y, Carpenter S. Expression of immunoreactive major histocompatibility complex products in human skeletal muscles. Ann Neurol 1988; 23:64-72.

13. Englund P, Lindroos E, Nennesmo I et al. Skeletal muscle fibers express major histocompatibility complex class II antigens independently of inflammatory infiltrates in inflammatory myopathies. Am J Pathol 2001; 159:1263-1273.
14. Andreetta F, Bernasconi P, Torchiana E et al. T-cell infiltration in polymyositis is characterized by coexpression of cytotoxic and T-cell-activating cytokine transcripts. Ann NY Acad Sci 1995; 756:418-420.
15. Lundberg I, Ulfgren AK, Nyberg P et al. Cytokine production in muscle tissue of patients with idiopathic inflammatory myopathies. Arthritis Rheum 1997; 40:865-874.
16. Nyberg P, Wikman A-L, Nennesmo I et al. Increased expression of interleukin-1 alpha and MHC class I in muscle tissue of patients with chronic, inactive polymyositis and dermatomyositis. J Rheumatol 2000; 27:940-948.
17. Englund P, Nennesmo I, Klareskog L et al. Interleukin-1alpha expression in capillaries and major histocompatibility complex class I expression in type II muscle fibers from polymyositis and dermatomyositis patients: Important pathogenic features independent of inflammatory cell clusters in muscle tissue. Arthritis Rheum 2002; 46:1044-1055.
18. Nagaraju K, Raben N, Loeffler L et al. Conditional up-regulation of MHC class I in skeletal muscle leads to self-sustaining autoimmune myositis and myositis-specific autoantibodies. Proc Natl Acad Sci USA 2000; 97:9209-9214.
19. Mantegazza R, Hughes SM, Mitchell D et al. Modulation of MHC class II antigen expression in human myoblasts after treatment with IFN-γ. Neurology 1991; 41:1128-1132.
20. Holhfeld R, Engel AG. Induction of HLA-DR expression on human myoblasts with interferon-gamma. Am J Pathol 1990; 136:503-508.
21. Goebels N, Michaelis D, Wekerle H et al. Human myoblasts as antigen-presenting cells. J Immunol 1992; 149:661-667.
22. Mantegazza R, Gebbia M, Mora M et al. Major histocompatibility complex class II molecule expression on muscle cells is regulated by differentiation: Implications for the immunopathogenesis of muscle autoimmune diseases. J Neuroimmunol 1996; 68:53-60.
23. Beauchamp JR, Abraham DJ, Bou-Gharios G et al. Expression and function of heterotypic adhesion molecules during differentiation of human skeletal muscle in culture. Am J Pathol 1992; 140:387-401.
24. Michaelis D, Goebels N, Hohlfeld R et al. Costitutive and cytokine-induced expression of human leukocyte antigens and cell adhesion molecules by human myotubes. Am J Pathol 1993; 143:1142-1149.
25. Hardiman O, Faustman D, Li X et al. Expression of major histocompatibility complex antigens in cultures of clonally derived human myoblasts. Neurology 1993; 43:604-608.
26. Carosella ED, Paul P, Moreau P et al. HLA-G and HLA-E: Fundamental and pathophysiological aspects. Immunol Today 2000; 21:532-534.
27. Carosella ED, Moreau P, Aractingi S et al. HLA-G: A shield against inflammatory aggression. Trends Immunol 2001; 22:553-555.
28. Wiendl H, Behrens L, Maier S et al. Muscle fibers in inflammatory myopathies and cultured myoblasts express the nonclassical major histocompatibility antigen HLA-G. Ann Neurol 2000; 48:679-684.
29. Wiendl H, Mitsdoerffer M, Hofmeister V et al. The nonclassical MHC molecule HLA-G protects human muscle cells from immune-mediated lysis: Implications for myoblast transplantation and gene therapy. Brain 2003; 126:176-185.
30. Wiendl H, Mitsdoerffer M, Weller M. Express and protect yourself: The potential role of HLA-G on muscle cells and in inflammatory myopathies. Hum Immunol 2003; 64:1050-1056.
31. Carreno BM, Collins M. The B7 family of ligands and its receptors: New pathways for costimulation and inhibition of immune responses. Annu Rev Immunol 2002; 20:29-53.
32. Nagaraju K, Raben N, Villalba ML et al. Costimulatory markers in muscle of patients with idiopathic inflammatory myopathies and in cultured muscle cells. Clin Immunol 1999; 92:161-169.
33. Bernasconi P, Confalonieri P, Andreetta F et al. The expression of costimulatory and accessory molecules on cultured human muscle cells is not dependent on stimulus by pro-inflammatory cytokines: Relevance for the pathogenesis of inflammatory myopathy. J Neuroimmunol 1998; 85:52-58.
34. Behrens L, Kerschensteiner M, Misgeld T et al. Human muscle cells express a functional costimulatory molecule distinct from B7.1 (CD80) and B7.2 (CD86) in vitro and in inflammatory lesions. J Immunol 1998; 161:5943-5951.
35. Murata K, Dalakas MC. Expression of the costimulatory molecule BB-1, the ligands CTLA-4 and CD28, and their mRNA in inflammatory myopathies. Am J Pathol 1999; 155:453-460.

36. Curnow SJ, Willcox N, Vincent A. Induction of primary immune responses by allogeneic human myoblasts: Dissection of the cell types required for proliferation, IFNgamma secretion and cytotoxicity. J Neuroimmunol 1998; 86:53-62.
37. Wiendl H, Mitsdoerffer M, Schneider D et al. Muscle fibres and cultured muscle cells express the B7.1/2-related inducible costimulatory molecule, ICOSL: Implications for the pathogenesis of inflammatory myopathies. Brain 2003; 126:1026-1035.
38. Beier KC, Hutloff A, Dittrich AM et al. Induction, binding specificity and function of human ICOS. Eur J Immunol 2000; 30:3707-3717.
39. Wiendl H, Mitsdoerffer M, Schneider D et al. Human muscle cells express a B7-related molecule, B7-H1, with strong negative immune regulatory potential: A novel mechanism of counterbalancing the immune attack in idiopathic inflammatory myopathies. FASEB J 2003; 17:1892-1894.
40. Garcia KC, Teyton L, Wilson IA. Structural basis of T cell recognition. Annu Rev Immunol 1999; 17:369-397.
41. Davis MM, Boniface JJ, Reich Z et al. Ligand recognition by $\alpha\beta$ T cell receptors. Annu Rev Immunol 1998; 16:523-544.
42. Mantegazza R, Andreetta F, Bernasconi P et al. Analysis of T cell receptor repertoire of muscle-infiltrating T lymphocytes in polymyositis. J Clin Invest 1993; 91:2880-2886.
43. Bender A, Ernst N, Iglesias A et al. T cell receptor repertoire in polymyositis: Clonal expansion of autoaggressive $CD8^+$ T cells. J Exp Med 1995; 181:1863-1868.
44. O'Hanlon TP, Dalakas MC, Plotz PH et al. Predominant TCR-$\alpha\beta$ variable and joining gene expression by muscle-infiltrating lymphocytes in the idiopathic inflammatory myopathies. J Immunol 1994; 152:2569-2576.
45. Mantegazza R, Bernasconi P, Torchiana E et al. Molecular analysis of T cell receptor repertoire of T cell infiltrates in sporadic and familial inclusion body myositis. Muscle Nerve 1994; 17(Suppl 1):117.
46. Lindberg C, Oldfors A, Tarkowski A. Restricted use of T cell receptor V genes in endomysial infiltrates of patients with inflammatory myopathies. Eur J Immunol 1994; 24:2659-2663.
47. O'Hanlon TP, Dalakas MC, Plotz PH et al. The $\alpha\beta$ T-cell receptor repertoire in inclusion body myositis: Diverse patterns of gene expression by muscle-infiltrating lymphocytes. J Autoimmun 1994; 7:321-333.
48. Fyhr IM, Moslemi AR, Mosavi AA et al. Oligoclonal expansion of muscle infiltrating T cells in inclusion body myositis. J Neuroimmunol 1997; 79:185-189.
49. Fyhr IM, Moslemi AR, Lindberg C et al. T cell receptor β-chain repertoire in inclusion body myositis. J Neuroimmunol 1998; 91:129-134.
50. Bender A, Behrens L, Engel AG et al. T-cell heterogeneity in muscle lesions of inclusion body myositis. J Neuroimmunol 1998; 84:86-91.
51. Amemiya K, Granger RP, Dalakas MC. Clonal restriction of T-cell receptor expression by infiltrating lymphocytes in inclusion body myositis persists over time: Studies in repeated muscle biopsies. Brain 2000; 123:2030-2039.
52. Nishio J, Suzuki M, Miyasaka N et al. Clonal biases of peripheral CD8 T cell repertoire directly reflect local inflammation in polymyositis. J Immunol 2001; 167:4051-4058.
53. Benveniste O, Chérin P, Maisonobe T et al. Severe perturbations of the blood T cell repertoire in polymyositis, but not in dermatomyositis patients. J Immunol 2001; 167:3521-3529.
54. Hofbauer M, Wiesener S, Babbe H et al. Clonal tracking of autoaggressive T cells in polymyositis by combining laser microdissection, single-cell PCR, and CDR3-spectratype analysis. Proc Natl Acad Sci USA 2003; 100:4090-4095.
55. Hengstman GJD, van Engelen BGM, Vree Egberts WTM et al. Myositis-specific autoantibodies: Overview and recent developments. Curr Opin Rheumatol 2001; 13:476-482.
56. Lieberman J. The ABCs of granule-mediated cytotoxicity: New weapons in the arsenal. Nat Rev Immunol 2003; 3:361-370.
57. Casciola-Rosen L, Andrade F, Ulanet D et al. Cleavage by granzyme B is strongly predictive of autoantigen status: Implications for initiation of autoimmunity. J Exp Med 1999; 190:815-825.
58. Levine SM, Rosen A, Casciola-Rosen LA. Anti-aminoacyl tRNA synthetase immune responses: Insights into the pathogenesis of the idiopathic inflammatory myopathies. Curr Opin Rheumatol 2003; 15:708-713.
59. Howard OMZ, Dong HF, Yang D et al. Histidyl-tRNA synthetase and asparaginyl-tRNA synthetase, autoantigens in myositis, activate chemokine receptors on T lymphocytes and immature dendritic cells. J Exp Med 2002; 196:781-791.
60. Ascherman DP, Oriss TB, Oddis CV et al. Critical requirement for professional APCs in eliciting T cell responses to novel fragments of histidyl-tRNA synthetase (Jo-1) in Jo-1 antibody-positive polymyositis. J Immunol 2002; 169:7127-7134.
61. Janeway CA, Bottomly K. Signals and signs for lymphocyte responses. Cell 1994; 76:275-285.

62. Andreetta F, Bernasconi P, Torchiana E et al. T-cell infiltration in polymyositis is characterized by coexpression of cytotoxic and T-cell-activating cytokine transcripts. Ann NY Acad Sci 1995; 756:418-420.
63. Lundberg I, Brengman JM, Engel AG. Analysis of cytokine expression in muscle in inflammatory myopathies, Duchenne dystrophy, and nonweak controls. J Neuroimmunol 1995; 63:9-16.
64. Lundberg I, Ulfgren AK, Nyberg P et al. Cytokine production in muscle tissue of patients with idiopathic inflammatory myopathies. Arthritis Rheum 1997; 40:865-874.
65. Tews DS, Goebel HH. Cytokine expression profile in idiopathic inflammatory myopathies. J Neuropathol Exp Neurol 1996; 55:342-347.
66. De Bleecker JL, Meire VI, Declercq W et al. Immunolocalization of tumor necrosis factor-alpha and its receptors in inflammatory myopathies. Neuromusc Disord 1999; 9:239-246.
67. Tateyama M, Nagano I, Yoshioka M et al. Expression of tumor necrosis factor-alpha in muscles in polymyositis. J Neurol Sci 1997; 146:45-51.
68. Nagaraju K, Raben N, Merritt G et al. A variety of cytokines and immunologically relevant surface molecules are expressed by normal human skeletal muscle cells under proinflammatory stimuli. Clin Exp Immunol 1998; 113:407-414.
69. Kuru S, Inukai A, Kato T et al.·Expression of tumor necrosis factor-α in regenerating muscle fibers in inflammatory and noninflammatory myopathies. Acta Neuropathol 2003; 105:217-224.
70. Uzel G, Pachman LM. Cytokines in juvenile dermatomyositis pathophysiology: Potential and challenge. Curr Opin Rheumatol 2003; 15:691-697.
71. Confalonieri P, Bernasconi P, Cornelio F et al. Transforming growth factor-beta1 in polymyositis and dermatomyositis correlates with fibrosis but not with mononuclear cell infiltrate. J Neuropathol Exp Neurol 1997; 56:479-484.
72. Gamble JR, Khew-Goodall Y, Vadas MA. Transforming growth factor-beta inhibits E-selectin expression on human endothelial cells. J Immunol 1993; 150:4494-4503.
73. Hurwitz AA, Lyman WD, Berman JW. Tumor necrosis factor α and transforming growth factor β up-regulate astrocyte expression of monocyte chemoattractant protein-1. J Neuroimmunol 1995; 57:193-198.
74. Zlotnik A, Yoshie O. Chemokines: A new classification system and their role in immunity. Immunity 2000; 12:121-127.
75. Confalonieri P, Bernasconi P, Megna P et al. Increased expression of β-chemokines in muscle of patients with inflammatory myopathies. J Neuropathol Exp Neurol 2000; 59:164-169.
76. De Bleecker JL, De Paepe B, Vanwalleghem IE et al. Differential expression of chemokines in inflammatory myopathies. Neurology 2002; 58:1779-1785.
77. Raju R, Vasconcelos O, Granger R et al. Expression of IFN-gamma-inducible chemokines in inclusion body myositis. J Neuroimmunol 2003; 141:125-131.
78. De Rossi M, Bernasconi P, Baggi F et al. Cytokines and chemokines are both expressed by human myoblasts: Possible relevance for the immune pathogenesis of muscle inflammation. Int Immunol 2000; 12:1329-1335.
79. Lieberman J. Mechanisms of granule-mediated cytotoxicity. Curr Opin Immunol 2003; 15:513-515.
80. Goebels N, Michaelis D, Engelhardt M et al. Differential expression of perforin in muscle-infiltrating T cells in polymyositis and dermatomyositis. J Clin Invest 1996; 97:2905-2910.
81. Nagaraju K, Casciola-Rosen L, Rosen A et al. The inhibition of apoptosis in myositis and in normal muscle cells. J Immunol 2000; 164:5459-5465.
82. Inukai A, Kobayashi Y, Ito K et al. Expression of Fas antigen is not associated with apoptosis in human myopathies. Muscle Nerve 1997; 20:702-709.
83. Behrens L, Bender A, Johnson MA et al. Cytotoxic mechanisms in inflammatory myopathies. Coexpression of Fas and protective Bcl-2 in muscle fibres and inflammatory cells. Brain 1997; 120:929-938.
84. Olive M, Martinez-Matos JA, Montero J et al. Apoptosis is not the mechanism of cell death of muscle fibers in human muscular dystrophies and inflammatory myopathies. Muscle Nerve 1997; 20:1328-1330.
85. Schneider C, Gold R, Dalakas MC et al. MHC class I-mediated cytotoxicity does not induce apoptosis in muscle fibers nor in inflammatory T cells: Studies in patients with polymyositis, dermatomyositis, and inclusion body myositis. J Neuropathol Exp Neurol 1996; 55:1205-1209.
86. Tews DS, Goebel HH. Cell death and oxidative damage in inflammatory myopathies. Clin Immunol Immunopathol 1998; 87:240-247.
87. Li M, Dalakas MC. Expression of human IAP-like protein in skeletal muscle: A possible explanation for the rare incidence of muscle fiber apoptosis in T-cell mediated inflammatory myopathies. J Neuroimmunol 2000; 106:1-5.
88. Greenberg SA, Sanoudou D, Haslett JN et al. Molecular profiles of inflammatory myopathies. Neurology 2002; 59:1170-1182.
89. Tezak Z, Hoffman EP, Lutz JL et al. Gene expression profiling in DQA1*0501^{+} children with untreated dermatomyositis: A novel model of pathogenesis. J Immunol 2002; 168:4154-4163.

Chapter 9

Hematologic Diseases:

Autoimmune Hemolytic Anemia and Immune Thrombocytopenic Purpura

Mattias Olsson, Sven Hagnerud, David U.R. Hedelius and Per-Arne Oldenborg

Summary

Autoimmune destruction of circulating blood cells in autoimmune hemolytic anemia (AIHA) and immune thrombocytopenic purpura (ITP) is often seen in autoimmune diseases and lymhoid malignancies. Erythrocytes or platelets that are recognized by autoantibodies are rapidly phagocytosed by macrophages. Although much is known about the mechanisms behind macrophage-mediated destruction of sensitized blood cells, less is known about the genetics behind AIHA and ITP. We here review what is known about the ethiology of AIHA and ITP, with particular emphasis on the role of genetic factors behind autoantibody production, T cell activation and apoptosis, and Fcγ receptor polymorphisms. The importance of inhibitory regulation of macrophages through CD47/SIRPα interaction, and its significance for autoimmune hematological disease is also discussed.

Autoimmune Hemolytic Anemia

Autoimmune hemolytic anemia (AIHA) is defined as an increased destruction of erythrocytes due to the presence of anti-erythrocyte autoantibodies (AEA) and can be classified as either autoimmune, alloimmune, or drug-induced depending on the type of antigen giving rise to the immune response.[1,2] General hemolytic anemia is estimated to occur in about 4 cases per 1000 per year, but for AIHA the annual incidence is estimated to about 1-3 cases per 100,000 per year.[3,4] Thus, AIHA is a rather rare disease, which can affect infants to the elderly but the majority of the patients are over the age of 40 years, with peak incidence at 70.[4] AIHA can appear either as a primary disease or, in about 20-80% of the cases, secondary to other autoimmune diseases, lymphoid malignancies, infections, immunodeficiencies, or tumors, where lymphoid malignancies are the most common reasons for secondary AIHA.[5,6] AEA are classified as cold or warm autoantibodies, as they react optimally at temperatures below 30°C or at 35°C to 40°C respectively.[1] Warm AEA are mostly IgG but sometimes IgA and/or IgM are also present, and are responsible for about 50-70% of AIHA cases.[1] The binding of warm IgG AEA to erythrocytes does not itself damage the erythrocytes, since erythrocyte bound IgG, in contrast to surface bound IgM, is a poor activator of the classical complement pathway.[1] Instead, surface bound IgG is usually recognized by Fcγ receptors of cells of the monocyte-macrophage phagocytic system, preferentially in the spleen and liver, resulting in uptake and destruction of IgG-opsonized erythrocytes (Fig. 1).[7-9] However, macrophage-mediated elimination of erythrocytes in AIHA is likely to be mediated by synergistic activity of macrophage Fcγ and complement receptors (recognizing complement

Immunogenetics of Autoimmune Disease, edited by Jorge Oksenberg and David Brassat.

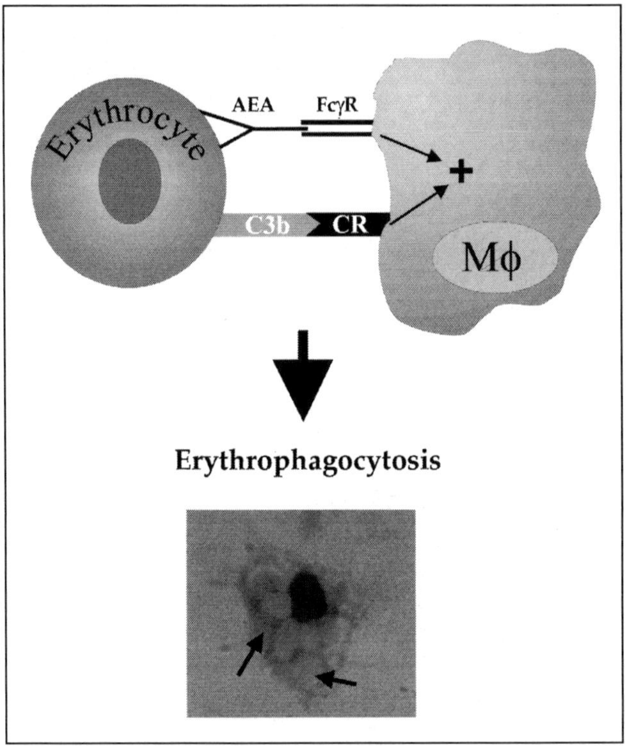

Figure 1. Macrophage Fcγ receptors and complement receptors act synergistically to stimulate erythrophagocytosis in AIHA. In AIHA, anti-erythrocyte autoantibodies (AEA) bound the erythrocytes are recognized by macrophage Fcγ receptors (FcγR), resulting in uptake and destruction of sensitized erythrocytes. Erythrocyte bound components of the complement system ($C3b/C3b_i$) are in a similar way reconized by macrophage complement receptors (CR). The synergistic effect of both FcγR and CR is thought to be a key component in erythrocyte phagocytosis by macrophages in vivo. The photograph shows a splenic macrophage, which has ingested several eryhtrocytes (exemplified by arrows).

factors C3b and $C3b_i$), since erythrocytes opsonized with very low levels of IgG are not eliminated in vivo in the absence of complement.[10] Furthermore, low levels of complement opsonization does not result in erythrocyte phagocytosis in the absence of IgG, whereas low levels of both complement and IgG-opsonization can induce efficient erythrocyte phagocytosis both in vivo and in vitro (Fig. 1).[10-12]

The etiology behind most AEA is poorly understood. However, it is likely to be the result of disrupted immune self-tolerance, or due to autoantibodies induced nonspecifically and transiently during microbial infections. A defective immune self-tolerance may be either due to a central defect during lymphocyte development, or due to a peripheral defect involving down-regulation of activated mature T and B cells.[2] Today, the most common treatments for AIHA are Fc receptor-competitive by intravenous infusion of IgG (IVIG), or immunosuppressive, such as cytotoxic drugs or splenectomy.[4]

Immune Thrombocytopenic Purpura

Immune thrombocytopenic purpura (ITP) is an autoimmune disease characterised by low platelet counts due to antibody-mediated destruction of platelets by macrophages.[13] ITP is classified as acute or chronic, where acute ITP has a rapid onset with typical petechiae and bruises, is often preceded by an infectious illness, mainly affects young children, and normally resolves spontaneously within six months.[13] Chronic ITP often has an adult onset that is more insidious than the acute form and is about two to three times as common among women as among men.[13]

A positive anti-platelet autoantibody test is found in about 70-80% of adults with ITP and in children with chronic ITP.[14] Platelet autoantibodies are of the IgG type and are mostly directed to platelet membrane glycoproteins, including GPIIb/IIIa, GPIb-IX, and GPIa-IIa.[15,16] Platelets coated with IgG autoantibodies undergo accelerated clearance through Fcγ receptor-mediated phagocytosis by macrophages, preferably in the spleen and liver.[13,17,18] The reasons for the initiation of antibody production are mostly unknown, however, association between anti-platelet glycoprotein antibodies and HLA class II has been described (see below). Most patients have antibodies directed to several different platelet surface proteins. In the acute form of ITP, one might expect molecular mimicry which means that antibodies produced as a response to a pathogen may be able to cross-react with the host tissue.[18] Of particular interest is the finding that some antiviral antibodies have been shown to cross-react with platelets, increasing the posibility of increased presentation of platelet antigens by MHC class II on phagocytic cells.[19]

Adults with diagnosed ITP are normally initially treated with corticosteroids,[20] whereas this treatment, albeit often sucessful and less risky, is used to a lesser extent in childhood ITP.[21] Intravenous gammaglobulin (IVIG) is another common approach in treatment of ITP, particularly for treatment of internal bleedings. IVIG has well known anti-inflammatory effects, generally attributed to the immunoglobulin G (IgG) Fc domain, which is thought to block pro-phagocytic Fc receptors on macrophages.[22] However, recent data from mouse models suggests that the inhibitory effect of IVIG is to a big extent dependent on binding to, and upregulation of, the inhibitory FcγRIIb receptor.[23] In more severe cases of ITP, and in cases of tolerance to corticosteroids, splenectomy may be required to reduce platelet destruction.[13]

Genetic Control of AEA in AIHA

The autoimmune-prone mouse strain New-Zealand Black (NZB) spontaneously develops AIHA, which is associated with production of AEA, splenomegaly and other clinical features such as reduced hematocrit and increased reticulocyte count.[24,25] Thus, due to its similarities with the human counterpart, and due to very limited knowledge on the immunogenetics behind human AIHA, this mouse strain has served as a model in attempts to dissect out the genetic peculiarities of AIHA. Autoimmune disease in NZB mice is inherited in a dominant fashion, but by studying crosses with nonautoimmune mouse strains, further knowledge on the genetics behind several AIHA-associated features has been generated. In this way, it was first suggested that production of AEA is under control of a single dominant gene.[26,27] Thus, the single dominant AIHA susceptibility allele *Aia-1* (autoimmune-anemia locus), loosely linked to the b locus of chromosome 4, was early associated with AEA.[27] However, later studies in crosses between NZB and nonautoimmune-prone mouse strains (e.g., C57BL/6) suggested that the contribution of *Aia-1*to expression of AEA production was under the control of suppresive genes such as *Aem-1* (anti-erythrocyte autoantibody modifying gene), mapped to the locus closely linked to *Mup-1* on chromosome 4.[28] More recently, data have been presented, which further supports that AIHA and AEA production are under multigenic control. By studying (C57BL/6 x NZB)F_1 x NZB, genotyped for chromosomal microsattelite markers polymorphic between C57BL/6 and NZB strains, two potential C57BL/6 suppressive loci for AEA were identified on chromosomes 7 and 10.[29] The locus on chromosome 7, designated *Aem-2* (anti-erythrocyte autoantibody modifying gene-2), was found located between microsomal sattelite markers *D7MIT30* and *D7MIT297*, and the locus *Aem-3* on chromosome 10 was significantly linked to the marker *D10MIT42*.[29] From this study it was concluded that production of AEA might be down-regulated by a combined effect of these potentially suppressive alleles.

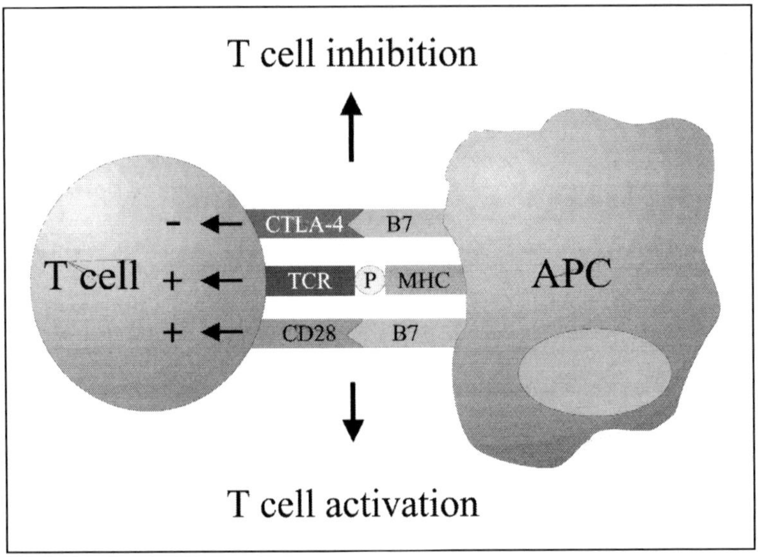

Figure 2. Receptor-mediated control of T cell activation. Activation of T cell antigen responses is stimulated by the T cell receptor (TCR) in contact with the antigen peptide (P) presented by major histocompatibility receptors (MHC) on the surface of antigen presenting cells (APC). For T cell activation, a second stimulatory signal is required, which is delivered by interaction between the APC costimulatory molecule B7 and T cell CD28. T cell response to antigen is also under control of inhibitory signaling through CTLA-4. CTLA-4 has a higher affinity than CD28 for B7, resulting in the capacity to inhibit T cell proliferation.

HLA Susceptibility Genes and ITP

Although the genetic factors that can influence the development of ITP may include genes coding for HLA, T cell receptors and immunoglobulin allotypes, the underlying predisposing causes for ITP are not completely understood. In a study of Caucasian patients with chronic primary ITP, no association could be found between HLA class I or II alleles and a single immunogenic susceptibility factor.[30] However, HLA-A2 appeared to be associated with ITP, particularly in female patients and in patients progressing to splenectomy.

In Japanese ITP patients, a strong association was found between anti-platelet glycoprotein autoantibodies and HLA class II genes. Anti-GPIIb-IIIa antibodies associated with DRB1*0405 and DQB1*0401, whereas anti-GPIb-IX antibodies associated with DRB1*0803 and DQB1*0601. Furthermore, a poor response to splenectomy was associated with DRB1*0405 and DQB1*0401 and anti-GPIIb-IIIa autoantibodies.[31] Another study of the same ethnic population showed a significan increase of the DRB1*0410 allele, but not of other DRB1*04 alleles, in ITP patients.[32] In this study, positivity for anti-GPIIb-IIIa autoantibodies was associated with HLA-DR4, but not with DRB1*0410.[32] This is in consistance with findings of GPIIb-IIIa autoreactive T cells in ITP patients, T cells which were capable to stimulate a HLA-DR-restricted B cell production of anti-platelet antibodies.[33]

Genetic Alterations in the Control of T Cell Activation

T cell antigen responses are activated by interaction between the T cell receptor (TCR) and peptide/MHC complex of the antigen presenting cell (APC), with additional costimulatory signals generated by T cell CD28 interacting with the costimulatory molecule B7 expressed by APCs. These two signals are both required for T cell activation (Fig. 2).[34,35] However, the T cell response to antigen is also under inhibitory control by CTLA-4, a molecule expressed on the surface of T cells following activation.[36] Due to a higher affinity for the costimulatory molecule

B7, CTLA-4 inhibits T cell proliferation by reducing CD28/B7 interactions. Since CTLA-4-deficient mice show severe autoimmune tissue destruction,[36] and CTLA-4 is deficiently expressed in the diabetes-prone nonobese diabetic mice,[37] it is likely that CTLA-4 is of major importance in the pathogenesis of autoimmune diseases. A high prevalence of an A to G polymorphism at position 49 of the CTLA-4 first exon, resulting in a Thr-Ala amino acid substitution at codon 17 of the CTLA-4 leader peptide, has been associated with increased susceptibility to autoimmune diseases such as insulin-dependent diabetes, Graves' disease, rheumatoid arthritis, multiple sclerosis, and also systemic lupus erythematosis.[38-40] More recently, the G allele of CTLA-4 was also found to predispose to the development of AIHA. This association was found to be highest in patients with chronic lymphocytic leukemia, who subsequently developed AIHA.[41] In contrast, A to G polymorphism has not been found to be associated with ITP.

Defective Lymphocyte Apoptosis

During early T cell differentiation in the thymus, self-reactive T cell clones are deleted on contact with thymic antigens. However, self-reactive mature T cells encountering self-antigens in the periphery must be deleted to avoid autoimmune disease. The elimination of self-reactive mature T cells is mediated by a number of pro-apoptotic pathways, of which Fas-mediated apoptosis is the most prominent.[42] T lymphocytes constitutively express Fas receptors, but the Fas ligand (FasL) is expressed only after repeated exposure to antigen or after nonspecific stimulation via the CD3/TCR complex.[43,44] Ligation of Fas by FasL results in so called activation-induced cell death (AICD).[42] A study of patients with chronic hematologic autoimmunity (having AIHA and/or ITP) showed a defective Fas-mediated AICD in 25% of these patients, which was not explained by reduced Fas expression, FasL function or Fas mutations.[45] However, another study was unable to find any defects in Fas function in patients with chronic ITP.[46] Fas-mediated AICD in mature T cells is controlled by IL-2, which primes activated T cells to undergo apoptosis via the Fas pathway.[47] Disruption of the interaction between the Fas and IL-2 pathways, as in IL-2 refractory cases of AIHA and ITP, will interfere with AICD, leading to expansion of self-reactive T cells that would normally be targeted for elimination.[45]

Fcγ Receptor Polymorphisms in ITP

As described above, the pathophysiology of ITP is dependent on the recognition of IgG-sensitized platelets by Fcγ receptors (FcγR) on macrophages in the spleen and liver. So far, three classes of Fcγ receptors have been characterized: FcγRI, FcγRII and FcγRIII, where each subclass exists in several different isoforms.[48] In humans, 12 FcγR transcripts are involved, all derived from eight genes (*FcγR Ia, FcγR Ib, FcγR Ic, FcγR IIa, FcγR IIb, FcγR IIc, FcγR IIIa* and *FcγR IIIb*) on chromosome 1.[49] FcγRI (CD64) is a high-affinity receptor with the capacity to bind monomeric IgG. FcγRII (CD32) and FcγRIII (CD16) are low-affinity receptors for immune complexes or multimeric IgG. Inherited functional single nucleotide polymorphisms in FcγRIIa and FcγRIIIa results in increased heterogeneity and randomly distributed allelic variants in populations, which may further vary between ethnic groups.[50] For FcγRIIa, the genetic polymorphism is the result of a single nucleotide histidine (H) or arginine (R) substitution at position 131, resulting in a marked increase in the binding affinity for IgG2 to FcγRIIa-131H as compared to FcγRIIa-131R.[51] In the same way, the binding affinity for IgG1 and IgG3 differs between FcγRIIIa having valine (V) or phenylalanine (F) at codon 158, where FcγRIIIa-158V has the highest affinity.[52] It is of interest to note, that a significant over-representation of the FcγRIIa-131H and FcγRIIIa-158V variants were found in children with acute or chronic ITP.[53] However, another study of children with chronic ITP failed to find an association between FcγRIIa genotype and disease incidence, but confirmed that the FcγRIIIa-158V variant was increased.[54] A similar finding was also reported in adults with chronic ITP.[55]

Erythrocyte CD47 and Autoimmune Hemolytic Anemia

CD47 (Integrin-associated protein/IAP) is a ubiquitously expressed cell surface glycoprotein, which maps to chromosome 3q13.1-q13.2 in humans and to chromosome 16 in mice.[56,57] It was first identified as a protein associated with $\alpha_v\beta_3$ integrins in placenta and in neutrophil granulocytes, and shown to regulate integrin function and leukocyte reponses to RGD-containing extracellular matrix proteins.[58,59] Erythrocytes do not express integrins, but still express high levels of CD47, which suggests important integrin-independent functions for CD47 in these cells. Interestingly, CD47 can function as a ligand for the inhibitory macrophage receptor Signal Regulatory Protein alpha (SIRPα/SHPS-1/BIT/P84).[60] This interaction was recently found to be important to prevent phagocytosis of circulating erythrocytes by splenic macrophages, since erythrocytes from CD47-deficient mice were rapidly cleared from the circulation of wild-type recipient mice.[61] Clearance of CD47 deficient erythrocytes was not dependent on complement activation, lymphocytes or antibodies, but entirely due to the absence of inhibitory CD47/SIRPα signaling.[61] Using CD47-deficient and CD47 wild-type erythrocytes, it was also shown that erythrocyte CD47 can reduce clearance and phagocytosis of IgG opsonized erythrocytes through interaction with macrophage SIRPα.[62] In this system, the inhibitory signal generated by CD47/SIRPα interaction is integrated with the prophagocytic Fcγ receptor signal proximal to the decision to phagocytose. Neither the SIRPα nor the Fcγ receptor signal seems to be dominant, rather the activation of phagocytosis is determined by the relative signaling strength of activating and inhibitory signals. In the same way, erythrocytes opsonized with the complement fragment $C3b_i$ are bound and phagocytosed via complement receptors (CR3/$\alpha_M\beta_2$ integrin),[63] and also complement-mediated phagocytosis of erythrocytes is regulated by the inhibitory CD47-SIRPα signal.[62] As mentioned earlier, Fcγ and complement receptors are known to act synergistically in stimulating phagocytosis of erythrocytes in AIHA. Therefore, it seems likely that phagocytosis of erythrocytes in AIHA is also based on the summation of the prophagocytic signals from Fcγ receptors and complement receptors with the negative signal from SIRPα (Fig. 3). A significant importance of the inhibitory CD47/SIRPα system in limiting erythrocyte destruction and severity of AIHA is emphasized by studies in the autoimmune-prone nonobese diabetic (NOD) mice. NOD mice that do not develop diabetes, may instead develop a mild form of AIHA at the age of 300-550 days.[64] When breeding CD47-deficient NOD mice, we found that a majority of these mice developed an acute lethal form of AIHA at the age of 180-280 days.[65] The exact ethiology behind the increased sensitivity of CD47-deficient NOD mice to develop this severe form of AIHA is not entirely clear. However, our recent results suggest that CD47-deficient erythrocytes are more susceptible to autoantibody-mediated immune destruction, since the absent interaction between CD47 and SIRPα enhances pro-phagocytic signals induced by Fcγ and complement receptors.[62] CD47-deficient NOD mice all have higher levels of antibody-opsonized erythrocytes than wild-type NOD mice of the same age. It is therefore suggested that the onset of anti-erythrocyte autoantibody production is accelerated in CD47-deficient NOD mice, which might be explained by the fact that phagocytosis of CD47-deficient erythrocytes occure already at very low levels of IgG opsonization, which may possibly promote antigen presentation of pathogenic self-peptides. In a more generalized perspective, during microbial infections, the inhibitory CD47/SIRPα interaction may be of importance to avoid autoimmune cellular damages to host cells by nonspecifically and transiently induced autoantibodies. Here, a low level of IgG opsonization might be enough to trigger phagocytosis of a foreign particle that do not express CD47, whereas a host cell, such as an erythrocyte, would not be phagocytosed due to its expression of CD47 and the resulting inhibitory signals generated upon contact with macrophage SIRPα. However, in autoimmune diseases such as AIHA, elevated erythrocyte IgG opsonization and Fcγ receptor activation will override the CD47-SIRPα signal, resulting in erythrocyte phagocytosis and clinically overt AIHA. Platelets do also express CD47 and investigations are underway to determine the role of inhibitory CD47/SIRPα signaling in the regulation of platelet clearance in ITP.

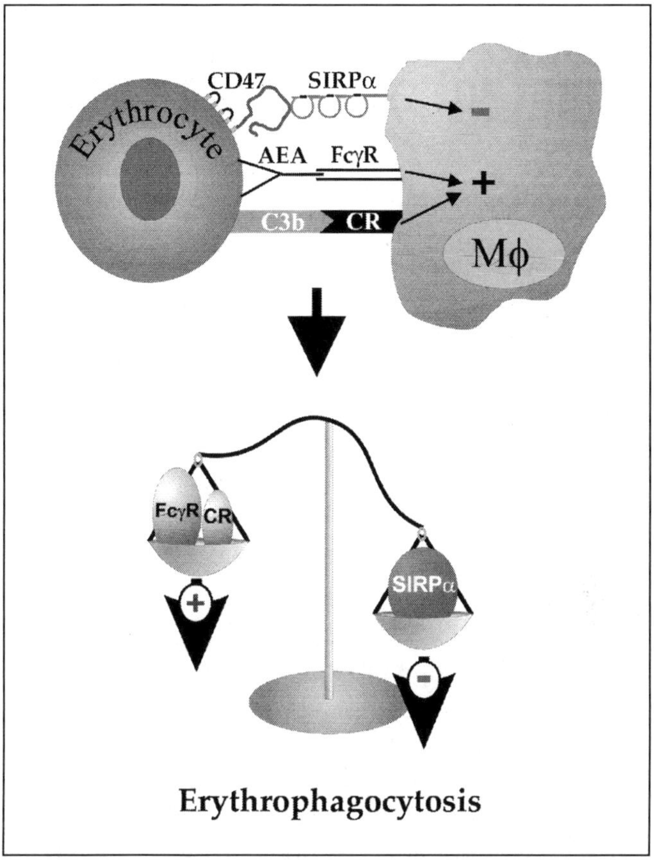

Figure 3. FcγR and CR-mediated erythrophagocytosis can be down-regulated by CD47/SIRPα interaction. The phagocytosis stimulating signals generated through ligation of FcγR and/or CR are counteracted by the inhibitory receptor SIRPα The ligand for SIRPα is the ubiquitously expressed cell surface glycoprotein CD47, which is expressed at high levels by erythrocytes. Neither the positive nor the inhibitory signals seems to be dominant, but are instead integrated to determine phagocytosis activation of the macrohage. The absence of this inhibitory signaling system results in severe sensitivity to AIHA in animal models.

Acknowlegements

Supported by grants from the Swedish Research Council for Medicine (06P-14098, 31X-14286), the NIH (GM57573-06), the Swedish Society of Medicine, the Åke Wiberg Foundation and the Faculty of Medicine, Umeå University.

References

1. Engelfriet CP, Overbeeke MAM, Kr.von dem Borne AEG. Autoimmune hemolytic anemia. Semin Hematol 1992; 29:3-12.
2. Gehrs BC, Friedberg RC. Autoimmune hemolytic anemia. Am J Hematol 2002; 69:258-271.
3. Bottinger LE, Westerholm B. Acquired haemolytic anemia. Acta Med Scand 1973; 193:223-226.
4. Packman CH, Leddy JP. Aquired hemolytic anemia due to warm-reacting autoantibodies. In: Williams WJ, Beutler E, Erslev AJ et al, eds. Hematology. New York: McGraw-Hill, Inc. 1990:666-675.
5. Bell CA, Zwicker H, Sacks HJ. Autoimmune hemolytic anemia: Routine serologic evaluation in a general hospital population. Am J Clin Pathol 1973; 60:903-911.
6. Sokol RJ, Hewitt S, Stamps BK. Autoimmune hemolysis: An 18-year study of 865 cases referred to a regional transfusion centre. Br Med J 1981; 282:2023-2027.

7. Clynes R, Ravaetch JV. Cytotoxic antibodies trigger inflammation through Fc receptors. Immunity 1995; 3:21-26.
8. Meyer D, Schiller C, Westermann J et al. FcγRIII (CD16)-deficient mice show IgG isotype-dependent protection to experimental autoimmune hemolytic anemia. Blood 1998; 92:3997-4002.
9. Pottier Y, Pierard I, Barclay A et al. The mode of action of treatment by IgG of haemolytic anaemia induced by an anti-erythrocyte monoclonal antibody. Clin Exp Immunol 1996; 106:103-107.
10. Logue GL, Kurlander RJ. Immunologic mechanisms of hemolysis in autoimmune hemolytic anemia. Pathobiol Annu 1978; 8:61-83.
11. Ehlenberger AG, Nussenzweig V. The role of membrane receptors for C3b and C3d in phagocytosis. J Exp Med 1977; 145:357-371.
12. Gigli I, Nelson RA. Complement dependent immune phagocytosis. Exp Cell Res 1968; 51:45-67.
13. Cines DB, Blanchette VS. Immune thrombocytopenic purpura. N Engl J Med 2002; 346:995-1007.
14. Berchtold P, McMillan R, Tani P et al. Autoantibodies against platelet membrane glycoproteins in children with acute and chronic immune thrombocytopenic purpura. Blood 1989; 74:1600-1602.
15. McMillan R, Tani P, Millard F et al. Platelet-associated and plasma anti-glycoproteins in chronic ITP. Blood 1987; 70:1040-1045.
16. Wadenvik H, Stockelberg D, Hou M. Platelet proteins as autoantibody targets in idiopathic thrombocytopenic purpura. Acta Paediatr 1998; 424:26-36.
17. Beardsley DS. Pathophysiology of immune thrombocytopenic purpura. Blood Rev 2002; 16:13-14.
18. Semple JW. Immune pathophysiology of autoimmune thrombocytopenic purpura. Blood Rev 2002; 16:9-12.
19. Wright JW, Chia WK, Freedman GJ. Characterization of platelet-reactive antibodies in children with varicella-associated acute immune thrombocytopenic purpura (ITP). Br J Haematol 1996; 95:145-152.
20. George JN, Woolf SH, Raskob GE et al. Idiopathic thrombocytopenic purpura: A practice guideline developed by explicit methods for the American Society of Hematology. Blood 1996; 88:3-40.
21. Lilleyman JS. Management of childhood idiopathic thrombocytopenic purpura. Br J Haematol 1999; 105:871-875.
22. Teeling JL, Jansen-Hendriks T, Kuijpers TW et al. Therapeutic efficacy of intravenous immunoglobulin preparations depends on the immunoglobulin G dimmers: Studies in experimental immune thrombocytopenia. Blood 2001; 98:1095-1099.
23. Samuelsson A, Towers TL, Ravetch JV. Anti-inflammatory activity of IVIG mediated through the inhibitory Fc receptor. Science 7; 291:484-486.
24. Helyer BJ, Howie JB. Spontaneous auto-immune disease in NZB/BL mice. Br J Haematol 1963; 9:119-131.
25. Howie JB, Helyer BJ. The immunology and pathology of NZB mice. Adv Immunol 1968; 9:215-266.
26. Bielschowsky M, Helyer BJ, Howie JB. Spontaneous hemolytic anemia in mice of the NZB/B1 strain. Proc Univ Otago Med Sch 1959; 37:9.
27. Knight JG, Adams DD. Genes determining autoimmune disease in New Zealand mice. J Clin Lab Immunol 1981; 5:165-170.
28. Ozaki S, Honda H, Maruyama N et al. Genetic regulation of erythrocyte autoantibody production in New Zealand Black mice. Immunogenetics 1983; 18:241-254.
29. Ochiai K, Ozaki S, Tanino A et al. Genetic regulation of anti-erythrocyte autoantibodies and splenomegaly in autoimmune hemolytic anemia-prone New Zealand Black mice. Int Immunol 2000; 12:1-8.
30. Stanworth SJ, Turner DM, Brown J et al. Major histocompatibility complex susceptibility genes and immune thrombocytopenic purpura in Caucasian adults. Hematology 2002; 7:119-121.
31. Kuwana M, Kaburaki J, Pandey JP et al. HLA class II alleles in Japanese patients with immune thrombocytopenic purpura. Associations with anti-platelet glycoprotein autoantibodies and response to splenectomy. Tissue Antigens 2000; 56:337-343.
32. Nomura S, Matsuzaki T, Okazi Y et al. Clinical significance of HLA-DRB1*0410 in Japanese patients with idiopathic thrombocytopenic purpura. Blood 1998; 91:3616-3622.
33. Kuwana M, Kaburaki J, Ikeda Y. Autoreactive T cells to platelet GPIIb-IIIa in immune thrombocytopenic purpura: Role in production of anti-platelet autoantibody. J Clin Invest 1998; 102:1393-1402.
34. Lafferty KJ, Gill RG. The maintenance of self-tolerance. Immunol Cell Biol 1993; 71:209-214.
35. Linsley PS, Ledbetter JA. The role of the CD28 receptor during T cell responses to antigen. Annu Rev Immunol 1993; 11:191-212.
36. Tivol EA, Borriello F, Schweitzer AN et al. Loss of CTLA-4 leads to massive lymphoproliferation and fatal multiorgan tissue destruction, revealing a critical negative regulatory role of CTLA-4. Immunity 1995; 3:541-547.

37. Colucci F, Bergman M-L, Penha-Gonçalves C et al. Apoptosis resistance of nonobese diabetic peripheral lymphocytes linked to the Idd5 diabetes succeptibility region. Proc Natl Acad Sci USA 1997; 94:8670-8674.
38. Ligers A, Xu C, Saarinen S et al. The CTLA-4 gene is associated with multiple sclerosis. J Neuroimmunol 1999; 97:182-190.
39. Marron MP, Raffel LJ, Garchon HJ et al. Insulin-dependent diabetes mellitus (IDDM) is associated with CTLA-4 polymorphisms in multiple ethnic groups. Hum Mol Genet 1997; 6:1275-1282.
40. Seidl C, Donner H, Fisher B et al. CTLA-4 codon 17 dimorphism in patients with rheumatoid arthritis. Tissue Antigens 1998; 51:62-66.
41. Pavkovic M, Georgievski B, Cevreska L et al. CTLA-4 exon 1 polymorphism in patients with autoimmune blood disorders. Am J Hematol 2003; 72:147-149.
42. Nagata S. Apoptosis by death factor. Cell 1997; 88:355-365.
43. Russell JH, White CL, Loh DY et al. Receptor-stimulated death pathway is opened by antigen in mature T cells. Proc Natl Acad Sci USA 1991; 88:2151-2155.
44. Russell JH, Rush BJ, Abrams SI et al. Sensitivity of T cells to anti-CD3-stimulated suicide is dependent of functional phenotype. Eur J Immunol 1992; 22:1655-1658.
45. Shenoy S, Mohanakumar T, Chatila TA et al. Defective apoptosis in lymphocytes and the role of IL-2 in autoimmune hematologic cytopenias. Clin Immunol 2001; 99:266-275.
46. Dianzani U, Bragardo M, DiFranco D et al. Deficiency of the Fas apoptosis pathway without Fas gene mutations in pediatric patients with autoimmunity/lymphoproliferation. Blood 1997; 89:2871-2879.
47. Lenardo M. Interleukin-2 programs mouse alpha beta T lymphocytes for apoptosis. Nature 1991; 353:858-861.
48. Ravetch JV, Bolland S. IgG Fc receptors. Annu Rev Immunol 2001; 19:275-290.
49. Van de Winkel JGJ, Capel PJA. Human IgG Fc receptor heterogeneity: Molecular aspects and clinical implications. Immunol Today 1993; 14:215-221.
50. Joutsi L, Javela K, Partanen J et al. Genetic polymorphism H131R of Fcγ receptor type IIA (FcγRIIA) in a Finnish population and in patients with or without platelet-associated IgG. Eur J Haematol 1998; 61:183-189.
51. Warmerdam PA, van de Winkel JG, Vlug A et al. A single amino acid in the second Ig-like domain of the human Fc gamma receptor II is critical for human IgG2 binding. J Immunol 1991; 147:1338-1343.
52. Wu J, Edberg JC, Redecha PB et al. A novel polymorphism of FcγRIIIa (CD16) alters receptor function and predisposes to autoimmune disease. J Clin Invest 1997; 100:1059-1070.
53. Carcao MD, Blanchette VS, Wakefield CD et al. Fcγ receptor IIa and IIIa polymorphisms in childhood immune thrombocytopenic purpura. Br J Haematol 2003; 120:135-141.
54. Foster CB, Zhu S, Erichsen HC et al. Polymorphisms in inflammatory cytokines and Fcγ receptors in childhood immune thrombocytopenic purpura: A pilot study. Br J Haematol 2001; 113:596-599.
55. Fujimoto T-T, Inoue M, Shimomura T et al. Involvement of Fcγ receptor polymorphisms in the therapeutic response of idiopathic thrombocytopenic purpura. Br J Haematol 2001; 115:125-130.
56. Lindberg FP, Lublin DM, Telen MJ et al. Rh-related antigen CD47 is the signal-transducer integrin associated protein. J Biol Chem 1994; 269:1567-1570.
57. Lindberg FP, Bullard DC, Caver TE et al. Decreased resistance to bacterial infection and granulocyte defects in IAP-deficient mice. Science 1996; 274:795-798.
58. Brown EJ, Hooper L, Ho T et al. Integrin-associated protein: A 50-kD plasma membrane antigen physically and functionally associated with integrins. J Cell Biol 1990; 111:2785-2794.
59. Lindberg FP, Gresham HD, Schwarz E et al. Molecular cloning of Integrin-Associated Protein: An immunoglobulin family member with multiple membrane spanning domains implicated in alpha-v, beta-3-dependent ligand binding. J Cell Biol 1993; 123:485-496.
60. Jiang P, Lagenaur CF, Narayanan V. Integrin-associated protein is a ligand for the P84 neural adhesion molecule. J Biol Chem 1999; 274:559-562.
61. Oldenborg P-A, Zheleznyak A, Fang Y-F et al. Role of CD47 as a marker of self on red blood cells. Science 2000; 288:2051-2054.
62. Oldenborg P-A, Gresham HD, Lindberg FP. CD47-SIRPα regulates Fcγ and complement receptor-mediated phagocytosis. J Exp Med 2001; 193:855-862.
63. Brown EJ. Complement receptors and phagocytosis. Curr Opin Immunol 1991; 3:76-82.
64. Baxter AG, Mandel TE. Hemolytic anemia in nonobese diabetic mice. Eur J Immunol 1991; 21:2051-2055.
65. Oldenborg P-A, Gresham HD, Chen Y et al. Lethal autoimmune hemolytic anemia in CD47-deficient NOD mice. Blood 2002; 99:3500-3504.

Chapter 10

Genetics of Autoimmune Myocarditis

Mehmet L. Guler, Davinna Ligons and Noel R. Rose

Abstract

Autoimmune heart diseases in humans are multifactorial and genetically complex. Fortunately a great deal has been learned from animal models. They have established that a variety of infectious or toxic insults can lead to autoimmune heart disease in genetically susceptible animals. These animal models suggest that autoimmune heart disease has multiple etiologies, with differing mechanisms but overlapping genetic determinants culminating in the same end stage inflammatory heart disease. In this review we will focus on autoimmune heart disease caused by two different infectious agents, *Trypanosoma cruzi* and *Coxsackievirus* B3. Both pathogens are known to infect the heart and are largely cleared after a brief illness. In certain susceptible individuals, however, a chronic, putative autoimmune attack is initiated. We review the evidence that post infectious chronic myocarditis is indeed autoimmune in nature and discuss our recent findings about the common genetic elements that may predispose to autoimmunity and autoimmune disease.

Introduction

A variety of insults can lead to autoimmune disease of the heart. Classic examples are infectious autoimmune endocarditis and valvulitis after pharyngeal streptococcal infection, well known as rheumatic heart disease, and myocarditis and dilated cardiomyopathy after infection with *Trypanosoma cruzi* (Chagas' disease) and certain viruses, most notably *Coxsackievirus* B3 (CB3). The mechanisms by which these infectious agents lead to autoimmune disease in the heart are not fully known. Indeed proving that these infections can lead to bona fide autoimmune disease in the heart has itself been challenging, especially since two of these infectious agents, *T. cruzi* and CB3, infect the heart and directly induce injury of the myocytes. Moreover, majority of individuals afflicted with these infections never develop chronic debilitating autoimmune heart disease. Yet astute clinical observations and work with a variety of animal models has firmly established a role for autoimmune disease in the chronic progression of post infectious heart disease and has opened the way for greater understanding of mechanistic processes. Early work has suggested that a variety of factors, including pathogen strain, environmental stress, and host genetic background all contribute to the likelihood that a chronic autoimmune disease will ensue. This review will focus on our current understanding of genetic influences on autoimmune heart disease, especially on CB3 induced autoimmune myocarditis. Excellent reviews covering the clinical aspects and immunobiology of rheumatic fever,[1-3] Chagas' disease,[4,5] and post viral myocarditis[6-9] can be found elsewhere. We will first discuss the evidence that post viral autoimmune myocarditis leading to dilated cardiomyopathy is an autoimmune disease, and then explore our current understanding of genetic factors leading to increased susceptibility.

Immunogenetics of Autoimmune Disease, edited by Jorge Oksenberg and David Brassat.

The Clinical Impact of Autoimmune Heart Disease

Heart failure affects nearly five million individuals each year in the United States at a cost of over $12 billion.[10] Dilated cardiomyopathy accounts for 25% of cases of heart failure[11] and is the primary cause of sudden death in adults less than 40 years of age.[12] Although the etiology of dilated cardiomyopathy is unidentified only half the time, over 10% of cases are associated with viral myocarditis – largely induced by *Coxsackievirus* B3 (CB3).[13] Yet the majority of people infected with CB3 virus suffer no more than flu-like symptoms. Since onset of heart failure is a late occurance and susceptibilility is relatively rare, a genetically determined autoimmune response has been implicated as its cause.

Coxsackievirus B3 (CB3) Induced Cardiomyopathy Is an Autoimmune Disease

Several lines of clinical evidence suggest that chronic myocarditis and dilated cardiomyopathy result from a progressive autoimmune process initiated by viral myocarditis.[14] During initial myocardial infection with CB3 virus, and after virus is cleared, it has been hypothesized that normal immunologic tolerance to heart tissue is broken, resulting in a chronic autoimmune response. The majority of patients suffer only a transient myocarditis and recover however, acute viral myocarditis can sometimes lead to fulminant heart failure and death. A small portion of the patients who recover subsequently develop chronic myocarditis and dilated cardiomyopathy, often many weeks after the initial infection, suggesting that the cardiac pathology is mediated by immune mechanisms, long after viral infection and anti-viral responses have subsided. Furthermore, patients with chronic myocarditis and dilated cardiomyopathy are often found to have circulating IgG-type autoantibodies to cardiac myosin and other heart antigens.[15,16]

The best line of evidence supporting the autoimmune pathogenesis of chronic myocarditis and dilated cardiomyopathy as a sequela of viral myocarditis has come from studies of animal models.[17,18] A disease resembling human myocarditis can be produced in mice utilizing a cardiotropic strain of *Coxsackievirus* B3 (CB3).[19] After infection with CB3, all strains of mice develop an acute viral myocarditis characterized by focal cardiomyocyte necrosis and infiltration by neutrophils and mononuclear cells. This initial phase begins on day 3 of infection, reaches a peak at day 7 and essentially resolves by day 21. It is associated with the presence of infectious virus; virus as well as viral neutralizing antibodies can be demonstrated during this phase of the disease both in the heart and serum. In a few strains of susceptibile mice, especially A/J and other strains sharing the A background, a second phase is found which is characterized by a diffuse mononuclear infiltrate and little myocyte necrosis. Infectious virus is not detectable, although some residual viral RNA is found in a few myocytes utilizing highly sensitive techniques.[20] Nevertheless, the magnitude of myocardial inflammation suggests reactivity to an abundant cardiac antigen. Reactivity to self antigens, a prerequisite for an autoimmune disease, is demonstrated by the production of anti-cardiomyocyte IgG autoantibodies and the expansion of cardiac myosin specific T cells.[15,16] Moreover, these autoreactive antibodies and cells are only demonstrable in genetically susceptible mice.[21-25]

In the study of autoimmunity it is important to distinguish between autoimmune phenomena and autoimmune disease. Demonstration of autoreactive antibodies and cells, collectively known as autoimmune phenomena, although necessary for disease, are not necessarily indicative of active disease. Evidence must be provided establishing that autoimmunity is the cause and not the consequence of the disease. Indeed, many seemingly normal individuals have autoantibodies and autoreactive T and B cells, but never develop disease.[26] Nevertheless, there is growing evidence to suggest that autoimmune phenomena forecast subsequent disease. For example, family members of individuals with autoimmune diseases are much more likely than average to have high titers of autoantibodies, and these individuals are more likely to develop subsequent autoimmune disease.[16]

To test the significance of autoimmune phenomena in animal models after CB3 infection, experiments fulfilling a version of Koch's postulates in autoimmune disease have been performed.[27] Autoreactive T cells derived from susceptible cardiac myosin immunized mice are able to transfer disease to naïve recipients after in vitro expansion,[28,29] estabishing the pathogenic role of autoreactive cells in this disease model. In most animal models of CB3 induced myocarditis, transfer of autoantibodies has not successfully transferred disease, except in the DBA/2 mouse strain which will be described later. These observations further suggest that there could be a variety of mechanisms that lead to autoimmune heart disease, including both T-cell-mediated or antibody-mediated pathways, and that each animal model is most likely representative of one or few of the multitude of mechanims that lead to the same final pathologic outcome of chronic myocarditis and dilated cardiomyopathy.

Chronic myocarditis in susceptible strains post *T. cruzi* infection (Chagas' disease) can also be due, at least in part, to an autoimmune attack on myocardium.[4] Conceptually, Chagas' disease and CB3 induced autoimmune myocarditis are very similar in that they are both thought to result from loss of self-tolerance to the heart after infection of myocardium. In both infections, the pathogen direcly infects heart tissue, but subsequently is all but cleared. Most hosts recover, but a few go on to develop a chronic myocarditis that is thought to be autoimmune. As will be more apparent later, Chagas' disease and CB3-induced autoimmune myocarditis also share the same genetic susceptibility patterns in the murine strains studied. The best evidence supporting an autoimmune pathogenesis of Chagas' disease comes from animal models. Syngeneic transplanted newborn hearts into susceptible BALB/c mice previously infected with *T. cruzi*, modeling Chagas' disease, are rejected and this is dependent on CD4+ T cells, lending strong support to the autoimmune hypothesis.[30] Utilizing different strains of mice (C57Bl/6 and C3H/HeSnJ), Tarleton et al later demonstrated that transplanted hearts were not rejected in mice unless there was active infection, and concluded that Chagas' disease does not have an autoimmune component. They failed to take into account, however, that C57Bl/6 and C3H/HeSnJ mice are resistant to autoimmune heart disease[32,33] and thus are not expected to have autoimmune disease that can be transferred and cause transplant rejection, thereby highlighting the importance of genetic background on disease susceptibility. C57Bl/6 mice are known to be resistant to chronic myocarditis induced by *T. cruzi* and CB3 virus, and C3H/HeSnj mice are well established to be resistant in the CB3 virus model; therefore the conclusions made in the original transplant study, utilizing BALB/c mice which are both susceptible to *T. cruzi* and CB3 induced chronic myocarditis, seem to validate the autoimmune pathogenesis of Chagas' disease in this murine model.

To further test the autoimmune pathogenesis of CB3 induced heart disease, our laboratory originated a virus-free mouse model for human myocarditis termed experimental autoimmune myocarditis (EAM).[24] Previous observations have lead to the hypothesis that initial infection with CB3 virus causes presentation of cardiac antigens in an inflamed, immunogenic context, leading to development of autoreactive lymphocytes in genetically susceptible mice. These autoreactive lymphocytes subsequently lead to autoimmune myocarditis and eventual dilated cardiomyopathy long after the acute viral myocarditis has been cleared. To test this hypothesis, we set out to mimic viral infection and cardiac injury through subcutanous immunization of mice with native cardiac myosin in complete Freund's adjuvant (CFA). Susceptible strains immunized with purfied cardiac myosin in CFA develop a chronic myocarditis characterized by a mononuclear infiltrate, cardiac specific autoantibodies, and dilated cardiomyopathy reproducing the second phase of CB3 virus induced myocarditis. Finally, and most important, cardiac myosin immunization breaks tolerance and produces pathology only in strains of mice that are susceptible to the later chronic phase of CB3 virus induced myocarditis. Thus it is likely that mechanisms leading to genetic predisposition to autoimmune myocarditis are similar in both the virus-induced and cardiac-myosin induced experimental models, making EAM an effective tool in the study of the pathogenesis of autoimmune myocarditis.[24]

Genetic Influence on Autoimmune Heart Disease

The role of genetic background in autoimmune heart disease has been difficult to establish in humans. Multiple environmental insults can lead to inflammatory heart disease which can cause debilitating heart failure. In most cases, the triggers are not known. *Streptococci* (rheumatic heart disease), *T. cruzi* (Chagas' disease), and *Coxsackieviruses* cause chronic autoimmune disease in a minority of patients and possibly by many different mechanisms. Furthermore, based on experience with other autoimmune diseases, autoimmune myocarditis is likely to be multifactorial and polygenic where susceptibility is controlled by complex multiple interacting loci and is dependent on several poorly characterized environmental factors. All these factors contribute to the difficulty in establishing the genes that influence autoimmune heart disease in humans. Nevertheless, observations pointing to the importance of genetic background have been reported. For example, increased susceptibility to rheumatic fever has been reported in families that have members afflicted with the disease.[34,35] In addition, families with members suffering from post-viral autoimmune myocarditis also seem to have a propensity to develop anti-myosin autoantibodies in unaffected individuals.[16] This again suggests that multiple loci probably contribute to acquisition of full disease, and different family members who have inherited only a portion of the susceptibility loci only manifest subclinical findings.

As before, animal models have contributed greatly to our appreciation of hereditary factors in autoimmune heart disease. Susceptibility to CB3 induced autoimmune myocarditis varies among different strains of mice and appears to be influenced by both MHC and nonMHC genes, and therefore is an ideal system for the study of genetic influence on autoimmune diseases.[24,33] Interestingly, among autoimmune disease models, autoimmune heart disease seems to be least influenced by MHC. For example, most A background mice such as A/J (H-2a), A.SW (H-2s) and A.CA (H-2f), differing only at the MHC locus, develop severe myocarditis upon infection with CB3 virus, while most B strains of mice, such as C57BL/6J, B10.A, B10.RIII, B10.S, B10.SM, B10.WB, B10.PL (H-2b, a, r, s, v, j, f, u respectively) , are resistant to the induction of chronic autoimmune myocarditis. Other strains such as BALB/c demonstrate intermediate susceptibility. These results highlight the importance of the non-MHC genes in the susceptibility to autoimmunity. Nevertheless, MHC genes still play an important role in autoimmunity as noted in all major models of autoimmune diseases. For instance, A.BY (H-2b) mice, harboring the ordinarily susceptible A background, display a mild phenotype, and B10.D2, B10.BR, and B10.Q (H-2d, H-2k, H-2q respectively) mice, harboring the ordinarily resistant B background, develop moderate myocarditis. C3H/HeSn and C3H.JK (H-2k, j) are resistant whereas C3H.NB and C3H.SW (H-2p, b) are susceptible.

T. cruzi induced autoimmune myocarditis also demonstrates a similar susceptibility pattern. A/J mice develop significant chronic autoimmune myocarditis and produce anti-myosin autoantibodies after infection with *T. cruzi* whereas C57Bl/6 mice are resistant.[4,32] These results suggest that both CB3 and *T. cruzi* infection induce autoimmune myocarditis by a similar set of mechanisms which most likely involve presentation of self antigens such as myosin in an inflammatory context induced by infection. This notion is supported by the experimental autoimmune myocarditis (EAM) model where strains susceptible to virus induced autoimmunity such as A/J and A.SW mice are also susceptible to myosin/CFA immunization induced myocarditis and strains resistant to virus induced autoimmunity like C57Bl/6 and B10.S mice are resistant to myosin/CFA immunization.[24]

Study of Mechanism of Autoimmunity through Identification of Susceptibility Genes

Several mechanisms that can be broadly grouped into two main categories have been proposed to explain how self tolerance is broken to self antigens. It is beyond the scope of this review to explore these proposed mechanisms in great detail; several other reviews have tackled these issues.[36,37] The first broad category is antigen based and the second is based on homeostasis and regulatory networks. During normal host development, the immune system is programmed to recognize the universe of antigens and yet effectively inhibit any self-reactivity. This is thought to be achieved in two ways. Initially, in a process known as central tolerance, immature T and B lymphocytes undergo apoptosis if they happen to express self-reactive antigen receptors. Even though this process eliminates the majority of potentially self-reactive cells, many autoimmunogenic cells are allowed to join the peripheral pool of lymphocytes which is actively engaged in host defense. Recently it is becoming clear that several regulatory networks involving cells and cytokines are actively engaged in suppressing the activation of these autoreactive cells. Theoretically, then, autoimmunity results when either central tolerance or peripheral regulatory mechanisms fail. In the antigen-based model for disruption of self-tolerance, it is hypothesized that certain intracellular antigens are either sequestered, or not processed in an immunogenic fashion, until an infection induces disruption of tissues, exposing antigens or releasing special enzymes which digest self antigen in new ways, effectively making self antigens targets for immune attack. Alternatively, antigens of the pathogen are hypothesized to mimic self antigens, and induce autoimmune disease through cross-reactive lymphocytes. Experimental evidence documenting cross reactivity, or "molecular mimicry," has been published; however, it has been difficult to prove that this mechanism actually causes disease.[38,39] In the second broad category, it is hypothesized that infections disrupt homeostatic mechanisms that are continually at work in suppressing self-reactivity. For example, infectious agents ordinarily cause inflammatory reactions through engagement of several innate, nonspecific receptors, like receptors of the Toll family, and complement, which greatly enhance and shape later, adaptive immune reactions.[40] In certain susceptible individuals, this enhanced immunogenicity during infections may disrupt mechanisms that normally suppress self-reactivity. Clearly, these mechanisms are not fully understood and much needs to be done to define the precise pathways that lead to autoimmune disease.

Fortunately, defining the genes, and their polymorphisms which may lead to susceptibility to autoimmune diseases does not require knowledge of pathogenesis of disease and, most important, will later be instrumental in identifying the key pathways that are involved in development of disease. For this reason, several groups are greatly interested in identifying the genes and their polymorphisms that are associated with autoimmune disease in a variety of models.

Loci Which Influence Autoimmune Myocarditis Are Also Involved in Other Autoimmune Diseases in the A vs. B (C57BL/6) Murine Model

In an effort to identify genetic loci which control susceptibility to CB3 virus induced autoimmune myocarditis, our laboratory initially compared inheritance of the susceptibility trait in all available AxB and BxA recombinant inbred strains (n=13, and n=9 respectively).[41] With the available genomic markers at the time, suggestive linkage to the T cell receptor-α locus on murine Chromosome 14 was identified. Current analysis, with the addition of more markers based on single strand length polymorphic (SSLP) markers has led us to conclude that these original observations were probably not significant and require analysis of many more meiotic combinations, beyond the limited number of meiotic combinations that are represented by recombinant inbred strains.

In a fresh approach, we decided to identify loci controlling differential susceptibility to experimentally induced (myosin/CFA induced) autoimmune myocarditis in the A.SW and B10.S strains.[42] We chose to study the experimentally induced model of autoimmune myocarditis because there is less variability in phenotype, perhaps due to diminished influence of infection. Despite standardization of methods, careful control of mouse living environment, diet and other controllable factors, there is still significant variability in phenotype in ordinarily susceptible strains of mice. For example, after infection with CB3 virus, only 40-50% of susceptible A/J mice develop chronic autoimmune myocarditis, demonstrating a significant environmental influence on disease penetrance.[43] This variability markedly diminishes, but is not entirely absent in the experimentally induced model. Furthermore, since we knew MHC loci influence disease, we chose to focus on non-MHC genes by fixing the MHC locus between susceptible and resistant model strains. We compared susceptibility to EAM in the H-2s congenic mice A.SW (A/J background) and B10.S (C57Bl/6 background). After immunization with cardiac myosin in CFA, A.SW mice were highly susceptible to autoimmune myocarditis, demonstrating chronic inflammation involving 26.5 +/- 9.2% of the myocardium after immunization. In contrast, B10.S mice were highly resistant, demonstrating inflammation involving only 4.5 +/- 7.5 % of the myocardium. Despite the considerable variability of phenotype from individual to individual, again demonstrating the influence of environment, the difference in susceptibility between A.SW mice and B10.S mice is highly significant ($p = 1.9 \times 10^{-17}$).[42]

In order to determine the loci controlling susceptibility to autoimmune myocarditis, we performed F1 (A.SW x B10.S), and F2 (F1 x F1) crosses. Interestingly F1 mice were intermediate in susceptibility to EAM and showed wide variance, demonstrating inflammation in 10.3 +/- 12.0 % of the myocardium. Despite this variability, the intermediate F1 phenotype is significantly different from the susceptible A.SW and resistant B10.S phenotypes ($p = 3.05 \times 10^{-6}$ and $p = 9.03 \times 10^{-5}$ respectively). This wide variance is surprising since all F1 mice are genetically identical, and may help to explain great variance in susceptibility to autoimmune disease even between identical twins in the human population. F1 x F1 mice (F2 mice, n= 296) demonstrated the complete range of phenotypes: B10.S-like resistant, F1-like intermediate and A.SW-like highly susceptible. Linkage analysis performed using 90 SSLP markers spanning the entire murine genome yielded highly significant contribution of a locus on distal murine chromosome 6 (named *Eam2*) and highly suggestive linkage on proximal Chromosome 1 (named *Eam1*). Weaker linkage to Chromosome 4 was also found.[42] The significance of Chr.1 especially and Chr.4 are currently being tested with additional experimental crosses. Interestingly, the Chr.6 locus was operative exclusively in male mice.

Both the Chr.1 and Chr.6 loci identified as influencing autoimmune myocarditis have been previously identified in other autoimmune diseases such as murine lupus, diabetes and autoimmune orchitis.[42] The human counterpart of the murine Chr.1 locus has also been implicated in diabetes and autoimmune thyroid disease. This strongly suggests that there are common mechanisms leading to autoimmune diseases, with other genetic and environmental influences determining tissue specificity of disease. Indeed, a recent survey of published linkage studies on autoimmune or immune-mediated diseases revealed several overlapping syntenic human and mouse chromosomal regions with a cluster of disease susceptibility loci.[44] These studies provide support for the hypothesis that autoimmune disorders in different species are controlled by a common set of susceptibility genes. Therefore, understanding the mechanisms that lead to the disease in animals may provide fresh insight into their human disease counterparts.

The immunologically important regulatory molecule CTLA-4, found in the Chr.1 locus, has been implicated in several autoimmune diseases.[45,46] CTLA-4 is a transmembrane protein expressed primarily on the surface of activated T cells. Upon T cell activation, CTLA-4 is up-regulated and interacts with B7.1 and B7.2 on antigen presenting cells, and is thought to deliver down-regulatory signals to the T cell. Some regulatory T cells (CD25+CD4+ cells) seem to express CTLA-4 constitutively.[47] Mutant mice lacking CTLA-4 display a lymphoproliferative disorder and succumb to a severe multi-organ autoimmune disorder.[48] The CTLA-4 locus has long been implicated in human autoimmune diseases like autoimmune thyroid disease and diabetes, and in the murine model of type-1 diabetes, NOD. Recently, it has been shown that polymorphisms within CTLA-4 genomic sequences influencing alternative splicing of CTLA-4 is most likely cause of linkage to this locus in human autoimmune thyroid disease and murine diabetes.[49] Human CTLA-4 is expressed in two main forms:

membrane bound, and secreted. The secreted form results from an alternative splice where the transmembrane domain is excluded. The secreted isoform of CTLA-4 seems to be decreased in susceptible individuals due to a mutation in the 3' region of the gene. In mice, CTLA-4 also has an additional isoform, where the ligand binding domain is spliced out, reportedly conferring constitutive activity on this form. Susceptible NOD mice express a mutation in a splice control motif in exon 2 which decreases the level of expression of this ligand-independent form of CTLA-4 compared to healthy mice. It is currently not known how changes in the relative expression of these splice forms influences autoimmune disease, but it is thought that these particular alterations in the expression of CTLA-4 isoforms can diminish the total inhibitory signal that is delivered to activated self-reactive T cells, thus increasing the likelihood of autoimmunity. We are currently investigating whether these polymorphisms or others influence CTLA-4 and its function in the pathogenesis of autoimmune myocarditis in the mouse.

Sensitivity to Apoptosis May Influence Development of Autoimmune Myocarditis

In addition to developing spontaneous diabetes, NOD mice display a multitude of immunologic peculiarities. For example, immature T cells in the thymus of NOD mice are relatively insensitive to induction of apoptosis by the stressor dexamethasone (Dxm), compared to disease-free control mice.[50,51] Decreased potential for apoptosis in NOD thymocytes could potentially lead to retention of autoreactive T cells and susceptibility to an autoimmune disease like diabetes. This trait, differential sensitivity to Dxm induced apoptosis, was mapped to the distal portion of murine Chr.6 – the same locus that already harbors a diabetes susceptibility locus, *idd6*. Interestingly, *Eam2*, the locus identified as influencing susceptibility to experimental autoimmune myocarditis also maps to this area.[42] Due to the colocalization of autoimmune susceptibility and apoptosis-sensitivity in NOD mice, we asked whether A.SW mice, which are susceptible to EAM, also demonstrate diminished susceptibility to dexamethasone induced thymocyte apoptosis. Indeed, like in NOD mice, A.SW thymocytes demonstrated diminished sensitivity to apoptosis compared to the autoimmune myocarditis resistant strain B10.S. Thymocytes from B10.S mice showed enhanced sensitivity to Dxm compared to A.SW mice: 28.6 % +/- 11.1 of B10.S thymocytes whereas 11.1% +/- 8.6 of A.SW thymocytes displayed signs of apoptosis ($p = 1.3 \times 10^{-5}$).[42]

A second immunologic peculiarity identified in NOD mice is the relative insensitivity of mature peripheral T lymphocytes to cyclophosphamide (Cy)-induced apoptosis compared to disease free control mice.[52] This trait, although similar to the thymic apoptosis trait described above, is controlled by a different locus, situated in the proximal portion of murine Chr.1. This is the same locus on Chr.1 that is shared between the diabetes susceptibility locus, *idd5*, and the autoimmune myocarditis susceptibility locus, *Eam1*. Again, like in NOD mice, A.SW lymphocytes demonstrate diminished sensitivity to Cy induced apoptosis.[42] Lymphocytes from B10.S mice showed enhanced sensitivity to Cy compared to A.SW mice: 46.2 % +/- 11.9 of B10.S lymphocytes whereas 21.4% +/- 6.1 of A.SW lymphocytes displayed signs of apoptosis ($p = 4.1 \times 10^{-6}$).[42]

Thus, NOD mice which develop diabetes and A.SW mice which are susceptible to experimentally induced autoimmune myocarditis not only share two susceptibility loci, but also demonstrate two abnormalities associated with apoptosis of T cells. These two loci affect apoptosis at different stages of T cell development: Chr.6 influencing immature thymocyte apoptosis and Chr.1 influencing mature peripheral T cell apoptosis. It remains to be demonstrated that the genetic elements which control sensitivity to drug induced apoptosis at either of these loci are the same genetic elements that control susceptibility to autoimmune disease. It will be very important to determine how polymorphisms at these loci influence apoptosis and how they control susceptibility to autoimmune diseases like diabetes and myocarditis.

Autoimmune Myocarditis in the DBA/2 Mouse Model—Same Phenotypic Disease via Different Mechanisms and Different Loci

As mentioned before, transfer of myocarditis from effected individuals to naïve recipients has been mostly successful through the transfer of lymphocytes, adding strong support to the autoimmune pathogenesis hypothesis of post-viral or experimentally induced autoimmune myocarditis.[28,29] These experiments have been mostly performed in the A or BALB/c model strains. Although autoantibodies are produced in parallel with the emergence of autoimmune myocarditis, transfer of antibodies in these model strains has not led to the transfer of disease to naïve hosts.[29,53] Contrary to these observations, DBA/2 mice which also demonstrate susceptibility to CB3 or experimentally induced autoimmune myocarditis can also develop disease merely through the passive transfer of IgG anti-myosin autoantibodies, suggesting that these mice develop disease that is phenotypically similar to autoimmune myocarditis in A and BALB/c mice, but the mechanisms may be different.[54,55]

Interestingly, DBA/2 mice express α-myosin, or a closely related antigen on the surface of cardiac myocytes, rendering these cells susceptible to autoantibody induced inflammation.[55,56] Indeed, α-myosin is an intracellular protein in most strains of mice, but DBA/2 mice are unique in this regard, and the mechanism for this differential localization is not understood. IgG autoantibodies, but not IgM autoantibodies can transfer disease.[57] This difference is thought to be due to the greater vascular permeability of IgG compared to IgM which is usually found as a pentameric complex in serum.

In an effort to understand the genetic basis of susceptibility to antibody-transfer mediated myocarditis, resistant BALB/c mice and susceptible DBA/2 mice were utilized in a standard mendelian study.[56] This genetic study prudently isolated the effect of autoantibodies through challenge with preformed autoantibodies, since both strains are susceptible to autoimmune myocarditis induced by virus or myosin/CFA immunization; however, only DBA/2 mice are susceptible to autoantibody-transfer induced disease. This approach greatly simplifies the problem by tackling the effector phase of the autoimmune response which is also under genetic control in this model system. Hopefully future studies will address the genetic loci which control the initial production of autoantibodies.

F1 (BALB/c x DBA/2) mice were resistant to autoantibody transfer mediated myocarditis, demonstrating that this trait is recessive. Incidentally, expression of extracellular myosin is also recessively controlled, since F1 (BALB/c x DBA/2) mice do not express myosin extracellularly. Backcross F1 x DBA/2 offspring displayed both resistant and susceptible phenotypes. Linkage analysis utilizing polymorphic SSLP markers throughout the murine genome lead to the discovery of several loci influencing autoantibody-transfer mediated myocarditis. There was highly significant linkage to a locus in the middle portion of Chr.12, and suggestive linkage to distal Chr.1 and Chr.9. Interestingly the Chr.1 linkage was only apparent in male mice.

These observations demonstrate that the same disease phenotype can manifest itself through a variety of different mechanisms. It is not known if extracellular expression of cardiac myosin is present in any human population leading to increased susceptibility to autoimmune myocarditis. However, it is plausible that rheumatic fever, induced by autoantibodies to extracellular valvular, endothelial and myocardial antigens after pharyngeal infection with *Streptococcus* in susceptible individuals may be controlled by some of the same susceptibility loci as in the autoantibody-transfer mediated myocarditis model in DBA/2 mice. Perhaps other mechanisms, not represented by any of the current animal models, also contribute to autoimmune myocarditis in humans. This reality reflects one of the difficulties of genetic mapping of complex diseases like autoimmune diseases, especially in humans, and underscores the importance of studying a multitude of animal models with the same disease phenotype.

Conclusions

Autoimmune myocarditis, like most other autoimmune diseases is multifactorial and genetically complex. Our understanding of the genetic factors which influence autoimmune myocarditis has grown tremendously owing largely to a variety of animal models. Even so, there is much progress to be made, not only in autoimmune myocarditis but in autoimmune diseases in general. Many loci controlling autoimmune disease have been identified, and many of these loci overlap, suggesting common mechanisms; however, the actual genes, their polymorphisms and how they cause disease is largely unknown. Even though the involvement of MHC genes in autoimmune diseases is well established, and their function in antigen presentation well characterized, we still do not understand why certain alleles predispose to disease. Identification of genes and their polymorphisms that predispose to autoimmune diseases will be the next challenge and should be facilitated with the advent of the genome projects and new technologies in gene identification. Identification of these genes and their function will not only help in diagnosing these disorders but lead to understanding of the mechanisms of autoimmune diseases which should further help in the establishment of rational therapies.

Acknowledgements

The authors' research is supported by NIH research grants RO1 HL67290 and RO1 HL70729 and a grant from MARRC (R21A151835). MG is supported by NIH training grant AI07-247.

References

1. Roberts S, Kosanke S, Terrence Dunn S et al. Pathogenic mechanisms in rheumatic carditis: Focus on valvular endothelium. J Infect Dis 2001; 183(3):507-511.
2. Cunningham MW. Pathogenesis of group A streptococcal infections. Clin Microbiol Rev 2000; 13(3):470-511.
3. Cunningham MW. Streptococcus-induced myocarditis in mice. Autoimmunity 2001; 34(3):193-197.
4. Engman DM, Leon JS. Pathogenesis of Chagas heart disease: Role of autoimmunity. Acta Trop 2002; 81(2):123-132.
5. Higuchi Mde L, Benvenuti LA, Martins Reis M et al. Pathophysiology of the heart in Chagas' disease: Current status and new developments. Cardiovasc Res 2003; 60(1):96-107.
6. Hill SL, Rose NR. The transition from viral to autoimmune myocarditis. Autoimmunity 2001; 34(3):169-176.
7. Fairweather D, Kaya Z, Shellam GR et al. From infection to autoimmunity. J Autoimmun 2001; 16(3):175-186.
8. Afanasyeva M, Rose NR. Immune Mediators in inflammatory heart disease: Insights from a mouse model. European Heart Journal 2002; 4(Supplement I):131-136.
9. Noutsias M, Pauschinger M, Poller WC et al. Current insights into the pathogenesis, diagnosis and therapy of inflammatory cardiomyopathy. Heart Fail Monit 2003; 3(4):127-135.
10. O'Connell JB, Bristow MR. Economic impact of heart failure in the United States: Time for a different approach. Journal of Heart and Lung Transplantation 1994; 13(4):S107-112.
11. Brown CA, O'Connell JB. Myocarditis and idiopathic dilated cardiomyopathy. American Journal of Medicine 1995; 99(3):309-314.
12. Drory Y, Turetz Y, Hiss Y et al. Sudden unexpected death in persons less than 40 years of age. American Journal of Cardiology 1991; 68(13):1388-1392.
13. Felker GM, Hu W, Hare JM et al. The spectrum of dilated cardiomyopathy. The Johns Hopkins experience with 1,278 patients. Medicine (Baltimore) 1999; 78(4):270-283.
14. Rose NR, Herskowitz A, Neumann DA et al. Autoimmune myocarditis: A paradigm of post-infection autoimmune disease. Immunology Today 1988; 9(4):117-120.
15. Caforio AL, Goldman JH, Haven AJ et al. Circulating cardiac-specific autoantibodies as markers of autoimmunity in clinical and biopsy-proven myocarditis. The Myocarditis Treatment Trial Investigators. European Heart Journal 1997; 18(2):270-275.
16. Caforio AL, Goldman JH, Haven AJ et al. Evidence for autoimmunity to myosin and other heart-specific autoantigens in patients with dilated cardiomyopathy and their relatives. International Journal of Cardiology 1996; 54(2):157-163.
17. Gauntt CJ, Tracy SM, Chapman N et al. Coxsackievirus-induced chronic myocarditis in murine models. European Heart Journal 1995; 16(Suppl O):56-58.

18. Wang Y, Afanasyeva M, Hill SL et al. Characterization of murine autoimmune myocarditis induced by self and foreign cardiac myosin. Autoimmunity 1999; 31(3):151-162.
19. Rose NR, Wolfgram LJ, Herskowitz A et al. Postinfectious autoimmunity: Two distinct phases of Coxsackievirus B3-induced myocarditis. Annals of the New York Academy of Sciences 1986; 475:146-156.
20. Reetoo KN, Osman SA, Illavia SJ et al. Quantitative analysis of viral RNA kinetics in Coxsackievirus B3-induced murine myocarditis: Biphasic pattern of clearance following acute infection, with persistence of residual viral RNA throughout and beyond the inflammatory phase of disease. Journal of General Virology 2000; 81(Pt 11):2755-2762.
21. Rose NR, Neumann DA, Herskowitz A et al. Genetics of susceptibility to viral myocarditis in mice. Pathology and Immunopathology Research 1988; 7(4):266-278.
22. Wolfgram LJ, Beisel KW, Herskowitz A et al. Variations in the susceptibility to Coxsackievirus B3-induced myocarditis among different strains of mice. Journal of Immunology 1986; 136(5):1846-1852.
23. Wolfgram LJ, Beisel KW, Rose NR. Heart-specific autoantibodies following murine Coxsackievirus B3 myocarditis. Journal of Experimental Medicine 1985; 161(5):1112-1121.
24. Neu N, Rose NR, Beisel KW et al. Cardiac myosin induces myocarditis in genetically predisposed mice. Journal of Immunology 1987; 139(11):3630-3636.
25. Neu N, Beisel KW, Traystman MD et al. Autoantibodies specific for the cardiac myosin isoform are found in mice susceptible to Coxsackievirus B3-induced myocarditis. Journal of Immunology 1987; 138(8):2488-2492.
26. Lam-Tse WK, Lernmark A, Drexhage HA. Animal models of endocrine/organ-specific autoimmune diseases: Do they really help us to understand human autoimmunity? Springer Semin Immunopathol 2002; 24(3):297-321.
27. Rose NR, Bona C. Defining criteria for autoimmune diseases (Witebsky's postulates revisited). Immunol Today 1993; 14(9):426-430.
28. Smith SC, Allen PM. The role of T cells in myosin-induced autoimmune myocarditis. Clinical Immunology and Immunopathology 1993; 68(2):100-106.
29. Smith SC, Allen PM. Myosin-induced acute myocarditis is a T cell-mediated disease. Journal of Immunology 1991; 147(7):2141-2147.
30. dos Santos RR, Rossi MA, Laus JL et al. Anti-CD4 abrogates rejection and reestablishes long-term tolerance to syngeneic newborn hearts grafted in mice chronically infected with Trypanosoma cruzi. J Exp Med 1992; 175(1):29-39.
31. Tarleton RL, Zhang L, Downs MO. "Autoimmune rejection" of neonatal heart transplants in experimental Chagas disease is a parasite-specific response to infected host tissue. Proc Natl Acad Sci USA 1997; 94(8):3932-3937.
32. Leon JS, Godsel LM, Wang K et al. Cardiac myosin autoimmunity in acute Chagas' heart disease. Infect Immun 2001; 69(9):5643-5649.
33. Beisel KW, Wolfgram L, Hershkowitz A et al. Differences in severity of Coxsackievirus B3 - induced myocarditis among H-2 congenic strains. In: Skamane E, ed. Genetic Control of Host Resistance to Infection and Malignancy: Alan R. Liss, Inc., 1985:195-201.
34. Wilson MGSM, Lubschez R. The familial epidemiology of rheumatic fever. Journal of Pediatrics 1943; 22:468-492.
35. Taranta ATS, Metrakos JD. Rheumatic fever in monozygotic and dizygotic twins. Circulation 1959; 20:778-792.
36. Leng Q, Bentwich Z. Beyond self and nonself: Fuzzy recognition of the immune system. Scand J Immunol 2002; 56(3):224-232.
37. Shevach EM. Regulatory T cells in autoimmmunity*. Annu Rev Immunol 2000; 18:423-449.
38. Rose NR. Infection, mimics, and autoimmune disease. J Clin Invest 2001; 107(8):943-944.
39. Rose NR, Mackay IR. Molecular mimicry: A critical look at exemplary instances in human diseases. Cell Mol Life Sci 2000; 57(4):542-551.
40. Janeway Jr CA, Medzhitov R. Innate immune recognition. Annu Rev Immunol 2002; 20:197-216.
41. Traystman MD, Beisel KW. Genetic control of Coxsackievirus B3-induced heart-specific autoantibodies associated with chronic myocarditis. Clinical and Experimental Immunology 1991; 86(2):291-298.
42. Guler ML, Ligons D, Wang Y et al. Two autoimmune diabetes loci influencing T cell apoptosis control susceptibility to experimental autoimmune myocarditis. J Immunol 2005; 174(4):216.
43. Neu N, Craig SW, Rose NR et al. Coxsackievirus induced myocarditis in mice: Cardiac myosin autoantibodies do not cross-react with the virus. Clin Exp Immunol 1987; 69(3):566-574.
44. Vyse TJ, Todd JA. Genetic analysis of autoimmune disease. Cell 1996; 85(3):311-318.

45. Chang TT, Kuchroo VK, Sharpe AH. Role of the B7-CD28/CTLA-4 pathway in autoimmune disease. Curr Dir Autoimmun 2002; 5:113-130.
46. Kristiansen OP, Larsen ZM, Pociot F. CTLA-4 in autoimmune diseases—a general susceptibility gene to autoimmunity? Genes Immun 2000; 1(3):170-184.
47. Shevach EM. CD4+ CD25+ suppressor T cells: More questions than answers. Nat Rev Immunol 2002; 2(6):389-400.
48. Tivol EA, Borriello F, Schweitzer AN et al. Loss of CTLA-4 leads to massive lymphoproliferation and fatal multiorgan tissue destruction, revealing a critical negative regulatory role of CTLA-4. Immunity 1995; 3(5):541-547.
49. Ueda H, Howson JM, Esposito L et al. Association of the T-cell regulatory gene CTLA4 with susceptibility to autoimmune disease. Nature 2003; 423(6939):506-511.
50. Bergman ML, Penha-Goncalves C, Lejon K et al. Low rate of proliferation in immature thymocytes of the nonobese diabetic mouse maps to the Idd6 diabetes susceptibility region. Diabetologia 2001; 44(8):1054-1061.
51. Bergman ML, Duarte N, Campino S et al. Diabetes protection and restoration of thymocyte apoptosis in NOD Idd6 congenic strains. Diabetes 2003; 52(7):1677-1682.
52. Colucci F, Bergman ML, Penha-Goncalves C et al. Apoptosis resistance of nonobese diabetic peripheral lymphocytes linked to the Idd5 diabetes susceptibility region. Proc Natl Acad Sci USA 1997; 94(16):8670-8674.
53. Neu N, Ploier B, Ofner C. Cardiac myosin-induced myocarditis. Heart autoantibodies are not involved in the induction of the disease. J Immunol 1990; 145(12):4094-4100.
54. Huber SA, Lodge PA. Coxsackievirus B-3 myocarditis. Identification of different pathogenic mechanisms in DBA/2 and Balb/c mice. Am J Pathol 1986; 122(2):284-291.
55. Liao L, Sindhwani R, Rojkind M et al. Antibody-mediated autoimmune myocarditis depends on genetically determined target organ sensitivity. J Exp Med 1995; 181(3):1123-1131.
56. Kuan AP, Chamberlain W, Malkiel S et al. Genetic control of autoimmune myocarditis mediated by myosin-specific antibodies. Immunogenetics 1999; 49(2):79-85.
57. Kuan AP, Zuckier L, Liao L et al. Immunoglobulin isotype determines pathogenicity in antibody-mediated myocarditis in naive mice. Circ Res 2000; 86(3):281-285.

Index

Symbols

A

B

C

T

U

V